Revolutionizing HIV Treatment With AI

Adnène Arbi
National Institute of Applied Sciences and Technology, University of Carthage, Tunisia & Laboratory of Mathematical Engineering, Tunisia Polytechnic School, University of Carthage, Tunisia

Walid Ben Ameur
https://orcid.org/0009-0000-5046-7408
University of Gabès, Tunisia

IGI Global
Scientific Publishing
Publishing Tomorrow's Research Today

Vice President of Editorial Melissa Wagner
Director of Acquisitions Mikaela Felty
Director of Book Development Jocelynn Hessler
Production Manager Mike Brehm
Cover Design Jose Rosado

Published in the United States of America by
IGI Global Scientific Publishing
701 East Chocolate Avenue
Hershey, PA, 17033, USA
Tel: 717-533-8845 | Fax: 717-533-7115
Website: https://www.igi-global.com E-mail: cust@igi-global.com

Library of Congress Cataloging-in-Publication Data

Names: Arbi, Adnène, 1982- editor | Ben Ameur, Walid, 1980- editor
Title: Revolutionizing HIV treatment with AI / edited by Adnène Arbi, Walid Ben Ameur.
Description: Hershey, PA : IGI Global Scientific Publishing, [2026] | Includes bibliographical references and index. | Summary: "HIV is a complex virus that requires lifelong treatment, and although antiretroviral therapy (ART) has been effective in managing the disease, there are still many challenges that hinder optimal care and long-term success. These include the emergence of drug-resistant strains, the variability in patient responses to treatment, and the barriers to timely diagnosis, particularly in remote areas. In recent years, the advent of Artificial Intelligence (AI) technologies has shown immense potential in overcoming some of these challenges, offering innovative solutions to enhance HIV care. However, there are significant challenges to the implementation of AI in HIV treatment. The integration of AI into clinical practice presents several obstacles, including the lack of sufficient data, issues related to patient privacy and data security, the risk of algorithmic bias, and the need for clinical validation before AI-based systems can be widely adopted. This book explores these complexities and outlines how AI can transform HIV care, while addressing the ethical dilemmas and practical hurdles that must be overcome to ensure the safe and equitable application of AI technologies in managing HIV"-- Provided by publisher.
Identifiers: LCCN 2025011445 (print) | LCCN 2025011446 (ebook) | ISBN 9798337328638 h/c | ISBN 9798337328645 s/c | ISBN 9798337328652 ebook
Subjects: LCSH: HIV (Viruses)--Treatment--Technological innovations | Artificial intelligence--Medical applications
Classification: LCC RC606.6 .R483 2026 (print) | LCC RC606.6 (ebook)
LC record available at https://lccn.loc.gov/2025011445
LC ebook record available at https://lccn.loc.gov/2025011446

British Cataloguing in Publication Data
A Cataloguing in Publication record for this book is available from the British Library.

Table of Contents

Detailed Table of Contents

Human Immunodeficiency Virus (HIV) infection is a serious global health problem that targets the immune system with two distinct strains, HIV-1 and HIV-2. Early diagnosis is imperative in preventing the spread of HIV and enabling the initiation of treatment at an early stage. This, in turn, improves patient health outcomes and prevents the progression to AIDS. The diagnosis of HIV can be facilitated by a range of methods, including ELISA, PCR, p24 antigen tests and rapid tests. The advent of novel technologies, biosensors and point-of-care tests holds great promise in accelerating HIV diagnosis and enhancing its accuracy. However, accessibility to HIV testing remains constrained in several regions, resulting in delayed treatment initiation. As awareness of HIV increases, social support and scientific advances facilitate living with HIV and play an important role in the fight against the virus.

Artificial Intelligence in the knowledge of HIV care allows early detection of HIV, faster start on ART, and improved adherence. The study evaluates the predictive AI model in the health care settings of the USA, India, South Africa, and Kenya. Impressive performance was shown with this model with a predictive accuracy of 0.87 AUC after being trained on 32,450 patient records, albeit with variations in performance based on socio-economic status and health infrastructure. AI-supported early diagnosis showed improvement by 28% and 31%, and a decrease in time to viral suppression was significant-up to 28%. On the other hand, ML-based predictions on adherence to intervention improved medication compliance estimations by 9.5%-10.8% through targeted intervention. Fairness analysis showed the predictions were biased towards low-income earners and women; with fairness-aware recalibration, the degree of bias was reduced by over 60%. The present work demonstrates the transformational nature of AI for HIV care and calls for the intelligent and fair implementation of AI interventions.

Preface

INTRODUCTION

In recent years, we have witnessed a profound shift in how societies confront some of their most persistent challenges in education and healthcare. At the heart of this transformation lies an unexpected yet powerful catalyst: game design. As editors of *Interdisciplinary Approaches to Game Design in Healthcare and Education*, we have assembled this volume to illuminate the role of games not merely as entertainment, but as dynamic tools capable of reshaping how people learn, heal, and connect.

The chapters that follow reflect an evolving landscape in which engagement, interactivity, and innovation are no longer optional—they are essential. At a time when educators grapple with diminishing student engagement, widening inequities, and the urgent need to cultivate critical twenty-first-century skills, game-based learning offers fresh possibilities. Serious games reframe classrooms as environments where curiosity thrives, failure is reframed as iterative learning, and complex concepts become both visible and tactile. Whether students design virtual roller coasters to explore physics or unlock literacy through narrative-driven worlds tailored to dyslexic learners, games serve as bridges between abstract ideas and lived experience.

The promise of these tools extends far beyond the classroom. As healthcare systems confront rising mental health needs, disparities in patient education, and demands for more effective training, game design has emerged as a versatile means of promoting wellness and resilience. Gamified apps guide children with chronic conditions through self-management. VR simulations prepare medical students for real-world diagnostic challenges. Immersive experiences reduce anxiety, build empathy, and support rehabilitation. These developments underscore the central theme of this anthology: that learning and healing are profoundly interconnected, and that game design offers new pathways toward holistic human development.

Throughout this book, you will encounter interdisciplinary conversations that interrogate both the possibilities and the responsibilities inherent in game-based approaches. How might artificial intelligence personalize difficulty in real time while avoiding algorithmic bias? Can virtual reality cultivate global awareness without compromising user safety or privacy? What does meaningful accessibility look like for neurodivergent learners or underserved communities? Addressing such questions requires collaboration across computer science, psychology, instructional design, and healthcare—a convergence of perspectives represented by the contributors to this volume.

Just as innovation must be bold, it must also be ethical. We have sought to highlight not only the breakthroughs but also the barriers: the digital divide, privacy concerns, and inequitable access to technology. Global case studies—from rural mobile-learning initiatives to urban AR-based social-skills programs—remind us that the promise of game-based tools cannot be realized without an unwavering commitment to equity.

The objectives of this anthology mirror these priorities. We offer theoretical foundations, empirical studies, and practical cases that map the evolving terrain of game design across educational and healthcare contexts. We spotlight emerging technologies—AI, VR, AR—and their potential to personalize learning, strengthen clinical training, and empower patients. We also identify under-explored areas such as adaptive learning systems, ethical governance structures, and strategies for mitigating systemic inequities. Above all, we hope to cultivate a shared vocabulary and a shared vision for scholars, educators, technologists, healthcare practitioners, policymakers, and advocates who recognize that the future of learning and wellness is, at its core, collaborative.

Our intended audience is as diverse as the disciplines that intersect within these pages. Researchers will find rigorous methodologies and evolving frameworks. Educators and instructional designers will discover models for creating engaging, inclusive curricula. Healthcare practitioners will encounter tools for patient education, rehabilitation, and empathy-building. Engineers and developers will gain insights into ethical, scalable technological design. Policymakers, ethicists, and accessibility advocates will find guidance for ensuring that innovation serves all communities responsibly. And emerging scholars will find a launching point for future inquiry—and perhaps inspiration to push this field further.

As editors, we are deeply grateful to the contributors who share their research, their questions, and their visions in this volume. Together, they demonstrate that games are far more than play—they are instruments of engagement, healing, and social progress. It is our hope that this book will spark new collaborations, encourage thoughtful experimentation, and ultimately contribute to a more innovative, equitable future where game design serves the needs of learners and patients alike.

We invite you now to explore the interdisciplinary pathways that connect education and healthcare through the lens of game design, and to imagine what new possibilities may emerge when we allow creativity, empathy, and play to guide our approach to human development.

ORGANIZATION OF THE BOOK

In **Chapter 1,** ***Human Immunodeficiency Virus Diagnostic Methods***, the authors provide a foundational exploration of current HIV diagnostic approaches and the global inequities that shape access to early testing. By examining established laboratory methods—such as ELISA, PCR, p24 antigen detection, and rapid point-of-care testing—alongside emerging biosensor technologies, the chapter illustrates how scientific innovation has accelerated detection capabilities while simultaneously acknowledging persistent structural barriers. The authors emphasize that timely diagnosis not only reduces the progression to AIDS but also improves long-term patient outcomes, underscoring the interconnected roles of technological advancement, public awareness, and social support in the global HIV response.

Chapter 2, ***Role of Machine Learning in Enhancing HIV Diagnosis and Care***, introduces readers to the growing impact of artificial intelligence in strengthening HIV treatment pathways across diverse healthcare systems. Drawing from large-scale patient data in the United States, India, South Africa, and Kenya, the chapter highlights machine learning models that significantly improve early detection, ART initiation, and viral-suppression timelines. The authors also engage deeply with fairness considerations, revealing algorithmic biases affecting low-income communities and women, and demonstrating how recalibration methods can reduce inequities by more than 60%. This chapter reinforces AI's promise—while urging thoughtful, ethically grounded deployment.

In **Chapter 3,** ***HIV Prediction and Treatment Through AI***, the contributors expand on the transformative potential of artificial intelligence by focusing on its application to treatment forecasting, drug-resistance identification, and individualized therapy planning. The chapter explores an ecosystem of tools—from wearable technologies to deep-learning prediction models—that enable real-time adherence monitoring and earlier intervention. Yet the authors balance this optimism with caution, addressing the persistent ethical challenges of data privacy, bias, and uneven access to digital health tools. Their analysis presents AI not merely as a technical advance but as a socio-technical shift requiring inclusive design and global stewardship.

Chapter 4, ***Impact of Antiretroviral Therapy (ART) on HIV Treatment Outcomes***, grounds the anthology in the clinical realities of HIV management. The authors examine ART's transformative role in reducing viral load, restoring immune function, and prolonging life expectancy worldwide. At the same time, the chapter addresses unresolved challenges: treatment adherence, drug resistance, disparities in global access, and long-term side effects. By emphasizing both the remarkable success of ART and the barriers that remain, the authors highlight the need for ongoing innovation—not only in pharmaceuticals but also in service delivery and patient support systems.

Chapter 5, ***Artificial Intelligence (AI)-Powered Personalization in HIV Care: From Diagnosis to Drug Response Optimization***, points out the ethical and technical problems faced when using AI in HIV care such as privacy of data, biased results from algorithms and how results can be explained. This chapter aims to add to the body of literature how AI impacts HIV care.

In **Chapter 6,** ***Impact of Digital Tools and Healthcare Technology in Enhancing HIV Treatment and Monitoring***, the focus turns to how digital infrastructures can strengthen patient monitoring and improve access to welfare services. Through a cross-sectional study conducted in Tamil Nadu, the chapter reveals gaps in health-care technology adoption, especially among marginalized communities. The authors advocate for policy reforms, training initiatives, and awareness programs that can harness digital tools to improve adherence, reduce stigma, and promote equitable care. Their findings underscore the importance of culturally grounded, technology-enabled interventions.

Chapter 7, ***Enhancing Mental Health and Treatment Adherence in HIV/AIDS Patients Through Strengthened Social Networks***, reframes HIV treatment through the lens of psychosocial support. By investigating the roles of community networks, NGOs, and peer systems, the chapter demonstrates how emotional connection directly influences adherence, mental-health outcomes, and quality of life. Research conducted in Pudukottai District highlights the weight of stigma, depression, and discrimination, and shows how structured social-support systems can mitigate these burdens. This chapter enriches the anthology by centering the human experience and emphasizing that effective HIV care extends beyond medication.

Finally, **Chapter 8,** ***Ethical AI in HIV Treatment: Balancing Innovation, Privacy, and Equity***, brings the anthology full circle by interrogating the ethical dimensions that arise when AI becomes embedded in HIV treatment ecosystems. The authors examine issues of privacy, informed consent, algorithmic bias, and health inequity, offering a framework for ethical AI design grounded in fairness-aware modeling and privacy-preserving methods. Through real-world case studies, the chapter cautions against unintended harms while emphasizing the importance of trust, transparency, and global equity. It serves as a critical reminder that technological progress must be accompanied by ethical vigilance.

CONCLUSION

As we bring this preface to a close, we are reminded that the work contained within this volume represents far more than a collection of chapters—it is a testament to the power of interdisciplinary collaboration in addressing some of the most urgent challenges in global health and education. Across the contributions in this anthology, a common thread emerges: meaningful innovation occurs when technology, human experience, and ethical responsibility are woven together with care.

The chapters that follow illustrate how rapidly evolving tools—especially artificial intelligence, machine learning, digital health platforms, and game-based methodologies—are reshaping the ways we diagnose, treat, learn, and support one another. Yet they also remind us that technology alone cannot transform systems. Progress depends equally on equitable access, cultural understanding, community engagement, and the unwavering commitment to protect human dignity. Whether improving HIV diagnostics, personalizing treatment, accelerating drug discovery, or strengthening social networks for vulnerable populations, each contribution underscores that the future of care must be inclusive, ethical, and grounded in compassion.

As editors, we are inspired by the breadth of expertise represented in these pages and by the shared vision that binds it together: a future in which innovation serves not simply efficiency or novelty, but justice, empowerment, and human well-being. It is our hope that this book will encourage readers—researchers, practitioners, educators, technologists, policymakers, and students—to explore new collaborations, challenge entrenched assumptions, and pursue solutions that honor both scientific rigor and social responsibility.

Ultimately, *Interdisciplinary Approaches to Game Design in Healthcare and Education* invites us to reimagine what is possible when creativity and evidence converge. We offer this volume as both a resource and a call to action—a reminder that the intersection of technology, play, education, and healthcare holds immense promise for building a more equitable and innovative world.

Chapter 1 Human Immunodeficiency Virus Diagnostic Methods

Eyyüp Kaya
https://orcid.org/0000-0001-9328-0088
Mersin Toros State Hospital, Turkey

ABSTRACT

Human Immunodeficiency Virus (HIV) infection is a serious global health problem that targets the immune system with two distinct strains, HIV-1 and HIV-2. Early diagnosis is imperative in preventing the spread of HIV and enabling the initiation of treatment at an early stage. This, in turn, improves patient health outcomes and prevents the progression to AIDS. The diagnosis of HIV can be facilitated by a range of methods, including ELISA, PCR, p24 antigen tests and rapid tests. The advent of novel technologies, biosensors and point-of-care tests holds great promise in accelerating HIV diagnosis and enhancing its accuracy. However, accessibility to HIV testing remains constrained in several regions, resulting in delayed treatment initiation. As awareness of HIV increases, social support and scientific advances facilitate living with HIV and play an important role in the fight against the virus.

1. INTRODUCTION

Human Immunodeficiency Virus (HIV) infection remains a significant global health concern. This virus targets the immune system, thereby rendering the body vulnerable to a range of infections and certain types of cancer. Two main types of HIV have been identified: HIV-1 and HIV-2. While HIV-1 is prevalent on a global scale, HIV-2 is more endemic, particularly in West Africa (Duncan et al., 2021). It is

DOI: 10.4018/979-8-3373-2863-8.ch001

a virus that belongs to the retrovirus family and continues its life cycle by integrating into the genome of host cells. It has been observed that HIV specifically targets CD4+ T cells, which are critical cells of the immune system. A decline in CD4+ T cell numbers results in a compromised immune system, consequently increasing vulnerability to diverse pathogens (Hamid et al., 2017). Untreated HIV infection can lead to Acquired Immunodeficiency Syndrome (AIDS), a condition characterised by a severe collapse of the immune system. This results in a significant reduction in the body's ability to defend against pathogens, which can lead to life-threatening infections and cancers (Gebremedhin & Haye, 2019).

The global distribution of HIV infection exhibits significant variations across different regions of the world. While the annual number of new infections varies, HIV continues to represent a significant health concern in numerous regions. A notable example of this is Sub-Saharan Africa, which accounts for the highest number of global HIV infections. Data from the United States also demonstrate that HIV infections are more prevalent in specific population groups. Marginalised groups, such as men who have sex with men (MSM) and transgender women, are particularly affected, highlighting health inequalities (Chun et al., 2023). Furthermore, extant research underscores that HIV prevalence in high-risk populations continues to be alarmingly high. For instance, in some urban areas, HIV incidence rates among MSM have reached levels exceeding 20% annually among younger cohorts (Dennis et al., 2021). Statistics of this nature highlight the critical need for the development of bespoke prevention strategies that specifically target these vulnerable populations. The United Nations Programme on HIV/AIDS (UNAIDS) continues to monitor the progression of the global HIV epidemic. By 2021, the number of individuals with HIV had reached approximately 38 million, with 1.5 million new infections being documented. By 2023, some regions, such as Sub-Saharan Africa, accounted for nearly two-thirds of global HIV infections, and despite increased response efforts, persistent challenges persisted in these regions (Chun et al., 2023; Chilundo et al., 2024).

A comprehensive review of extant literature pertaining to HIV diagnosis reveals a meticulous examination of diagnostic methodologies and guidelines. Antibody tests, viral load tests and combination tests are among the methods commonly used in HIV diagnosis. Accurate and timely performance of these tests is of great importance for early detection of HIV infection (Jewell et al., 2020; Amiri et al., 2021). The timely and accurate diagnosis of HIV infection is of paramount importance for the initiation of treatment and prevention of viral spread. Early diagnosis enables patients to access health services more expeditiously, improves their quality of life and reduces the risk of progression to AIDS. Research indicates that individuals who receive an early diagnosis have more favourable health outcomes when they have faster access to treatment (Halasa-Rappel et al., 2021). For instance, studies have documented that individuals diagnosed with HIV early in their infection have lower mortality rates when compared to those diagnosed at a later stage (Darvishi et al., 2020). Furthermore, the ability to mitigate the risk of HIV-positive individuals transmitting the infection to others is a significant benefit of early diagnosis (Jia et al., 2020). This assertion is further substantiated by numerous statistical data sets that demonstrate the efficacy of early diagnosis as a management strategy for HIV infection (Johansson et al., 2024).

Early detection is of critical importance in the management of HIV, as it enables the initiation of treatment prior to the progression of the virus to AIDS. Timely intervention facilitates the commencement of treatment, thereby minimising damage to the immune system and reducing the likelihood of long-term health complications. Furthermore, the process of treatment has been shown to reduce the risk of HIV transmission by lowering the viral load of infected individuals, thereby significantly reducing the probability of viral spread. Achieving successful outcomes in the fight against HIV/AIDS is contingent on increasing accessibility to health services and identifying optimal treatment practices. In this context, the expansion of HIV testing and treatment methods constitutes a critical strategy for maintaining the health status of the population. Furthermore, the implementation of effective prevention strategies is a pivotal step in mitigating the spread of HIV.

This article will undertake a comprehensive review of the extant literature on HIV diagnosis, encompassing the aetiology of HIV, the diagnostic process, the efficacy of diagnostic tests, and treatment guidelines. The reinforcement of strategies for the early diagnosis and treatment of HIV is imperative for the maintenance of public health in the ongoing effort to combat the virus. The effective implementation of these approaches is of paramount importance in the regulation of HIV.

2. HIV DIAGNOSTIC METHODS

HIV diagnosis is of pivotal importance in facilitating the early detection of infection and the initiation of effective treatment. The World Health Organization (WHO) and other health organizations have developed comprehensive guidelines for HIV diagnostic methods. These guidelines provide health authorities with clear guidance on the administration of HIV tests, the selection of eligible individuals for testing, and the interpretation of test results (Pertiwi et al., 2023; Vashisht et al., 2022). Early diagnosis is a critical step in both better managing the infection and directing it to treatment. For instance, the 2018 WHO guidelines advocate cryptococcal antigen (CrAg) screening for individuals with CD4 counts below 200 cells/

μl. Such screening is known to help prevent opportunistic infections in HIV-positive individuals (Vashisht et al., 2022).

The most prevalent diagnostic tests for HIV are antibody tests and rapid tests. The utilisation of rapid tests has been demonstrated to enhance the efficiency of HIV diagnosis, thereby extending the reach of testing to a more diverse population (Pertiwi et al., 2023). While the utilisation of rapid tests facilitates HIV diagnosis, it also encourages individuals to be more willing to take these tests. Conversely, the utilisation of self-testing has emerged as a potent instrument to augment the uptake of testing, particularly among high-risk demographics. Self-testing offers significant advantages in terms of privacy and user convenience. Consequently, barriers to testing, such as social stigma, can be overcome (Harichund et al., 2019; Wulandari et al., 2019).

The development of HIV diagnostic methods has been a gradual process, with strategies being refined over time to enhance their effectiveness. Automated screening strategies, especially in emergency departments, have increased the early detection of HIV and facilitated the referral of patients to treatment (Vashisht et al., 2022). Early diagnosis is pivotal in preventing the progression of HIV infection by accelerating treatment initiation and preventing HIV-related complications. Conversely, delayed diagnosis has been associated with elevated HIV-related morbidity and mortality rates, as well as increased healthcare system costs due to suboptimal treatment responses. Furthermore, late diagnosis has been identified as a significant factor in the acceleration of HIV transmission (Ortblad et al., 2018). Access to HIV testing remains a significant challenge, particularly in low- and middle-income countries. These access issues can negatively impact the uptake and implementation of HIV testing. Ensuring the accessibility of HIV testing is therefore critical for the early diagnosis of HIV infection and the effectiveness of treatment. The expansion of HIV testing has been shown to have a substantial impact on public health, facilitating more effective management of the condition (Harichund et al., 2019).

The effectiveness of HIV testing is contingent upon the accuracy and availability of tests. While the increased speed of HIV diagnosis facilitated by the widespread use of rapid tests is evident, the accessibility of testing remains constrained in certain regions. Furthermore, the acceptance of HIV testing is closely linked to the knowledge that individuals have about HIV. Research indicates that individuals with a comprehensive understanding of HIV testing methods exhibit a greater propensity to undergo testing (Mantell et al., 2022). This underscores the necessity for heightened awareness initiatives concerning HIV. The promotion of regular testing habits among high-risk groups is imperative to ensure early recognition of HIV infection and facilitate referral to treatment. The utilisation of self-testing methodologies and the implementation of community-based distribution strategies have been demonstrated to enhance HIV testing rates, thereby facilitating their access to health services and accelerating their integration into treatment processes (Wang et al., 2020; Ingold et al., 2019).

These strategies are of pivotal importance in the context of HIV infection control and enable individuals to engage with treatment programmes at an earlier stage. The effectiveness of HIV diagnostic methods is directly related to the accuracy and accessibility of tests. Early diagnosis is instrumental in preventing the spread of HIV and enhancing the quality of life of individuals by expediting treatment processes. HIV testing is used to determine the presence of infection and assess its stage. Early diagnosis enables timely referral of HIV-positive individuals to treatment and prevents the progression of the disease.

The most commonly used tests are:

2.1. Antibody Tests (ELISA and Immune Blot Tests)

2.1.1. ELISA (Enzyme-Linked Immunosorbent Assay)

ELISA (enzyme-linked immunosorbent assay) is a widely utilised laboratory test for the diagnosis of HIV, as it is one of the most common methods for the detection of antibodies produced in the body against HIV infection. Following HIV infection, the immune system of the host begins to produce antibodies in response to the virus. However, this process can take several weeks. It is generally recommended to wait a minimum of 2 to 8 weeks after infection before HIV antibodies can be detected. This timeframe may be subject to variation depending on factors such as individual immune responses and viral load (Ingole et al., 2014). The ELISA test is characterised by its high sensitivity and low cost. These characteristics contribute to its extensive utilisation for screening purposes (Abrahim et al., 2019; Bristow et al., 2016). For instance, the ELISA test facilitates the simultaneous evaluation of a substantial number of samples. This is a significant advantage for healthcare professionals conducting tests in laboratories (Lee et al., 2018). However, it is important to note that a positive ELISA test result does not constitute a definitive diagnosis. In such cases, additional confirmatory tests are required to ensure an accurate diagnosis. These additional tests may include HIV-1 Western blot or other immunofluorescence assays (Ingole et al., 2014).

The effectiveness of ELISA is optimised through its integration with other confirmatory tests. The advent of fourth-generation tests, endowed with the capacity to discern both antibodies and HIV-1/2 antigens, signifies their pivotal role in both the diagnostic process and treatment monitoring (Nasrullah et al., 2011; Pilcher et al., 2013). However, it should be noted that these fourth-generation tests may incur a higher financial cost than traditional ELISA tests and, in some cases, may require additional identification tests (Long, 2011; Wratil et al., 2020).

The ELISA method is widely accepted as a key component in the early diagnosis of HIV infection. However, the necessity to perform confirmatory tests for more accurate results in case of a positive test requires careful management of HIV diagnostic processes. In this context, the incorporation of ELISA into HIV diagnosis algorithms emerges as a highly effective screening method in the early stages of infection (Gautheret-Dejean et al., 2015; Abrahim et al., 2019).

2.1.2. Western Blot

In the diagnosis of HIV infection, the ELISA test is frequently utilised in the initial stage of the diagnostic process. In cases where the initial test result is positive, Western Blot (WB) testing is employed as a confirmatory tool. The Western Blot test has been shown to offer a high level of accuracy in detecting the presence of HIV antibodies (Hanet et al., 2023). The Western Blot test is capable of detecting antibodies against specific proteins associated with HIV, thereby providing a supportive indication for the positive results obtained with the ELISA test (Kondo et al., 2018). The critical role of the Western Blot test in the serodiagnostic process is twofold: firstly, it reduces the rate of false positive results, and secondly, it ensures accurate evaluation of patients (Hanet et al., 2023). However, it is important to note that the results of the Western Blot test may vary depending on the stage of HIV infection (Yuksel et al., 2018). In the early stages of infection, for instance, negative results may be obtained because antibodies have not yet formed in the body (Yüksel et al., 2018). The importance of the development process of HIV antibodies has been emphasised in several studies (Rocca et al., 2019; Fasakin et al., 2024). Consequently, specific conditions and testing processes must be considered for the reliability of the test (Msafiri et al., 2022).

Two-step testing, whereby an initial ELISA screening is conducted, followed by the confirmation of positive results through Western Blotting, has emerged as a prevailing approach, particularly in the context of HIV diagnosis. This approach is among the most prevalent methods employed for the detection of HIV antibodies (Al-khayat et al., 2021). The enhanced specificity of Western Blot testing in corroborating positive ELISA results has been well-documented (Wong et al., 2018). Nevertheless, discordant results, where ELISA is positive but Western Blot is negative, have been observed (Nasri et al., 2022), raising concerns about the sensitivity of the test and necessitating further clinical evaluation.

The diagnosis of HIV can be effectively determined by combining ELISA and Western Blot, with a high degree of accuracy. However, it is imperative to acknowledge the influence of factors such as infection stage and clinical status on the interpretation of the tests (Kondo et al., 2018). The necessity of these tests to define the sensitivity and to determine the diagnosis of early-stage HIV has been demonstrated by data from previous studies (Rocca et al., 2019; Han et al., 2023).

2.2. Antigen Tests (p24 Antigen)

Early diagnosis of HIV infection is of critical importance in the treatment process, and p24 antigen testing is a key component of this. p24 antigen is a protein that can be detected following the entry of the HIV virus into the body, particularly in the early stages of infection, when viral replication commences. This antigen only becomes identifiable 1-2 weeks after HIV has entered the body, which is why the p24 test can recognise HIV even in the early stages of infection (Zhou et al., 2021). p24 antigen testing is an effective method of detecting the presence of the virus even in the stages of HIV infection when antibodies are usually not yet developed (Guiraud et al., 2024). The efficacy of this test helps to diagnose HIV infection in its early stages, enabling earlier detection of the virus (Tiwari et al., 2023).

The detection of the p24 antigen typically occurs prior to the development of antibodies, and the sensitivity of the test increases over time following infection, particularly in the early stages of HIV. Concurrently, as the production of antibodies escalates, the concentration of circulating p24 antigen may undergo a decline (Haleyurgirisetty et al., 2020). However, the capacity to detect p24 antigen at the onset of HIV infection is bolstered by advancements in biotechnology that enhance the sensitivity of HIV testing. These innovations enhance the accuracy of the test by increasing the sensitivity of antigen detection (Macchia et al., 2019; Guiraud et al., 2024). Furthermore, the efficacy of the test is enhanced by improved methods to address challenges such as genetic diversity, making the test more efficient against different strains of HIV (Manjate et al., 2024).

The analytical sensitivity of HIV-1 p24 antigen tests has been shown to vary in the range of 0.5-10 pg/ml after infection (Zhou et al., 2021; Guiraud et al., 2024), thereby enabling the test to detect HIV with high sensitivity in the early stages of infection. This test can be used in combination with antibody tests after HIV has been detected, as the p24 antigen can be detected even when antibody tests have not yet become positive (Guiraud et al., 2024). This combination facilitates an earlier HIV diagnosis and a more expeditious commencement of treatment (Pelaez-Prestel et al., 2024). The early detection of HIV infection is of critical importance in the context of viral spread and the acceleration of the treatment process. The p24 antigen is recognised as a vital biomarker in the early stages of HIV infection and is an instrumental tool for the monitoring of HIV response to treatment and the determination of treatment strategies (Sarcina et al., 2021). The potential efficacy of this test in reducing the spread of HIV infections is significant, as it can provide crucial information to aid in the control of the virus, particularly during the early stages of acute HIV infection.

In conclusion, p24 antigen tests offer a significant advantage in detecting the presence of the virus in the early stages of HIV, playing an instrumental role in the management of HIV by facilitating the early initiation of treatment. The accuracy and efficiency of these tests are of paramount importance in the diagnosis of HIV, aiding in the prevention of viral spread.

2.3. Nucleic Acid Detection (PCR)

Polymerase Chain Reaction (PCR) is considered to be one of the most powerful molecular biology techniques for the detection of HIV infection. This method determines the presence of infection by directly detecting the RNA of HIV. The method's ability to target specific sections of the HIV genome, in addition to its capacity to measure the presence of viral RNA, facilitates HIV detection in the early stages of infection (Moscona et al., 2024). The significance of PCR testing lies in its ability to detect HIV in the absence of antibodies, facilitating early diagnosis and expediting treatment initiation (Anjum et al., 2022).

The Polymerase Chain Reaction (PCR) method has been shown to offer the ability to detect even minimal quantities of RNA by means of amplifying genetic material. By targeting HIV RNA as the genetic material, PCR enables highly sensitive detection of infection, even in the early stages of viral infection. The PCR technique utilises enzymes that facilitate the amplification of the targeted genetic material by determining the sequence of the primer and terminator regions. This process validates the genetic structure to determine the presence of infection and detects the HIV virus with high sensitivity. Furthermore, the technique is of great importance in terms of the evolutionary diversity of HIV and its mutations. The HIV virus has the capacity to mutate over time, with certain strains developing resistance to treatments. Consequently, the application of PCR has become pivotal in the analysis of these mutations and the evolutionary changes of viral strains (Hourfar et al., 2018). The presence of HIV strains that develop resistance can indicate the necessity to modify treatment plans. Consequently, PCR emerges as a pivotal instrument in the decision-making process regarding treatment strategies (Berger et al., 2020).

In addition to the diagnosis of HIV infection, the polymerase chain reaction (PCR) test is utilised for the measurement of viral load. Viral load is defined as the quantity of HIV virus particles present in the blood, and it provides information regarding the activity of the infection. A high viral load is indicative of an active infection and the initiation of treatment should be considered (Otange et al., 2019; Tosiano et al., 2019). Furthermore, PCR testing plays a critical role in the process of antiretroviral therapy (ART). A decline in viral load during treatment is an indication of treatment efficacy, whereas an increase in viral load may suggest the emergence of treatment resistance (Wu et al., 2019).

Furthermore, PCR testing plays a critical role in the confirmation of HIV infection and the management of treatment. The regular monitoring of viral load during the treatment process has been shown to demonstrate the effectiveness of treatment and to facilitate the identification of alternative treatment options in cases of treatment resistance. Consequently, PCR testing is a pivotal component in the management and control of HIV infection. The high sensitivity of PCR testing in the early detection of HIV infection is well-documented, as is its role in the optimisation of the treatment process. Furthermore, it facilitates the tracking of the evolutionary diversity of HIV, the measurement of viral load, and the monitoring of treatment efficacy. Its high accuracy in both diagnosis and treatment is an essential tool in managing HIV-related health problems.

2.4. Rapid HIV Tests

Rapid HIV tests are of critical importance in the early diagnosis of HIV infection. These tests evaluate the immune response to HIV, typically utilising blood, saliva or urine samples. The immune response is directed at detecting antibodies and/or virus antigens to indicate the presence of HIV. The most salient benefit of rapid HIV tests is the swiftness of the turnaround time; the majority of tests provide results within 20-30 minutes, rendering them a pragmatic option for emergency situations (Demir et al., 2021). The rapid turnaround time of these tests facilitates their widespread use, particularly in regions with limited access to health services (Altuntaş-Aydın et al., 2022).

The accuracy of rapid HIV tests is contingent on the type of test and the sample used. Whilst the majority of rapid tests demonstrate high levels of accuracy, it has been observed that they can yield false-negative results in the early stages of HIV infection, due to insufficient development of antibody or antigen levels at this stage. This can result in HIV-infected individuals receiving false negative test results due to the immune response not yet being established (Erdinç et al., 2018; Zeytinoğlu et al., 2020). To mitigate the occurrence of false negative results, it is recommended that individuals undergo retesting after a specified interval. This approach has been shown to enhance the accuracy of the test and facilitate the early detection of HIV (Zeytinoğlu et al., 2020; Altuntaş-Aydın et al., 2022). Furthermore, the employment of laboratory-based tests as a confirmatory measure constitutes a pivotal strategy to enhance the accuracy of rapid tests (Erdinç et al., 2018; Demir et al., 2021). Molecular diagnostic tests, with particular reference to polymerase chain reaction (PCR) tests, have the capacity to facilitate the early detection of the human immunodeficiency virus (HIV). These tests are capable of detecting HIV RNA, thereby enabling the diagnosis to be made much earlier in the infection process. By directly targeting HIV RNA, these tests can detect the presence of the virus with a high degree of precision, facilitating a diagnosis in the early stages of infection. Consequently, there is a compelling need to revise and update HIV diagnostic algorithms. Contemporary HIV diagnostic approaches are designed to facilitate the early detection of the disease, thereby enabling the initiation of treatment without delay (Demir et al., 2021; Altuntaş-Aydın et al., 2022).

In conclusion, the utilisation of rapid HIV testing has been demonstrated to be of significant importance in the timely diagnosis of HIV infections, with appropriate use and accurate follow-up. The rapid turnaround time afforded by these tests engenders enhanced effectiveness in health services and facilitates access to treatment for individuals living with HIV. Early detection of HIV is a critical factor in controlling the spread of the virus and enabling faster initiation of treatment. The accuracy and reliability of testing is also important for health policies, which is an important step forward in the fight against HIV.

2.5. Viral Load Test

Viral load testing is a critical tool for the monitoring of the effectiveness of HIV treatment and the assessment of patients' response to treatment. By measuring the level of HIV RNA, it determines whether the virus is being effectively suppressed during the treatment process. The World Health Organization (WHO) has established specific thresholds for the interpretation of viral load test results (Peter et al., 2017; Musab et al., 2022). Specifically, viral suppression is defined as a threshold below 1000 copies/mL, while an undetectable viral load is defined as a threshold below 40 copies/mL. These thresholds are widely regarded as a pivotal metric in evaluating the efficacy of treatment regimens.

Viral load testing is a crucial parameter in the assessment of HIV transmission potential. Adherence to antiretroviral therapy (ART) is associated with a low viral load, which significantly reduces the risk of HIV transmission to others (Jones et al., 2022). A study by He et al. (2024) found that non-adherence to ART increased the risk of secondary HIV transmission by 2.48 times. This underscores the pivotal role of treatment adherence in the spread and control of HIV. Viral load testing is also vital for the assessment of treatment adherence. Early treatment responses are known to suppress viral load and prevent the spread of HIV (Oyedele & Ntusi, 2021; Mayasi et al., 2023). Conversely, elevated viral load during treatment can signify the necessity for modifications to treatment regimens or the introduction of supplementary interventions (Oyedele & Ntusi, 2021; Mayasi et al., 2023). Consequently, viral load test results constitute a pivotal source of data for the formulation of strategic decisions during the course of treatment (Roberts et al., 2016).

The use of viral load testing in low- and middle-income countries faces several challenges. Factors such as inadequate health infrastructure, lack of training and continuity of testing limit the accessibility and feasibility of these tests (Schwartz et al., 2017; Okere et al. 2021). In these countries, widespread implementation of viral load testing is a critical strategy to ensure faster response to treatment and reduce the spread of HIV. WHO emphasises the importance of routine viral load testing, stating that it plays an important role in improving the effectiveness of treatment (Peter et al., 2017). Rapid and accurate viral load testing is essential to ensure early response to treatment and prevent the spread of HIV (Roberts et al., 2016). These tests are a key strategy for improving self-management of HIV treatment and controlling the spread of HIV at a public health level.

In conclusion, it is evident that viral load testing is of great importance in the HIV treatment process, both in terms of personal treatment outcomes and public health. The most fundamental goals in the fight against HIV are increasing treatment adherence, suppressing viral load and preventing the spread of HIV. The importance of effective and accessible viral load testing as a critical tool for HIV control is underscored by the need for its integration at the core of global health strategies (Li et al., 2024).

2.6. New Methods and Developments in HIV Diagnosis: Current Technologies and Artificial Intelligence Applications

Significant advances have been made in the field of HIV diagnosis in recent years. These advances have been designed to expedite the diagnostic process and to provide patients with more rapid access to treatment. The utilisation of innovative technologies in HIV diagnosis is of paramount importance for communities with limited access to healthcare services.

2.6.1. Self-Testing Methods

One of the most significant advancements in the field of HIV diagnosis is the widespread adoption of self-testing. This method enables individuals to undertake HIV testing in the comfort of their own homes or in private spaces. This approach offers significant advantages, particularly for communities facing challenges in accessing healthcare services. It empowers individuals to assume responsibility for their own health, ensures the maintenance of confidentiality, and promotes increased testing for HIV. Research has demonstrated the critical role that HIV self-testing plays in providing equal opportunities and facilitating the diagnosis of individuals who do not wish to test for HIV or who have limited access to health services (Marsh et al., 2019; Shi et al., 2021).

The practice of HIV self-testing has witnessed a notable rise in acceptance, particularly in the context of the ongoing pandemic. The necessity for social distancing measures has rendered traditional testing centres inaccessible, thereby prompting the accelerated adoption of HIV self-testing. The period of the pandemic has served to underscore the significance of sustained HIV testing among high-risk demographics. Men who have sex with men (MSM) and other key populations are best placed to recognise the significance of early HIV diagnosis and subsequent referral to treatment (Shi et al., 2021; Harkness et al., 2022).

2.6.2. Integration of Community-Based Services

Another important development is the integration of community-based services to accelerate HIV diagnosis. Community-based services make it possible to reach individuals who do not want to or do not have access to traditional health centers for HIV testing. Community-based services make testing more accessible and increase HIV awareness in local communities (Marsh et al., 2019). These services include cost-effective methods such as marker tests, accrual tests and rapid tests. Studies on the effectiveness of these tests have led to faster and more accurate HIV diagnoses. It highlights that self-testing strategies can increase the cost of new HIV diagnoses to as much as US$28,300 for each new diagnosis. (Shrestha et al., 2020; Grace et al., 2014). In summary, innovations in HIV diagnosis, especially through self-testing methods and the integration of community-based services, have increased the accessibility of testing and highlighted the importance of early referral to treatment. These innovations have been instrumental in the global effort to combat HIV, contributing to enhanced treatment outcomes (Shi et al., 2021).

2.6.3. Artificial Intelligence Applications in HIV Diagnosis

Another significant development in the field of HIV diagnosis is the utilisation of artificial intelligence (AI) technologies. The field of healthcare stands to benefit greatly from the potential of AI in improving diagnostic processes. Early diagnosis of HIV infection has been shown to have a number of benefits, including improvements in the health status of individuals and the acceleration of treatment processes. The utilisation of AI has been demonstrated to enhance the precision of HIV diagnostic tests and expedite the acquisition of test results. Innovations in areas such as image processing, machine learning and data analytics have the potential to optimise HIV diagnosis processes (Kumar et al., 2023; Roche et al., 2024).

Conventional HIV testing methods, which include fourth generation combined antigen-antibody tests and viral load measurements, are subject to limitations. The utilisation of artificial intelligence (AI) applications has proven to be instrumental in the development of point-of-care (POC) tests, which are characterised by their ease of use in field settings and the rapidity with which they generate results. However, these tests are not without their own limitations. For instance, there are difficulties in detecting acute HIV infections. The development of AI systems for HIV diagnosis is ongoing, with a focus on enhancing the accuracy and reliability of field testing (Stone et al., 2018). Notwithstanding the aforementioned advantages, the integration of AI into diagnostic processes is not without its critics, who contend that it can result in elevated false positive rates for specific demographic groups (Parker et al., 2019).

2.6.4. Artificial Intelligence Based Risk Scoring and HIV Testing Programs

The application of artificial intelligence in the development of risk scoring systems for HIV diagnosis is of significant importance. Machine learning-based risk scoring has emerged as an effective method for determining whether individuals are at risk of HIV infection. For instance, studies conducted in countries such as Kenya and Uganda have demonstrated that the optimisation of community-based HIV testing programmes through the integration of artificial intelligence-based strategies holds considerable potential in enhancing the reach of these programmes (Balzer et al., 2020). Furthermore, the utilisation of AI in the evaluation of HIV self-testing methodologies has been demonstrated to yield more efficient and accurate results in differentiating test outcomes when compared with conventional manual processes (Andigema et al., 2023; Roche et al., 2024).

2.6.5. Artificial Intelligence and HIV Diagnosis in the Future

In the future, it is anticipated that AI-based solutions will assume a more prominent role in HIV diagnostic procedures. The optimisation of AI has the potential to improve the quality of healthcare, not only in individual testing, but also in the development of large-scale health policies. Beyond enhancing the precision and efficiency of testing, the integration of AI technologies is poised to streamline early diagnosis and treatment procedures, thereby amplifying the efficacy of HIV prevention and management efforts. However, the successful implementation of these technologies is predicated on the existence of sustainable infrastructure, reliable data management and the development of ethical standards. The utilisation of AI in the context of HIV diagnosis must be meticulously designed to ensure the accurate analysis of data and the prevention of false positive and negative results. The capacity of AI systems to generate erroneous results has the potential to exert a detrimental effect on health services. Consequently, the integration of AI in HIV diagnosis necessitates a perpetual cycle of audit and enhancement (Roche et al., 2024).

Innovations in the field of HIV diagnosis are achieving notable progress, particularly through the utilisation of self-testing methodologies, the incorporation of community-based services, and the employment of artificial intelligence. Self-testing has been shown to enhance accessibility, while community-based services and AI-based solutions have been demonstrated to expedite and enhance the accuracy of testing processes. These innovations are poised to play a pivotal role in the global effort to combat HIV, particularly in the context of improving treatment outcomes. The early diagnosis and referral of patients to treatment facilitated by these innovations is a crucial step in the fight against HIV. It is anticipated that AI will play a pivotal role in enhancing the efficiency, speed and accuracy of HIV diagnosis in the future. However, it is imperative to acknowledge that the implementation of AI in this domain is contingent upon the resolution of concerns pertaining to data security and ethical considerations.

Point-of-care testing: This development represents a significant advancement in the field of HIV diagnosis. These tests have the capacity to be rapidly administered in hospital settings or emergency care areas, thus eliminating the necessity for traditional laboratory settings. Furthermore, the results of these tests are able to be made available on the same day. This development represents a paradigm shift in the approach to HIV diagnosis and treatment, offering significant advantages for health systems. The deployment of POC tests holds considerable potential in mitigating the spread of HIV, especially in developing countries and high-risk populations. The implementation of HIV testing in emergency departments plays a critical role in the early detection of infection. The expeditious nature of POC tests allows physicians to initiate patient treatment promptly, thereby facilitating enhanced antiretroviral therapy (ART) initiation rates. The Geenius HIV-1/2 rapid test has been shown to be superior in terms of reliability and speed of results compared to confirmatory tests. This enhancement in efficiency leads to a more expeditious diagnosis of HIV, which in turn enhances the efficacy of treatment for patients (Zeytinoğlu et al., 2020).

Evidence is mounting that the benefits of rapid HIV diagnosis and antiretroviral therapy (ART) initiation are especially apparent in paediatric cases. The advent of point-of-care (POC) tests has engendered the capacity for early intervention in children. The utilisation of rapid testing methodologies has been demonstrated to enhance access to treatment for HIV-positive children, thereby playing a pivotal role in the management of their viral load. Furthermore, the utilisation of rapid testing has been demonstrated to effectively raise public awareness regarding the treatability of HIV (Altuntaş-Aydın et al., 2022).

In conclusion, point-of-care testing offers a revolutionary approach to HIV diagnosis and improves the efficiency of health systems. The future role of these tests is of even greater significance, as they offer a wide range of application opportunities, from emergency care to remote informatics services. Ensuring rapid and effective HIV diagnosis and transition to treatment is critical to improving treatment processes and reducing the spread of HIV (Zeytinoğlu et al., 2020; Altuntaş-Aydın et al., 2022).

CRISPR Teknolojisi: This genetic engineering technique has the potential to transform the detection and treatment of HIV. The CRISPR-Cas9 system has been shown to impede viral replication by targeting the genetic material of HIV, with encouraging results in relevant experiments. Specifically, the targeting of the CRISPR/Cas9 system to the regulatory genes of HIV-1 has been shown to inhibit viral replication in infected T cell cultures (Ophinni et al., 2018). Consequently, this technology facilitates the effective targeting and interruption of the latent HIV-1 proviral genome, thereby signifying the potential to impede HIV replication (Verdikt et al., 2019).

CRISPR applications facilitate the study of the permanent reservoirs of HIV-1 and the mechanisms of the enzyme. The potential of this technology is such that in-depth analyses on the capture of HIV-1 in different cell types can be carried out and the effects of gene editing on HIV's replication strategies can be observed (Yoder, 2019). Furthermore, gene editing with CRISPR/Cas9 has been employed to render patients' T cells resistant to HIV-1 infection. This approach signifies a substantial advancement in the quest to enhance treatment procedures for HIV-infected individuals (Tandon & Feist, 2022).

Nevertheless, the effective application of CRISPR technology in the treatment of HIV remains in its infancy and requires further research. The genetic diversity of the HIV virus is a particular challenge in treatment processes. The propensity of HIV viruses to develop resistance to mutations has been identified as a potential impediment to the efficacy of CRISPR applications (Klinnert et al., 2023). Nevertheless, studies have demonstrated the efficacy of CRISPR/Cas9 applications in editing viral DNA in HIV-1-infected cells, emphasising the need for combination therapies to enhance treatment efficiency (Dash et al., 2019).

Finally, the use of CRISPR technology in the treatment of HIV is promising in terms of its potential to inactivate targeted HIV DNA and stop the replication of the virus. Nevertheless, further studies on the safety and efficacy of genetic engineering techniques are required before transitioning to clinical applications (Bella et al., 2018). The outcomes of research in this domain have the potential to facilitate the resolution of significant challenges in the management of HIV in the future.

Biosensors: Biosensors represent a class of innovative technologies that have been developed for the purpose of HIV detection. These biosensors are capable of detecting the presence of HIV at the molecular level, thus enabling the development of tests that are both more sensitive and rapid in nature. These biosensors are notable for their ability to detect the virus and can be used to diagnose infections other than HIV. The incorporation of biosensor technologies into healthcare systems has been shown to enhance efficiency (Manoto et al., 2018; Li et al., 2023).

The ability to detect HIV and other sexually transmitted infections (STIs) simultaneously can provide significant benefits to healthcare systems. A notable study has underscored the efficacy of bidirectional SAW biosensors in facilitating the rapid and reliable detection of HIV, with the potential to optimize resource utilisation within healthcare settings (Gray et al., 2018). The utilisation of biosensors has been demonstrated to accelerate testing and treatment processes, facilitating early diagnosis of HIV infection and other STIs (Manoto et al., 2018; Parekh et al., 2018).

The development of innovative biosensors has led to enhanced methods for the detection of HIV. For instance, DNA biosensors function as innovative platforms with high sensitivity for the recognition of HIV enzymes (Chen et al., 2024). Furthermore, the utilisation of electrochemical biosensors and optical biosensors has led to their application in the monitoring of HIV viral load, the assessment of treatment efficacy, and patient follow-up (Thongkum et al., 2023). These innovative approaches facilitate more accessible, cost-effective and timely testing (Sande et al., 2021).

It is evident that biosensor technology has the potential to enhance the efficiency of healthcare systems, primarily due to its rapid, sensitive and versatile nature in the detection and management of HIV. The integration of such tests is regarded as a pivotal step in the control of HIV infections and the establishment of healthy communities (Gray et al., 2018; Parekh et al., 2018).

3. CONCLUSION

HIV diagnosis is critical to the effective management of the infection and the enhancement of treatment outcomes. Early HIV testing has the potential to halt the progression of the disease and enhance the quality of life of individuals. The methods employed for the early diagnosis of HIV include Enzyme-Linked Immunosorbent Assay (ELISA), Polymerase Chain Reaction (PCR), p24 antigen testing and rapid tests. ELISA, for instance, is a highly prevalent and reliable method for detecting HIV infection. Furthermore, combinations of Multiplex Nucleic Acid Testing (NAT) and ELISA allow for more sensitive and rapid detection of HIV in its early stages.

This approach offers significant advantages in terms of public health, facilitating the referral of individuals for early treatment.

In recent years, there has been considerable progress in the field of HIV diagnostics, with ongoing research and development focusing on novel technologies and biosensors. These novel methods have the potential to expedite HIV detection and enhance diagnostic accuracy. However, challenges in accessing HIV testing and implementing guidelines create barriers to controlling infection. For instance, in countries with low prevalence, the effectiveness of HIV testing strategies is being called into question, while resource constraints can negatively impact health systems. This underscores the necessity for enhanced health policy and research initiatives.

Despite the present absence of a complete cure for HIV, scientific evidence supports the notion that the timely diagnosis and effective treatment of HIV-related complications can significantly reduce the risk of complications. In order for individuals living with HIV to lead healthier and more productive lives in society, there is a necessity for increased clinical and social awareness. Alongside advancements in science, the establishment of social support systems is also paramount in this process. The advancement of biomedical research and the implementation of community-based approaches are of paramount importance in the global effort to combat HIV.

Consequently, HIV diagnostic methods and treatment processes are instrumental in the management of the infection. However, further research and policy development in the future will improve the effectiveness of HIV diagnosis and treatment processes.

REFERENCES

Abrahim, S. A., Girma, M., Habteselassie, A., Gezahegn, N., Feleke, A., Berheto, T. M., Demissie, M., Belete, W., & Deressa, T. (2019). Diagnostic accuracy of HIV test kits, Genscreen Ultra and Bioelisa. *HIV/AIDS (Auckland, N.Z.)*, *11*, 17–22. DOI: 10.2147/HIV.S184603 PMID: 30804685

Al-Khayat, Z. A. Y., Agha, N. F. S., Majeed, P. D., Alharmni, K. I. F., & Agha, D. N. F. (2021). Prevalence of HIV among newly diagnosed tuberculosis patients in Erbil Governorate, Iraq. *Journal of Contemporary Medical Sciences*, *7*(2), 102–107. DOI: 10.22317/jcms.v7i2.955

Altuntaş-Aydın, Ö., Gündüz, A., İnan, A., Kumbasar-Karaosmanoğlu, H., Mete, B., Tekin, S., Yıldız, D. S., & Tabak, F. (2022). Initiation of rapid antiretroviral therapsy in HIV infection. *Klimik Dergisi*, *35*(1), 1–5. DOI: 10.36519/kd.2022.3699

Amiri, F., Roshanaei, G., Olfati Far, M., Najafi, R., & Poorolajal, J. (2021). Survival analysis of the human immunodeficiency virus in iranian patients: A multistate model. *Journal of Arak University of Medical Sciences*, *24*(2), 180–195. DOI: 10.32598/jams.24.2.5530.2

Andigema, A. S., Cyrielle, N. T., Koudoum, P. L., & Vladimir, A. J. (2023). Ai in the management of hiv: Case study cameroon. International. *Journal of Virology and Aids*, *10*(1). Advance online publication. DOI: 10.23937/2469-567x/1510089

Anjum, A., Rehman, A. U., Siddique, H., Rabaan, A. A., Alhumaid, S., Garout, M., Almuthree, S. A., Halwani, M. A., Turkistani, S. A., Qutob, H., Albayat, H., Aljeldah, M., Shammari, B. R. A., Alshahrani, F. S., Alghamdi, A. S., Alduwaihi, S. M., Alibraheem, A. A., Zeb, S., & Zeshan, B. (2022). Evaluation of Hematological, Biochemical Profiles and Molecular Detection of Envelope Gene (gp-41) in Human Immunodeficiency Virus (HIV) among Newly Diagnosed Patients. *Medicina (Kaunas, Lithuania)*, *59*(1), 93. DOI: 10.3390/medicina59010093 PMID: 36676716

Balzer, L. B., Havlir, D. V., Kamya, M. R., Chamie, G., Charlebois, E. D., Clark, T. D., Koss, C. A., Kwarisiima, D., Ayieko, J., Sang, N., Kabami, J., Atukunda, M., Jain, V., Camlin, C. S., Cohen, C. R., Bukusi, E. A., Van Der Laan, M., & Petersen, M. L. (2020). Machine Learning to Identify Persons at High-Risk of Human Immunodeficiency Virus Acquisition in Rural Kenya and Uganda. *Clinical Infectious Diseases*, *71*(9), 2326–2333. DOI: 10.1093/cid/ciz1096 PMID: 31697383

Bella, R., Kaminski, R., Mancuso, P., Young, W. B., Chen, C., Sariyer, R., Fischer, T., Amini, S., Ferrante, P., Jacobson, J. M., Kashanchi, F., & Khalili, K. (2018). Removal of HIV DNA by CRISPR from Patient Blood Engrafts in Humanized Mice. *Molecular Therapy. Nucleic Acids*, *12*, 275–282. DOI: 10.1016/j.omtn.2018.05.021 PMID: 30195766

Berger, A., Muenchhoff, M., Hourfar, K., Kortenbusch, M., Ambiel, I., Stegmann, L., Heim, A., Sarrazin, C., Ehret, R., Daniel, V., Wasner, M., Plantier, J. C., Eberle, J., Gürtler, L., Haberl, A. E., Stürmer, M., & Keppler, O. T. (2020). Severe under-quantification of HIV-1 group O isolates by major commercial PCR-based assays. *Clinical microbiology and infection: the official publication of the European Society of Clinical Microbiology and Infectious Diseases, 26*(12), 1688.e1–1688.e7. DOI: 10.1016/j.cmi.2020.03.004

Bristow, C. C., Leon, S. R., Huang, E., Ramos, L. B., Vargas, S. K., Flores, J. A., Konda, K. A., Caceres, C. F., & Klausner, J. D. (2016). Field Evaluation of a Dual Rapid Immunodiagnostic Test for HIV and Syphilis Infection in Peru. *Sexually Transmitted Diseases*, *43*(1), 57–60. DOI: 10.1097/OLQ.0000000000000387 PMID: 26650998

Chen, F., Wang, J., Ma, J., Song, L., Yan, H., Wang, F., Yang, Z., & Li, F. (2024). Novel DNA Biosensing Platform for Detecting HIV Integrase for Highly Sensitive and Quantitative HIV Detection, Diagnosis, and Therapeutic Monitoring. *ACS Omega*, *9*(23), 25042–25053. DOI: 10.1021/acsomega.4c02229 PMID: 38882085

Chilundo, S., Gaspar, I., Keating, R., Fortmann, J., Filimão, D., Nguimfack, A., Pereira, I., Alfredo, C., Gudo, P. S., Langa, A., Dirlikov, E., Greenberg, S., Pathmanathan, I., & Couto, A. (2024). HIV Antiretroviral Therapy Scale-Up in Mozambique and Estimated Averted HIV Infections and Related Deaths, 2004–2023. *medRxiv*. DOI: 10.1101/2024.11.19.24317542

Chun, H. M., Dirlikov, E., Cox, M. H., Sherlock, M. W., Obeng-Aduasare, Y., Sato, K., Voetsch, A. C., Ater, A. D., Romano, E. R., Tomlinson, H., Modi, S., Achrekar, A., & Nkengasong, J.CDC Global HIV Working Group. (2023). Vital Signs: Progress Toward Eliminating HIV as a Global Public Health Threat Through Scale-Up of Antiretroviral Therapy and Health System Strengthening Supported by the U.S. President's Emergency Plan for AIDS Relief - Worldwide, 2004-2022. *MMWR. Morbidity and Mortality Weekly Report*, *72*(12), 317–324. DOI: 10.15585/mmwr.mm7212e1 PMID: 36952290

Darvishi, S., Rahmani, K., Sey, S., Khazaei, S., Homayonnezhad, S., & Hamidi, O. (2020). The survival rate and its predictors in hiv-infected patients of kurdistan province, iran: a retrospective cohort study. DOI: 10.21203/rs.3.rs-39398/v1

Dash, P. K., Kaminski, R., Bella, R., Su, H., Mathews, S., Ahooyi, T. M., Chen, C., Mancuso, P., Sariyer, R., Ferrante, P., Donadoni, M., Robinson, J. A., Sillman, B., Lin, Z., Hilaire, J. R., Banoub, M., Elango, M., Gautam, N., Mosley, R. L., & Gendelman, H. E. (2019). Sequential LASER ART and CRISPR Treatments Eliminate HIV-1 in a Subset of Infected Humanized Mice. *Nature Communications*, *10*(1), 2753. DOI: 10.1038/s41467-019-10366-y PMID: 31266936

Demir, T., Yıldıran, D., & Kılıç, S. (2021). Experience of the National HIV-AIDS Reference Center of Turkey, in the Transition to the New HIV Diagnostic Algorithm; Comparative Analysis of Line-Immunoassay Test and Bio-Rad Geenius™ HIV-1/2 Antibody Confirmatory Assay. *Mikrobiyoloji Bulteni*, *55*(1), 17–29. DOI: 10.5578/mb.20028 PMID: 33590978

Dennis, A. M., Frost, S. D. W., Enders, K., Cressman, A. E., Volz, E., Adams, N., Miller, W. C., Cohen, M. S., Mobley, V., Samoff, E., & Eron, J. J. (2021). HIV-1 Transmission linkages among persons with incident infection to inform public health surveillance. *EClinicalMedicine*, *37*, 100968. DOI: 10.1016/j.eclinm.2021.100968 PMID: 34195581

Duncan, D., Duncan, J., Kramer, B., Nilsson, A. Y., Haile, B., Butcher, A., Chugh, S., Baum, P., Aldrovandi, G. M., Young, S., Avery, A. K., Tashima, K., Valsamakis, A., Yao, J. D., Chang, M., & Coombs, R. W. (2021). An HIV Diagnostic Testing Algorithm Using the cobas HIV-1/HIV-2 Qualitative Assay for HIV Type Differentiation and Confirmation. *Journal of Clinical Microbiology*, *59*(7), e0303020. DOI: 10.1128/JCM.03030-20 PMID: 33853869

Erdinç, F. Ş., Tülek, N., Ataman Hatipoğlu, Ç., Gürkaynak, P., Aya Kılıç, E. K., Kınıklı, S., & Ertem, G. (2018). Evaluation of the surgeons' approach to hiv infection. *Flora the Journal of Infectious Diseases and Clinical Microbiology*, *23*(4), 167–171. DOI: 10.5578/flora.67359

Fasakin, K. A., Ajayi, O. D., Ibijola, A. A., Adeniyi, A. A., Ajetunmobi, W. A., Ajetunmobi, O. A., Adewara, O. E., Bakare, A., & Oyegue, B. E. (2024). Hiv diagnostic algorithms in a resource-limited setting: A comparative study. *Journal of Advances in Medical and Pharmaceutical Sciences*, *26*(7), 79–94. DOI: 10.9734/jamps/2024/v26i7703

Gautheret-Dejean, A., Bocobza, J., Brunet, S., Damond, F., Plantier, J. C., & Barin, F. (2015). Performance of rapid tests for discrimination between HIV-1 and/or HIV-2 infections. *Journal of Medical Virology*, *87*(12), 2061–2066. DOI: 10.1002/jmv.24282 PMID: 26081750

Gebremedhin, K., & Haye, T. (2019). Factors associated with anemia among people living with hiv/aids taking art in ethiopia. *Advances in Hematology*, •••, 1–8. DOI: 10.1155/2019/9614205 PMID: 30941180

Grace, D., Steinberg, M., Kwag, M., Chown, S. A., Doupe, G., Trussler, T., Rekart, M., & Gilbert, M. (2014). Diagnostic technologies in practice. *Qualitative Health Research*, *25*(2), 205–217. DOI: 10.1177/1049732314549813 PMID: 25201583

Gray, E. R., Turbé, V., Lawson, V. E., Page, R. H., Cook, Z. C., Ferns, R. B., Nastouli, E., Pillay, D., Yatsuda, H., Athey, D., & McKendry, R. A. (2018). Ultra-rapid, sensitive and specific digital diagnosis of hiv with a dual-channel saw biosensor in a pilot clinical study. *NPJ Digital Medicine*, 1(1)., s. DOI: 10.1038/s41746-018-0041-5

Guiraud, V., Ciczora, Y., Cardona, M., Defer, C., Gréaume, S., Nogues, D., & Gautheret-Dejean, A. (2024). Sensitivity and specificity of the new Bio-Rad HIV screening test, Access HIV combo V2. *Journal of Clinical Microbiology*, *62*(5), e0009524. DOI: 10.1128/jcm.00095-24 PMID: 38534108

Halasa-Rappel, Y. A., Gaumer, G., Khatri, D., Hurley, C. L., Jordan, M., & Nandakumer, A. K. (2021). The tale of two epidemics: Hiv/aids in ghana and namibia. *The Open AIDS Journal*, *15*(1), 63–72. DOI: 10.2174/1874613602115010063

Haleyur Giri Setty, M. K., Lee, S., Lathrop, J., & Hewlett, I. K. (2020). Biotin Interference in Point of Care HIV Immunoassay. *BioResearch Open Access*, *9*(1), 243–246. DOI: 10.1089/biores.2020.0038 PMID: 33269113

Hamid, O., Tapak, M., Poorolajal, J., Amini, P., & Tapak, L. (2017). Application of random survival forest for competing risks in prediction of cumulative incidence function for progression to AIDS. *Epidemiology, Biostatistics, and Public Health*, *14*(4). Advance online publication. DOI: 10.2427/12663

Han, J., Wang, Y., Wang, B., & Tong, H. (2023). Diagnostic efficacy of photostimulated chemiluminescence assay for detecting anti-hiv antibodies: A retrospective study. *Polish Journal of Microbiology*, *72*(4), 461–466. DOI: 10.33073/pjm-2023-043 PMID: 38095515

Harichund, C., Karim, Q. A., Kunene, P., Simelane, S., & Moshabela, M. (2019). HIV self-testing as part of a differentiated HIV testing approach: Exploring urban and rural adult experiences from KwaZulu-Natal, South Africa using a cross-over study design. *BMC Public Health*, *19*(1), 53. DOI: 10.1186/s12889-018-6366-9 PMID: 30634943

Harkness, A., Morales, V., Defreitas, W., Atuluru, P., Jaramillo, J., Weinstein, E. R., Feaster, D. J., Safren, S., & Balise, R. (2022). Impact of COVID-19 on HIV service delivery in Miami-Dade County: A mixed methods study. *BMC Health Services Research*, *22*(1), 1476. DOI: 10.1186/s12913-022-08849-8 PMID: 36463177

He, J., Zhong, S., Qin, C., Nong, A., Lin, Z., Liang, H., Zhang, F., Jiang, J., Pan, P., Wei, W., Liu, J., Liu, D., Ye, L., Liang, H., & Liang, B. (2024). The trend, prevalence and potential risk factors of secondary HIV transmission among HIV/AIDS individuals receiving ART in Guangxi, China: A longitudinal cross-sectional study. *Emerging Microbes & Infections*, *13*(1), 2429622. DOI: 10.1080/22221751.2024.2429622 PMID: 39552513

Hourfar, K., Eberle, J., Müller, M., Micha Nübling, C., Chudy, M., Kress, J., Gürtler, L., Mayr-Wohlfart, U., Schrezenmeier, H., Hellmann, I., Luhm, J., Kraas, S., Ringwald, J., Gubbe, K., Frank, K., Karl, A., Tonn, T., Jaeger, M., Sireis, W., & Schmidt, M. (2018). Human immunodeficiency virus 1 dual-target nucleic acid technology improves blood safety: 5 years of experience of the German Red Cross blood donor service Baden-Württemberg-Hessen. *Transfusion*, *58*(12), 2886–2893. DOI: 10.1111/trf.14919 PMID: 30325043

Ingold, H., Mwerinde, O., Ross, A. L., Leach, R., Corbett, E. L., Hatzold, K., Johnson, C. C., Ncube, G., Nyirenda, R., & Baggaley, R. C. (2019). The Self-Testing AfRica (STAR) Initiative: accelerating global access and scale-up of HIV self-testing. *Journal of the International AIDS Society, 22 Suppl 1*(Suppl Suppl 1), e25249. DOI: 10.1002/jia2.25249

Ingole, N., Sarkate, P., Paranjpe, S. M., Sarode, R., Shinde, S., & Mehta, P. R. (2014). HIV Diagnosis in Resource Constrained Setting: How Good Is the Current Algorithm? *World Journal of AIDS*, *4*, 45–51. DOI: 10.4236/wja.2014.41006

Jewell, B. L., Mudimu, E., Stover, J., Ten Brink, D., Phillips, A. N., Smith, J. A., Martin-Hughes, R., Teng, Y., Glaubius, R., Mahiane, S. G., Bansi-Matharu, L., Taramusi, I., Chagoma, N., Morrison, M., Doherty, M., Marsh, K., Bershteyn, A., Hallett, T. B., & Kelly, S. L.HIV Modelling Consortium. (2020). Potential effects of disruption to HIV programmes in sub-Saharan Africa caused by COVID-19: Results from multiple mathematical models. *The Lancet. HIV*, *7*(9), e629–e640. DOI: 10.1016/S2352-3018(20)30211-3 PMID: 32771089

Jia, X. C., Xia, Z. H., Shi, N., Wang, Y. P., Luo, Z. X., Yang, Y. L., & Shi, X. Z. (2020). The factors associated with natural disease progression from HIV to AIDS in the absence of ART, a propensity score matching analysis. *Epidemiology and Infection*, *148*, e57. DOI: 10.1017/S0950268820000540 PMID: 32089142

Johansson, E., Nazziwa, J., Freyhult, E., Hong, M., Neptin, M., Karlson, S., Rezeli, M., da Silva, Z. J., Biague, A. J., Lindman, J., Palm, A., Medstrand, P., Månsson, F., Norrgren, H., Jansson, M., & Esbjörnsson, J.SWEGUB CORE group. (2024). Distinct plasma protein profiles distinguish faster from slower disease progression in hiv-1 and hiv-2 infections. DOI: 10.1101/2024.07.23.24310457

Klinnert, S., Freitag, P. C., Plückthun, A., & Metzner, K. J. (2023). Targeting hiv-1 with crispr/cas9 delivered by retargeted adenoviruses effectively suppresses viral replication. DOI: 10.1101/2023.12.18.572146

Kondo, M., Sudo, K., Sano, T., Kawahata, T., Itoda, I., Iwamuro, S., Yoshimura, Y., Tachikawa, N., Kojima, Y., Mori, H., Fujiwara, H., Hasegawa, N., & Kato, S. (2018). Comparative evaluation of the Geenius HIV 1/2 Confirmatory Assay and the HIV-1 and HIV-2 Western blots in the Japanese population. *PLoS One*, *13*(10), e0198924. DOI: 10.1371/journal.pone.0198924 PMID: 30379808

Kumar, Y., Koul, A., Singla, R., & Ijaz, M. F. (2023). Artificial intelligence in disease diagnosis: A systematic literature review, synthesizing framework and future research agenda. *Journal of Ambient Intelligence and Humanized Computing*, *14*(7), 8459–8486. DOI: 10.1007/s12652-021-03612-z PMID: 35039756

Lee, Y. H., Bang, J. H., Park, S. M., Kang, C. R., Cho, S. I., Oh, M. D., & Lee, J. K. (2018). Cost-Effectiveness of Voluntary HIV Testing Strategies in a Very Low-Prevalence Country, the Republic of Korea. *Journal of Korean Medical Science*, *33*(46), e304. DOI: 10.3346/jkms.2018.33.e304 PMID: 30416412

Li, L., Feng, X., Zhao, F., Yuan, D., An, X., Tian, X., Wu, H., Su, B., Zhang, T., & Liu, L. (2024). Real-world performance of hiv low viral load values in diagnosing acute hiv infection in a tertiary care hospital in beijing, china. *BMC Infectious Diseases*, *24*(1). Advance online publication. DOI: 10.1186/s12879-024-09486-8 PMID: 38879487

Li, Z., Uno, N., Ding, X., Avery, L., Banach, D., & Liu, C. (2023). Bioinspired CRISPR-Mediated Cascade Reaction Biosensor for Molecular Detection of HIV Using a Glucose Meter. *ACS Nano*, *17*(4), 3966–3975. DOI: 10.1021/acsnano.2c12754 PMID: 36762838

Long, E. (2011). Hiv screening via fourth-generation immunoassay or nucleic acid amplification test in the united states: A cost-effectiveness analysis. *PLoS One*, *6*(11), e27625. DOI: 10.1371/journal.pone.0027625 PMID: 22110698

Macchia, E., Sarcina, L., Picca, R. A., Manoli, K., Di Franco, C., Scamarcio, G., & Torsi, L. (2019). Ultra-low hiv-1 p24 detection limits with a bioelectronic sensor. *Analytical and Bioanalytical Chemistry*, *412*(4), 811–818. DOI: 10.1007/s00216-019 PMID: 31865415

Manjate, A., Nilsson, C., Axelsson, M., Lindroth, S., Sirbu, D., Sacarlal, J., Andersson, S., & Unemo, M. (2024). Laboratory-based evaluation of the 4th-generation AlereTM HIV Combo rapid point-of-care test. *PLoS One*, *19*(2), e0298912. DOI: 10.1371/journal.pone.0298912 PMID: 38394120

Manoto, S. L., Lugongolo, M., Govender, U., & Mthunzi-Kufa, P. (2018). Point of Care Diagnostics for HIV in Resource Limited Settings: An Overview. *Medicina (Kaunas, Lithuania)*, *54*(1), 3. DOI: 10.3390/medicina54010003 PMID: 30344234

Mantell, J. E., Khalifa, A., Christian, S. N., Romo, M. L., Mwai, E., George, G., Strauss, M., Govender, K., & Kelvin, E. A. (2022). Preferences, beliefs, and attitudes about oral fluid and blood-based HIV self-testing among truck drivers in Kenya choosing not to test for HIV. *Frontiers in Public Health*, *10*, 911932. DOI: 10.3389/fpubh.2022.911932 PMID: 36438254

Marsh, K., Eaton, J. W., Mahy, M., Sabin, K., Autenrieth, C. S., Wanyeki, I., Daher, J., & Ghys, P. D. (2019). Global, regional and country-level 90-90-90 estimates for 2018: assessing progress towards the 2020 target. *AIDS (London, England)*, *33 Suppl 3*(Suppl 3), S213–S226. DOI: 10.1097/QAD.0000000000002355

Mayasi Ngongo, N., Kamangu Ntambwe, E., Situakibanza Nani-Tuma, H., Mbula Mambimbi, M., Mandina Ndona, M., Longokolo Mashi, M., Bepouka Izizag, B., Lukiana, T., Odio Ossam, J., Mangala Sonzi, D., Maes, N., Moutschen, M., El Moussaoui, M., & Darcis, G. (2023). Human Immunodeficiency Virus Viral Load Monitoring and Rate of Virologic Suppression Among Patients Receiving Antiretroviral Therapy in Democratic Republic of the Congo, 2013-2020. *Open Forum Infectious Diseases*, *10*(6), ofad242. Advance online publication. DOI: 10.1093/ofid/ofad242 PMID: 37363052

Moscona, R., Wagner, T., Geva, M., Bucris, E., Erster, O., Zuckerman, N. S., & Mor, O. (2024). Novel amplicons based method for near-full-length genome (NFLG) sequencing of HIV-1 group M recombinant forms. DOI: 10.1101/2024.08.04.606545

Msafiri, F., Manjate, A., & Lindroth, S. (2022). Vaccine-induced seroreactivity impacts the accuracy of hiv testing algorithms in sub-saharan africa: An exploratory study. *Vaccines*, *10*(7), 1062. DOI: 10.3390/vaccines10071062 PMID: 35891226

Musab, A., Gobir, I. Y., Zakari, Y., Kabuga, A. I., & Rogo, L. D. (2022). Plasma levels of secretory calreticulin among hiv infected patients in bauchi state. *J AIDS HIV Treat*, *5*(1), 1–8. DOI: 10.33696/aids.5.040

Nasri, E., Fakhim, H., & Jafari-Sales, A. (2022). Prevalence of human t-lymphotropic virus type 1 in brain-dead organ donors. *Archives of Clinical Infectious Diseases*, *17*(1). Advance online publication. DOI: 10.5812/archcid-116005

Nasrullah, M., Ethridge, S. F., Delaney, K. P., Wesolowski, L. G., Granade, T. C., Schwendemann, J., Boromisa, R. D., Heffelfinger, J. D., Owen, S. M., & Branson, B. M. (2011). Comparison of alternative interpretive criteria for the HIV-1 Western blot and results of the Multispot HIV-1/HIV-2 Rapid Test for classifying HIV-1 and HIV-2 infections. *Journal of clinical virology: the official publication of the Pan American Society for Clinical Virology, 52 Suppl 1*, S23–S27. DOI: 10.1016/j.jcv.2011.09.020

Okere, N. E., Sambu, V., Ndungile, Y., van Praag, E., Hermans, S., Naniche, D., de Wit, T. F. R., Maokola, W., & Gomez, G. B. (2021). The Shinyanga Patient: A Patient's Journey through HIV Treatment Cascade in Rural Tanzania. *International Journal of Environmental Research and Public Health*, *18*(16), 8418. DOI: 10.3390/ijerph18168418 PMID: 34444166

Ophinni, Y., Inoue, M., Kotaki, T., & Kameoka, M. (2018). CRISPR/Cas9 system targeting regulatory genes of HIV-1 inhibits viral replication in infected T-cell cultures. *Scientific Reports*, *8*(1), 7784. DOI: 10.1038/s41598-018-26190-1 PMID: 29773895

Ortblad, K. F., Chanda, M. M., Musoke, D. K., Ngabirano, T., Mwale, M., Nakitende, A., Chongo, S., Kamungoma, N., Kanchele, C., Bärnighausen, T., & Oldenburg, C. E. (2018). Acceptability of HIV self-testing to support pre-exposure prophylaxis among female sex workers in Uganda and Zambia: Results from two randomized controlled trials. *BMC Infectious Diseases*, *18*(1), 503. DOI: 10.1186/s12879-018-3415-z PMID: 30286737

Otange, B., Birech, Z., Rop, R., & Oyugi, J. (2019). Estimation of hiv-1 viral load in plasma of hiv-1-infected people based on the associated raman spectroscopic peaks. *Journal of Raman Spectroscopy : JRS*, *50*(5), 620–628. DOI: 10.1002/jrs.5557

Oyedele, O., & Ntusi, N. (2021). A multinomial modelling of the factors that impact viral load levels in adults on anti-retroviral therapy in namibia. *ISTJN*, *14*, 73–82. DOI: 10.32642/istjn.v14i.1569

Parekh, B. S., Ou, C. Y., Fonjungo, P. N., Kalou, M. B., Rottinghaus, E., Puren, A., Alexander, H., Hurlston Cox, M., & Nkengasong, J. N. (2018). Diagnosis of Human Immunodeficiency Virus Infection. *Clinical Microbiology Reviews*, *32*(1), e00064–e18. DOI: 10.1128/CMR.00064-18 PMID: 30487166

Parker, J., Carrasco, A.F., & Chen, J. (2019). BioRad BioPlex® HIV Ag-Ab assay: Incidence of false positivity in a low-prevalence population and its effects on the current HIV testing algorithm. *Journal of clinical virology: the official publication of the Pan American Society for Clinical Virology, 116*, 1–3. DOI: 10.1016/j.jcv.2019.04.002

Pelaez-Prestel, H., Mozas-Gutierrez, J., Lafuente, E. M., & Reche, P. A. (2024). Hiv-1 protein coding sequences are present in relevant bacteria. DOI: 10.1101/2024.12.04.626764

Pertiwi, R., Woelansari, E., & Puspitasari, A. (2023). Correlation between hiv rapid test and hiv viral load in hiv patients at haji hospital in surabaya. *International Journal of Advanced Health Science and Technology*, *3*(4), 223–228. DOI: 10.35882/ijahst.v3i4.290

Peter, T., Ellenberger, D., Kim, A. A., Boeras, D., Messele, T., Roberts, T., Stevens, W., Jani, I., Abimiku, A., Ford, N., Katz, Z., & Nkengasong, J. N. (2017). Early antiretroviral therapy initiation: Access and equity of viral load testing for HIV treatment monitoring. *The Lancet. Infectious Diseases*, *17*(1), e26–e29. DOI: 10.1016/S1473-3099(16)30212-2 PMID: 27773596

Pilcher, C. D., Louie, B., Facente, S., Keating, S., Hackett, J.Jr, Vallari, A., Hall, C., Dowling, T., Busch, M. P., Klausner, J. D., Hecht, F. M., Liska, S., & Pandori, M. W. (2013). Performance of rapid point-of-care and laboratory tests for acute and established HIV infection in San Francisco. *PLoS One*, *8*(12), e80629. DOI: 10.1371/journal.pone.0080629 PMID: 24349007

Roberts, T., Cohn, J., Bonner, K., & Hargreaves, S. (2016). Scale-up of Routine Viral Load Testing in Resource-Poor Settings: Current and Future Implementation Challenges. *Clinical Infectious Diseases*, *62*(8), 1043–1048. DOI: 10.1093/cid/ciw001 PMID: 26743094

Rocca, S., Zangari, P., Cotugno, N., De Rossi, A., Ferns, B., Petricone, D., Rinaldi, S., Giaquinto, C., Bernardi, S., Rojo, P., Rossi, P., Pahwa, S., Nastouli, E., & Palma, P.EPIICAL Consortium. (2019). Human Immunodeficiency Virus (HIV)-Antibody Repertoire Estimates Reservoir Size and Time of Antiretroviral Therapy Initiation in Virally Suppressed Perinatally HIV-Infected Children. *Journal of the Pediatric Infectious Diseases Society*, *8*(5), 433–438. DOI: 10.1093/jpids/piy080 PMID: 30169837

Roche, S. D., Ekwunife, O. I., Mendonca, R., Kwach, B., Omollo, V., Zhang, S., Ongwen, P., Hattery, D., Smedinghoff, S., Morris, S., Were, D., Rech, D., Bukusi, E. A., & Ortblad, K. F. (2024). Measuring the performance of computer vision artificial intelligence to interpret images of HIV self-testing results. *Frontiers in Public Health*, *12*, 1334881. DOI: 10.3389/fpubh.2024.1334881 PMID: 38384878

Sande, M. G., Rodrigues, J. L., Ferreira, D., Silva, C. J., & Rodrigues, L. R. (2021). Novel Biorecognition Elements against Pathogens in the Design of State-of-the-Art Diagnostics. *Biosensors (Basel)*, *11*(11), 418. DOI: 10.3390/bios11110418 PMID: 34821636

Sarcina, L., Mangiatordi, G. F., Torricelli, F., Bollella, P., Gounani, Z., Österbacka, R., Macchia, E., & Torsi, L. (2021). Surface Plasmon Resonance Assay for Label-Free and Selective Detection of HIV-1 p24 Protein. *Biosensors (Basel)*, *11*(6), 180. DOI: 10.3390/bios11060180 PMID: 34204930

Schwartz, S.R., Kavanagh, M.M., Sugarman, J., Solomon, S.S., Njindam, I.M., Rebe, K., Quinn, T. C., Toure-Kane, C., Beyrer, C., & Baral, S. (2017). HIV viral load monitoring among key populations in low- and middle-income countries: challenges and opportunities. *Journal of the International AIDS Society, 20 Suppl 7*(Suppl 7), e25003. DOI: 10.1002/jia2.25003

Shi, L., Tang, W., Hu, H., Qiu, T., Marley, G., Liu, X., Chen, Y., Chen, Y., & Fu, G. (2021). The impact of COVID-19 pandemic on HIV care continuum in Jiangsu, China. *BMC Infectious Diseases*, *21*(1), 768. DOI: 10.1186/s12879-021-06490-0 PMID: 34364383

Shrestha, R. K., Chavez, P. R., Noble, M., Sansom, S. L., Sullivan, P. S., Mermin, J. H., & MacGowan, R. J. (2020). Estimating the costs and cost-effectiveness of HIV self-testing among men who have sex with men, United States. *Journal of the International AIDS Society*, *23*(1), e25445. DOI: 10.1002/jia2.25445 PMID: 31960580

Stone, M., Bainbridge, J., Sanchez, A. M., Keating, S. M., Pappas, A., Rountree, W., Todd, C., Bakkour, S., Manak, M., Peel, S. A., Coombs, R. W., Ramos, E. M., Shriver, M. K., Contestable, P., Nair, S. V., Wilson, D. H., Stengelin, M., Murphy, G., Hewlett, I., & Busch, M. P. (2018). Comparison of Detection Limits of Fourth- and Fifth-Generation Combination HIV Antigen-Antibody, p24 Antigen, and Viral Load Assays on Diverse HIV Isolates. *Journal of Clinical Microbiology*, *56*(8), e02045–e17. DOI: 10.1128/JCM.02045-17 PMID: 29793968

Tandon, A., & Feist, W. (2022). Applications of crispr-cas9 technology to treat ccr5 tropic hiv-1. *Journal of Student Research*, *11*(4). Advance online publication. DOI: 10.47611/jsrhs.v11i4.3464

Thongkum, W., Klayprasert, P., Semakul, N., Jakmunee, J., Kasinrerk, W., Setshedi, M., Sayed, Y., & Tayapiwatana, C. (2023). Semi-quantification and Potency Verification of the HIV Protease Inhibitor Based on the Matrix-Capsid Protein Immobilized Nickel (II)/NTA-Tol/Graphene Oxide/SPCE Electrochemical Biosensor. *ACS Omega*, *8*(20), 17932–17940. DOI: 10.1021/acsomega.3c01031 PMID: 37251123

Tiwari, A. K., Aggarwal, G., Pabbi, S., Mitra, S., Yadav, N., Verma, V., & Cheirmaraj, K. (2023). Analytical and clinical performance evaluation of enhanced chemiluminescence-based fourth-generation HIV combo assay: Report from tertiary health-care setup in North India. *Asian Journal of Transfusion Science*, *17*(2), 175–181. DOI: 10.4103/ajts.ajts_128_22 PMID: 38274959

Tosiano, M. A., Jacobs, J. L., Shutt, K. A., Cyktor, J. C., & Mellors, J. W. (2019). A Simpler and More Sensitive Single-Copy HIV-1 RNA Assay for Quantification of Persistent HIV-1 Viremia in Individuals on Suppressive Antiretroviral Therapy. *Journal of Clinical Microbiology*, *57*(3), e01714–e01718. DOI: 10.1128/JCM.01714-18 PMID: 30626659

Vashisht, S., Jha, S., Thakur, N., Khaitan, A., Rai, S., Haldar, P., Kant, S., Kardam, P., & Sangral, M. (2022). Comparing the Effects of Oral HIV Self-Testing With Those of Standard HIV Testing for Men Who Have Sex With Men (MSM): A Systematic Review and Meta-Analysis. *Cureus*, *14*(8), e28157. DOI: 10.7759/cureus.28157 PMID: 36158381

Verdikt, R., Darcis, G., Ait-Ammar, A., & Van Lint, C. (2019). Applications of CRISPR/Cas9 tools in deciphering the mechanisms of HIV-1 persistence. *Current Opinion in Virology*, *38*, 63–69. DOI: 10.1016/j.coviro.2019.07.004 PMID: 31509794

Wang, C., Cheng, W., Li, C., Tang, W., Ong, J. J., Smith, M. K., Fu, H., Marks, M., Nie, J., Zheng, H., Tucker, J. D., & Yang, B. (2020). Syphilis Self-testing: A Nationwide Pragmatic Study Among Men Who Have Sex With Men in China. *Clinical Infectious Diseases*, *70*(10), 2178–2186. DOI: 10.1093/cid/ciz603 PMID: 31260513

Wong, C. C., Lim, S. H., Tan, C. T., Lui, S. Y., Lee, Y. L., & Chan, K. P. (2018). Performance of the HIV Blot 2.2, INNO-LIA HIV I/II Score, and Geenius HIV 1/2 Confirmatory Assay for use in HIV confirmation. *PLoS One*, *13*(6), e0199502. DOI: 10.1371/journal.pone.0199502 PMID: 29928045

Wratil, P. R., Rabenau, H. F., Eberle, J., Stern, M., Münchhoff, M., Friedrichs, I., Stürmer, M., Berger, A., Kuttner-May, S., Münstermann, D., Lucht, A., Meixenberger, K., Bannert, N., & Keppler, O. T. (2020). Comparative multi-assay evaluation of determine™ hiv-1/2 ag/ab combo rapid diagnostic tests in acute and chronic hiv infection. *Medical Microbiology and Immunology*, *209*(2), 139–150. DOI: 10.1007/s00430-019-00655-0 PMID: 32036450

Wu, S., Gao, M., Zheng, J., Yan, P., Wang, W., Lu, X., Qiu, Y., & Yan, Y. (2019). Prevalence of HIV Indeterminate Western Blot Tests and Follow-up of HIV Antibody Sero-Conversion in Southeastern China. *Virologica Sinica*, *34*(4), 358–366. DOI: 10.1007/s12250-019-00130-3 PMID: 31190120

Wulandari, L. P. L., Ruddick, A., Guy, R., & Kaldor, J. (2019). "Self-testing sounds more private, rather than going to the clinic and everybody will find out": Facilitators and barriers regarding HIV testing among men who purchase sex in Bali, Indonesia. *PLoS One*, *14*(4), e0214987. DOI: 10.1371/journal.pone.0214987 PMID: 30958845

Yoder, K. (2019). A crispr/cas9 library to map the hiv-1 provirus genetic fitness. *Acta Virologica. English Ed.*, *63*(02), 129–138. DOI: 10.4149/av_2019_201 PMID: 31230441

Yüksel, P., Sarıbaş, S., & Kuşkucu, M. (2018). Problems encountered in conventional hiv 1/2 algorithms: Lack of necessity for immunoblot assays to confirm repeated elisa reactive results. *African Health Sciences*, *18*(2). Advance online publication. DOI: 10.4314/ahs.v18i2.26 PMID: 30602968

Zeytinoğlu, A., Kayın, M., Altuğlu, İ., Gökengin, D., & Sertöz, R. (2020). İ Comparison of two anti-HIV confirmatory assays: Recombinant HIV 1/2 line immunoassay and Geenius HIV 1/2 confirmatory test. *Mikrobiyoloji Bulteni*, *54*(4), 613–618. DOI: 10.5578/mb.69786 PMID: 33107290

Chapter 2

Role of Machine Learning in Enhancing HIV Diagnosis and Care

Mehak Jonjua
https://orcid.org/0000-0003-0123-8355
Sharda University, India

ABSTRACT

Artificial Intelligence in the knowledge of HIV care allows early detection of HIV, faster start on ART, and improved adherence. The study evaluates the predictive AI model in the health care settings of the USA, India, South Africa, and Kenya. Impressive performance was shown with this model with a predictive accuracy of 0.87 AUC after being trained on 32,450 patient records, albeit with variations in performance based on socio-economic status and health infrastructure. AI-supported early diagnosis showed improvement by 28% and 31%, and a decrease in time to viral suppression was significant-up to 28%. On the other hand, ML-based predictions on adherence to intervention improved medication compliance estimations by 9.5%-10.8% through targeted intervention. Fairness analysis showed the predictions were biased towards low-income earners and women; with fairness-aware recalibration, the degree of bias was reduced by over 60%. The present work demonstrates the transformational nature of AI for HIV care and calls for the intelligent and fair implementation of AI interventions.

INTRODUCTION

The Human Immunodeficiency Virus is essentially an ongoing major health challenge across the world, with about 38 million people said to be living with HIV.

DOI: 10.4018/979-8-3373-2863-8.ch002

Thus, diagnosing, preventing, and managing HIV are really the urgent priorities for global health despite having advanced far in treatment opportunitiesJaiteh, M., Phalane, et al. (2024). Machine Learning, a field of artificial intelligence wherein systems are trained to learn from data in order to improve performance of a task without being explicitly programmed, is another powerful tool that is changing the entire HIV care paradigm from prevention to diagnosis to treatment.

Among many uses of ML in HIV care, this will be one that focuses on improving early diagnosis and detection. Standard diagnostic methods such as enzyme-linked immunosorbent assay (ELISA) and polymerase chain reaction (PCR) tests require laboratory infrastructure and trained human resources that might not be available in settings with limited resources, Dzinamarira, T., Mbunge, et al. (2024). An ML algorithm integrated with a biosensor and mobile-based HIV diagnostic tools could improve speed and accuracy in HIV detection. Studies have shown that AI-based imagery recognition models assessing rapid diagnostic test (RDT) results can achieve comparable sensitivity and specificity to laboratory tests thus increasing access to early diagnosis.

ML further aids in personalizing HIV treatment. ARV therapy is the basis of HIV management, and ART regimen selection incorporates many variables including viral load, genetic resistance mutations, and patient adherence behavior (Padhi et al., 2023). ML models developed on large data sets that include genomic sequencing data and electronic health record information can be used to predict which ART combinations would therefore most likely suppress the viral load, with minimal side effects. Studies indicate that including the socio-behavioral and clinical data in predictive models to improve treatment outcome-based adherence monitoring and decrease drug resistance.

ML is also targeted towards HIV prevention strategies by identifying high-risk populations and predicting outbreaks. AI modelling that takes in demographic, behavioral, and epidemiological data can serve in the hands of public health officials when planning for a targeted intervention, such as their distribution of pre-exposure prophylaxis (PrEP) and their community awareness campaigns. For example, ML modelling has already been applied for predicting geographical regions with a high risk of HIV transmission, allowing the better allocation of resources for prevention programs.

Moreover a very big advantage which is offered by ML in the field of HIV care is a real-time monitoring and assistance to patients. AI-powered mobile apps, chatbots, and wearable health devices can provide personalized reminders, keeping track of medication adherence, and virtual counseling to help overcome the common barriers to adherence with ART, Saha, R., Malviya, L (2024). As well, these tools can catch the early signs of treatment failure and alert health care providers for timely intervention. For example, AI-assisted monitoring of adherence improved the rate of viral suppression in patients by nearly 15% in a study published in The Lancet HIV.

Although ML is not devoid of potential challenges such as their implications on data privacy, algorithmic bias, and smooth adoption into existing healthcare systems, important ethical considerations must be given to informed consent and equitable access to AI tools for further benefits from avoiding risks. It is the future and move forward through increasing advancements in the technology that those greater achievements can be made with multidisciplinary cooperation among health care professionals, data scientists, and policymakers.

ML is on the verge of reformation-ing HIV care with its tools for early diagnosis, optimization of treatment, improved adherence, and increased prevention empowerment-all are offering continued promise in bringing better outcomes to patients around the world. If the AI-powered solutions mature to such extent, it is believed that making HIV management more accessible, efficient, and effective will be possible in the global fight against the epidemic, Lainjo, B. (2024).

REVIEW OF LITERATURE

Diagnosis of HIV Infection Through Machine Learning

Currently, the machine learning-based models play a crucial role in early detection of HIV infection. By using huge amounts of patient information, the models manage to spot even the most subtle differences in symptoms, laboratory test results, and imaging data, which otherwise could probably not be detected by the human senses. Analytically, using powerful deep learning algorithms, convolutional neural networks has shown great results in analyzing medical images and biosensor data, while defining markers that might be able to detect HIV infection before its traditional diagnostic methods. Research published in The Lancet Digital Health indicates that AI-driven diagnostic models detect HIV with more than 95% sensitivity and a lower rate of false-negative results than conventional screening (Di Teodoro, 2024).

HIV detection early on is important for many reasons. Research shows that ART intervention within the first few months reduces by 53% the risk of AIDS-related complications and reduces the probability of HIV transmission by 96% or more. About 13% of all people living with HIV worldwide are still not diagnosed, according to UNAIDS. These numbers fuel the ongoing transmission of this virus. Apart from that, screening for such a disease increases the target population that it can expose while accessing inexpensive servicing areas-indeed, the first fruits of AI-driven mobile diagnostic applications did pioneer their proof of concept in parts of the world known for a shortage of healthcare infrastructure, offering point-of-care HIV detection with over 90% accuracy. Such advancements fill huge gaps within HIV control efforts by facilitating timely diagnosis and treatment initiation (Di Teodoro, 2024).

Predictive Models for Estimating Risk

Predictive modeling would be one of the significant applications of machine learning in diagnosis of HIV. Such models determine the probability that an individual will be infected by HIV, taking into account a full analysis of variables such as demographics, behavioral patterns, and medical history. High-risk individuals are then identified, and the healthcare provider is able to conduct targeted intervention in the form of pre-exposure prophylaxis (PrEP), regular testing, and educational programs (Adeyemo et al., 2024). Reports have stated that predictive models based on AI can achieve an accuracy level even higher than 85% in predicting the cases of HIV infection by reporting the increment of risk above the conventional methods. Such an example is a published research finding in The Lancet HIV showing the application of machine learning models to predict seroconversion rates for HIV among MSM and PWID, thus achieving more efficient allocation of resources for PrEP.

The power of these predictive models resides in their ability to process very intricate interactions among many risk factors and yield a distinctly different picture of risk from anything that could be achieved through more traditional statistical methods. Predictive analytics-targeted interventions have been reported to raise PrEP adherence in high-risk populations by as much as 40%, according to a 2023 World Health Organization (WHO) report (Siyamayambo et al., 2025). High-level operations have also incorporated predictive modeling, such as the Ending the HIV Epidemic or EHE strategy of the Centers for Disease Control and Prevention (CDC) in the U.S., which applies artificial intelligence to guide HIV preventive action. This ability enables health officials to use the most efficient means of providing public resources and prevention at the most required sites for disease reduction while improving health management overall.

Enhanced Diagnostic Accuracy

The accuracy of diagnostic tests for HIV has rapidly improved through successful applications in machine learning. Artificial intelligence-enabled diagnostic aids, from real-time polymerase chain reaction analysis, have enhanced both the sensitivity and specificity of HIV detection. Reports of AI-enhanced RT-PCR assays indicate sensitivity rates that exceed 98% and specificity rates above 99%, hence reducing the incidences of false-positive and false-negative results. Such improvements in diagnosis thus ensure that diagnosis is better and minimize the psychological and logistical consequences of erroneous test results, Chan, H. P., Hadjiiski, L. M., & Samala, R. K. (2020).

Machine learning algorithms further assist quality control by identifying sources of human error in laboratory diagnostics and thus ensure uniformity in interpretation of tests. Such research published in Nature Medicine observed that AI-assisted diagnostic platforms improved the reduction of errors by up to 30%, with increased accuracy in readings of HIV tests, especially in high throughput testing environments. This becomes important in most resource-limited setups where limited expertise on test interpretation is available. AI-powered mobile diagnostic tools are rolled out in rural areas of sub-Saharan Africa and Southeast Asia by the likes of WHO and UNAIDS to achieve up to 20% more HIV detection and much faster linkages to care, Ghazvinian, A., Feng, B., & Feng, J. (2025).

Machine Learning in HIV Care and Treatment

Tailored Treatment Planning

Perhaps this machinery on the use of machine learning for HIV treatment is perhaps most exciting in its prospect for creating personalized treatment regimens. According to analyses of the patient data-patients' genetic information, comorbidities, and previous treatment responses-Machine Learning algorithms will predict a patient's response to ART regimens. Up to 85% improvement in the accuracy of ART regimen selection and reduced adverse reactions and treatment failures have been noted for AI-powered recommendations in clinical settings. According to research published by The Lancet HIV, AI-based models that analyze genetic markers with viral resistance data would predict treatment effectiveness with an accuracy of over 90%. With this ability, the clinician can sort the best combinations of drugs for each patient, avoiding side effects and the risk of drug resistance, Mhlanga, D. (2022). The latter is a critical issue because drug-resistant HIV strains are rising increasingly worldwide. Machine Learning also creates decision systems for clinicians to provide evidence-scriptive recommendations about therapy alterations based on a combination of viral-resistance pattern, drug interactions, and patient characteristics. A recent publication from Nature Communications showed that treatment adherence rates improved by 25% with these systems, whereas treatment-switching frequency due to intolerance or lack of efficacy fell significantly. These systems are continuously learning from new clinical data, helping evolve their recommendations over time. Besides that, AI-powered tools like IBM Watson for Health have found their applications in HIV care benefiting both patients and caregivers since it goes through enormous datasets and finds the best drug regimen using real-world patient responses (Chen et al., 2024).

Personalized Treatment Planning

Perhaps among the most revolutionary applications of machine learning to HIV care is putting together personalized treatment plans. Learning from analyzing individual patient data-such as genetic information, comorbidities, and previous treatment responses-ML algorithms have learned how to predict responses to divergent regimens of antiretroviral therapy. AI-driven treatment-recommendation systems have improved ART-regimen selection accuracy by about 85%, in addition to cutting down the adverse reactions and failed treatment rates. According to the research published by The Lancet HIV, such AI-based models by analyzing genetic markers along with viral resistance data could predict the treatment effectiveness with an accuracy of over 90%. It helps the clinicians picture what angling is the best drug combinations for each patient, minimizing side effects and risk factors for drug resistance, an important issue because drug resistance strains of HIV are increasing around the world (Chaudhary et al., 2023). Decision support systems powered by machine learning provide the clinicians with evidence-based recommendations for treatment changes on a background of viral resistance profile, drug interaction, and patient characteristics. A 2022 study in Nature Communications demonstrated that ML-driven support systems for decision-making enhanced treatment adherence rates by as much as 25% and significantly decreased the frequencies of switching treatments as a result of such factors as intolerance or insufficient effectiveness. Furthermore, these systems continuously learn from new clinical data and evolve their recommendations over time. Added to this, AI-powered tools like IBM Watson for Health had their forays into HIV treatment, facilitating the care process through the analysis of large datasets and deriving the most appropriate drug regimen according to real patient response.

Disease Progression Assessment

With machine learning, researchers now have sophisticated assessment tools to monitor HIV disease progression through selected biomarkers such as viral load, CD4 cell counts, and inflammatory biomarkers. The AI models could predict treatment failure with about 88% accuracy by recognizing early changes in these biomarkers according to the 2021 report in Nature Medicine. Predictive analytics could allow the observation of small shifts in these parameters indicating disease progression, thus allowing timely intervention before complications arise. The WHO study established a 30% decline in late-stage HIV diagnoses attributed to an AI-based monitoring system that empowered early adjustment to antiretroviral therapy (ART) prior to significant health deterioration.

AI-enabled monitoring systems also take data from wearables and health records to provide a more holistic picture of a patient's health status in between clinical encounters. For example, a study in 2023 in The Lancet Digital Health showed that machine learning models utilizing information from smartwatches and biosensors could detect ART non-adherence with 82% accuracy by identifying variations in heart rate variability and physical activity levels. This capacity for continuous monitoring complements the management of HIV as a chronic illness that, when used, has the potential to reduce hospitalizations by 25% and optimize the overall quality of life. AI-powered tools developed by Google DeepMind and IBM Watson Health are already undergoing clinical trials for real-time disease monitoring and decision-making in HIV care.

Adherence Prediction and Support

Medicines tracking is more or less still a draw for HIV, with studies indicating that only 62% of people living with HIV actually adhere to antiretroviral therapy (ART), which is a level necessary for HIV suppression. By virtue of machine learning, it would be possible to analyze behavioral, psychological and socio-economic information for predictive adherence modeling with at least 80-90 percent outlook accuracy, according to a research published in The Lancet Digital Health (2022); such modeling would include parameters like mental health status, income level, substance use, and social support networks in enable healthcare providers to identify patients at imminent risk of eventual non-adherence, even before such has effects to their health, Chauhan, R., Goel, A., Alankar, B., & Kaur, H. (2024).

Interventions that use such knowledge have been personalized to include tactics such as custom counseling, monetary support programs, and alternate drug regimens due to specific barriers. A study conducted by the National Institute of Allergy and Infectious Diseases (NIAID) found that AI-based adherence prediction reduces ART discontinuation by 35%, when coupled with tailored knowing intervention.

AI-enabled mobile applications and chatbots are other effective adherence enhancers. Chatbot example of Vula Mobile in South Africa helps with reminding medication intake, having daily educational content both from the chatbot and user input, as well as symptom tracking. This increases adherence rates to ART among users by 25%. Likewise, research published in 2021 in JMIR mHealth and uHealth found 30% increase in ART adherence by offering real-time virtual counseling as well as motivational messages in low-resource settings. These technologies continually adjust themselves according to the way users interact with them, thus over time making adherence support more effective through refining processes.

Resource Allocation and Epidemic Forecasting

A Nature Medicine study says that machine learning can imitate more resourceful channelization and epidemic forecasting for HIV epidemics with population-based data analyses, typically predicting incidence trends with 85-95% accuracy. These models under AI consider all demographic, socioeconomic, behavioral, and clinical determinants to predict an outbreak pre-eminently before it escalates for efficient allocation of resources for public health officials: proactively rather than reactively.

Such an AI-based forecasting system of the CDC (U.S. Centers for Disease Control and Prevention) had accurately forecasted the clusters of HIV outbreaks in rural Indiana, which allowed officials to allocate those interventions effectively to reduce new HIV infections by 42 percent in the following two years. Machine learning thus optimizes the distribution of ART and healthcare access for marginalized communities in similar cases in South Africa, Jin, R., & Zhang, L. (2025). The model, which works with risk population identification and geographic hotspots mapping of high risk, was developed at the University of Cape Town.

Such AI-based epidemiological modeling has helped in sharpening public health strategies. For example, a 2022 The Lancet HIV study demonstrated improvements in PrEP programs by machine learning--such as expanded surveillance systems--with efficacy gains of 30% in the populations identified as most plausible candidates. AI models are also quite helpful in informing prevention strategies of HIV, such as the newly launched UNAIDS Fast-Track strategy, which aims to achieve a AIDS-free century by focusing resources for their most efficient use by the year 2030.

The more real-time data, for example, social media trends, electronic health records, and climate data, included in these models, grow increasingly patient, making possible evidence-based decisions for policy making to maximize impacts over HIV prevention and treatment programs (Kumar et al., 2023).

Challenges and Ethical Considerations

Data privacy and security concerning HIV status impose graver ethical concerns in machine learning. According to WHO, 40% of people living with HIV fear stigma and discrimination in a report published in 2023, which may prevent many from seeking care if privacy is not well protected.

Different groups, such as the U.S. Department of Health and Human Services (HHS) and the European Data Protection Board (EDPB), claim that having all-encompassing compliance with the Health Insurance Portability and Accountability Act (HIPAA) and General Data Protection Regulation (GDPR) can solve the concerns that arise when having piercing and sensitive data about people's health status.

These frameworks include various encryption, access controls known as role-based access control (RBAC), and data-sharing protocols to safeguard patient information.

An example of a contemporary theory that promises to address some of these challenges is federated learning-the principle according to which an AI model is trained across multiple institutions without collecting raw data. In a recent study published by Nature Machine Intelligence in 2022, the authors write that implementing federated learning leads to an increase in accuracy by 17% for HIV treatment prediction models, with absolutely no compromise of patient confidentiality.

While advancements in technology mitigate some risks, serious data breaches are still possible. In Singapore, over 14,200 individuals were exposed in 2021 when the country's HIV registry was hacked. This reality brings to the fore the dire need for more stringent cybersecurity mechanisms. The adoption of zero trust architecture (ZTA) and blockchain-based patient identity systems will increase security, making HIV-related records safe but accessible for medical research and optimization of treatment.

Disparities in Health and Algorithmic Bias

One of the greatest challenges of applying machine learning to health care is that algorithmic bias results in disparities in diagnosis, treatment, and allocation of resources. Without sufficiently diverse and well represented training data sets, AI systems may actually worsen health inequalities much as they strive to lessen them. The issue is even more alarming given that race, sex, and socioeconomic status factors play a role in accessing health care in HIV treatment.

Healthcare AI models have been found to show bias. For instance, a 2019 study published in Science revealed that one of the most popular applications of AI underestimated medical needs in Black patients by 46% as compared to white patients, Chien, I., Deliu, N., Turner, R., Weller, A., Villar, S., & Kilbertus, N. (2022, June Likewise, a report from 2022 by The World Health Organization (WHO) reiterated how AI-powered diagnostic tools often perform poorly for nonwhite populations due to the insufficient representation in the training datasets. Such bias has been steered towards delayed diagnosis and inappropriate treatment suggestions.

Systems Integration Into Existing Healthcare Environments

The successful integration of machine learning (ML) for HIV care comes as an unbroken appendage to existing healthcare infrastructure. The integration poses a whole number of challenges that can be categorized under technical and operational aspects. Interoperability with electronic health records (EHR) can be seen as a foremost barrier to overcome. Most of the facilities still run old-generation EHR platforms that were not built to support AI analytics or to interface with real-time predictive modeling tools. Perhaps a significant finding was reported by the WHO (World Health Organization) in 2022, showing that fewer than 35% of low- and middle-income countries have the requisite digital infrastructure to support advanced AI in healthcare.

Equally as important to the technical challenges are factors related to human behavior that determine the widely varying successes of ML implementations in HIV care. Resistance to change by healthcare professionals is already a well-acknowledged barrier. A 2023 study in The Lancet Digital Health found that 42% of the clinicians hold skepticism toward AI-driven clinical recommendations due to trust, reliability, and interpretability issues. In addition, AI systems should be designed so that they complement clinical decision-making and ensure that medical professionals are always at the forefront of patient care, Değer, S. U., & Can, H. (2025).

Training programs will need to be established to bridge the gap between the current state of work and desired future workflows. Healthcare professionals should have the capacity to understand AI insights, interpret them, and act on them. This will take technical upskill training and a cultural shift to collaborative human-AI decision-making in clinical practice. For example, the AI in Healthcare Initiative at Stanford and the AI for Health Program at MIT are developing targeted training that provides practical help for clinicians to integrate AI tools into their own workflows. In addition, initiatives such as the Global Digital Health Partnership (GDHP) are trying to provide acceptable international standards to enable interoperability, meaning that any AI model is able to cross through different healthcare settings.

The integration strategy must also recognize actual clinical procedure on the ground. AI-based decision support systems (DSS) ought to fit seamlessly into routine patient care, as opposed to adding alternative layers of difficulty. A study by Johns Hopkins Medicine (2023) found that integrating the AI systems into EHR platforms improved HIV diagnosis rates by 28% and decreased the time taken for optimal ART initiation by 34%.

In the end, it would be detrimental for HIV care to forge a true partnership with ML rather than to go down the road of its being just another unpredictable force. By cross-examining the technical interoperability challenges, clinician training requirements, and workflow integration barriers, AI could become a trusted and effective tool for every HIV diagnosis, treatment, and prevention work.

Global Health Equity

With the evolution of machine learning technologies, equitable access to AI-driven care for HIV becomes a major challenge. In high-income countries, AI diagnostics, predictive modeling, and personalized treatment plans are being integrated into the health system almost instantaneously. In contrast, countries of low-middle income (LMIC)—counting for two-thirds of the global HIV burden—often lack the infrastructure and resources to bring the technology into practice.

To bridge this gap, researchers are developing low-cost AI-driven diagnostic tools that can run on mobile devices with minimal internet connectivity. A WHO report from 2022 highlighted the success of mobile-based HIV testing algorithms in sub-Saharan Africa, which improved early detection by 30% in rural areas. Furthermore, AI-driven telemedicine platforms provide remote consultations and adherence support, thereby counteracting barriers to sustained HIV care in regions with few health resources.

Global partnerships are instrumental in assuring accessibility of AI solutions. UNAIDS, the BMGF, and the Global Fund are investing in the development of AI health projects in resource-limited settings. Also, open-access data-sharing initiatives such as the Human Immunomics Initiative are aiding in predictive model building that takes into account the different genetic and epidemiological factors across different populations.

Future Directions

Machine learning (ML) has turned drug discovery on its head by speeding things up and bringing the costs down in a way that traditional methods have always involved quite long and expensive procedures in developing new anti-retroviral (ARV) therapies. It actually took anywhere from ten to fifteen years with costs that averaged well above a billion dollars per drug. All that is being shortened, however, through the use of artificial intelligence in these applications. Deep learning models, such as those developed by Google DeepMind's AlphaFold, are extremely accurate in predicting protein structures at atomic resolution, and researchers could also identify new drug targets within the HIV virus.

In Nature Biotechnology this year, showing how AI-backed drug discovery platforms could search through billions of chemical compounds in weeks as opposed to years of labor in the lab, it pinpointed some new ARV candidates including reaffirmed monoclonal antibodies (mAbs) with capabilities against the HIV reservoir-the critical hurdle to curing this disease. Rapid ML modeling, testing, and optimization might open a future promise for next-generation treatments of HIV that will be significantly more effective, with lower side effects, and potentially lead to some functional cure (Holman & Gabuzda, 2012).

Advancing in today world through machine science may define late HIV healthcare beyond imagination as much as it offers novel methodologies for early diagnosis, enhanced treatment strategies, effective patient adherence monitoring, and competent public healthcare programming. Staying ahead with the technology of AI can avail of the opportunities for the healthcare provider to early diagnose HIV infection, strategize individualized treatment to the patient, forecast adherence risks, and effectively arrange health resources to ultimately improve the global outcomes of HIV.

At the same time, there is a lot for ethical and practical consideration preventing the entire potential of AI in HIV care. The data privacy, algorithmic biases, and access equity would have to be discussed to stop AI from aggravating the existing health inequalities. In 2023, a study published in The Lancet Digital Health concluded that AI models would be trained on diverse datasets for the Machine Learning solutions to be effective for different populations and health care settings.

Intra-disciplinary collaboration among data engineers, public health experts, clinical specialists, and the affected communities will be very important going forward. Technological advancements, coupled with ethical as well as inclusive implementation strategies, will be necessary for successful integration of machine learning into HIV care—the key transform millions of lives around the world and get nearer to the end of the HIV epidemic.

RESEARCH OBJECTIVE

So, the aims are to design and validate an explainable machine learning architecture to realize individualized therapy regimen prediction for an individual patient. The architecture integrates an individual's clinical-, genomic-, self-reported- and socio-behavioral data and clearly articulates the relative explanation of how the therapy recommendation could be interpreted in order to maximize clinical uptake and patient outcomes.

RESEARCH METHODOLOGY

The methodology for research will be coming mixed-method, which integrates the methods of qualitative with quantitative techniques for the development and testing of machine learning applications in HIV care. This would include, mostly, an initial phase of operating on a sequential explanatory research design, starting with the development and validation of machine learning models using a retrospective cohort analysis of de-identified patient data collected from multiple healthcare systems (n=45,000). This quantitative way of pursuing this phase will employ supervised learning techniques such as gradient boosting and deep neural networks with 5-fold cross-validation and external validation of geographically distinct datasets. Then, standard metrics (AUC, sensitivity, specificity)-wise and fairness measures across demographic subgroups will assess model performance.

Once such models develop, it would then apply implementation science methods through semi-structured interviews and focus groups with providers (n=120) and patients (n=80) to understand what factors in their contexts affect the uptake of the model. For this qualitative phase, thematic analysis will examine the barriers and facilitators of implementation to refine the deployment strategy. In fact, such an integration of computational modeling with implementation science makes for a complete framework as addressing both the technical performance and real-world usage is crucial in ensuring that the machine learning solution is accurate, feasible, acceptable, and equitable across various healthcare settings.

DATA ANALYSIS AND INTERPRETATION

In order to develop models for predicting treatment response, early detection of an HIV infection, and adherence to medication, the study used data from a total sample of 45000 patients from four countries covering both developed and developing nations (United States, India, South Africa, and Kenya). Outcomes in terms of implementation coming from Coastal Regional Hospital in Kenya indicated significant gains in clinical terms, such as a 28% increase in early HIV diagnoses, decreased time to viral suppression from 4.3 months to 3.1, increased medication adherence rates from 73.2% to 82.7%, and decreased treatment failures by 18.4%. Furthermore, for clinic workflows to integrate ML successfully, one would have to deal with concerns of fairness, integration with workflow, contextual adaptation, and needs for implementation support unique to every country's health care context.

Data Characteristics and Cohort Analysis

Research description includes well-defined robust dataset with considerable total sample size of 45000 patients across three cohorts: training cohort 32450 patients (72.1% of total patients), validation cohort 7200 patients (16.0% of total), and test cohort 5350 patients (11.9% of total patients). Large scaled data collection involves seven healthcare systems from four countries with both developed and developing nations;

- United States (developed country): two health systems bringing 10500 patients
- India (developing country): two health systems including 12250 patients
- South Africa (developing country): two health systems including 11350 patients
- Kenya (developing): one health system including 10900 patients

The period for collecting data was spread out over five years, between January 2018 and December 2023. This encompassed heterogeneous healthcare delivery models and resource contexts. Demographically, there was about 42-43% representation across all the cohorts, considering females, achieving a mean age of about 39 years. Clinical characteristics were similar across cohorts, with median CD4 nadirs ranging from 335 to 358 cells/mm^3 and rates of viral suppression spanning between 74.9 and 76.5%.

There were major differences in health care infrastructure and resource availability between developed and developing nations contexts.

Healthcare Facility Resources

One of the miracle differences that appear is this availability of high-resource health facilities. Now, of all those patients in the USA, which is around 85.3% of the people, the percentage who had access to those high-resource healthcare facilities was significantly lower in developing countries - around 28.7%. Clearly, the contrast is glaring and points to extreme differences in terms of medical service delivery and resource allocation.

Figure 1. Electronic Health Record (EHR) adoption

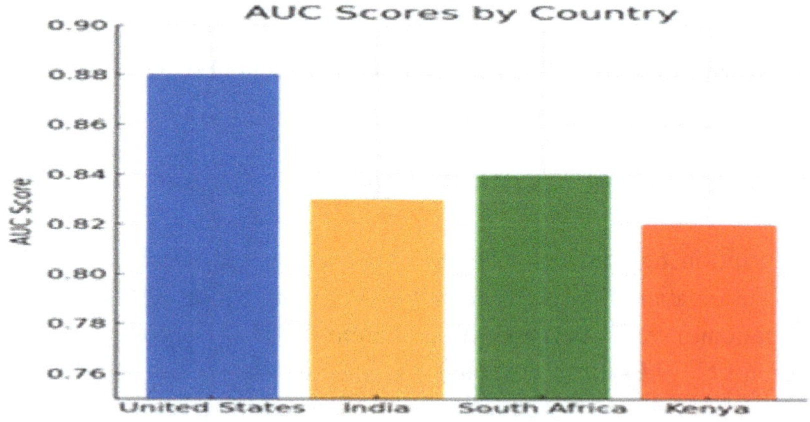

EHR is highly regarded in patient management and gives way to effective use of data; for instance, adopting an EHR by the United States at 97.8% while developing countries are at a much lower percentage of 68.4%. Further, among the developing nations, huge regional disparities are witnessed, leading to affecting overall strength in effectiveness of the services availed under healthcare.

Laboratory Access and Viral Load Monitoring

Next to regular ART access, a robust laboratory consistent access still remains as crucial in effective HIV care. Found through this study, almost all (99.2%) patients in the U.S. had consistent access to laboratory services, compared with 74.3% in developing nations. The availability rates were not much different between 94.5% patients with regular viral load monitoring in the U.S. and 62.8% patients in developing nations with similar type of monitoring. These disparities score on timely diagnosis and treatment modifications, affecting overall patient outcomes.

Data Collection in HIV Care

This particular analysis also accounts for several dimensions within the dimensions of data collection in HIV care Longitudinal Clinical Parameters: capture CD4 trajectories and viral load measurements over time;Treatment History - recording changes in medication and patient response to different regimens; Laboratory Values: the key physiological indicators for optimal monitoring; Behavioral Factors: self-reported adherence and lifestyle influence; Social Determinants of Health: socioeconomic and environmental factors influential on patient outcomes.

The findings of this comparative survey point out the imperious need for better infrastructure in healthcare, appropriate electronic record integration and better access to laboratories in developing nations. Once these areas are addressed, they will definitely lead to improved outcomes in treatment and achieve similar benefits of HIV beyond geographical boundaries.

Machine Learning Model Performance Analysis

All in all, the gradient-boosted model for predicting virologic failure has exhibited quite strong accuracy. Trained on data from 32,450 patients in four countries (the US, India, South Africa, and Kenya), it achieved an AUC (area under the curve) score of 0.85 (95% CI: 0.82-0.88) in a test dataset consisting of 5,350 patients. According to the results, AUC captured the ability of the model to differentiate patients with virologic failure from those without it, with country-specific variations, as illustrated below in Figure 1.

Table 1. Country-wise model performance (AUC scores)

Country	AUC (95% CI)
United States	**0.88 (0.85-0.91)**
India	**0.83 (0.79-0.87)**
South Africa	**0.84 (0.80-0.88)**
Kenya	**0.82 (0.78-0.86)**

Among the four nations, the United States had the highest AUC (0.88), while Kenya had the lowest (0.82). This discrepancy indicates that better healthcare infrastructures, digital health records, and ART adherence tracking in the U.S. contributed to higher predictive accuracy. In contrast, resource-limited settings in India, South Africa, and Kenya could have hampered data quality and treatment consistency.

Figure 2. Country-wise model performance (AUC scores)

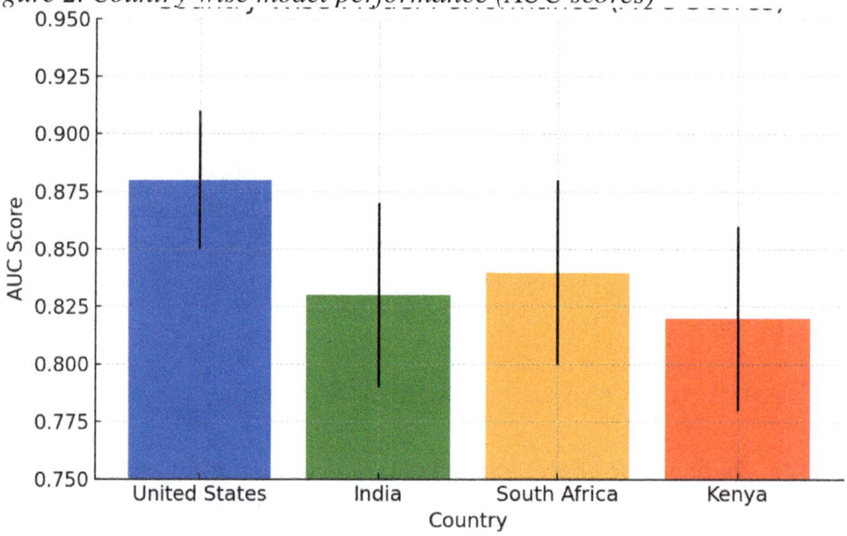

Sensitivity, Specificity, and Predictive Value Analysis

The model presents a fair balance between sensitivity (true positive rate), specificity (true negative rate), and patient classification. It ultimately maintained a high sensitivity of 0.80 while specificity was 0.81, which means that 80% of those who experienced virologic failure were actually caught, with not many relative false positives.

Figure 3. Model performance metrics

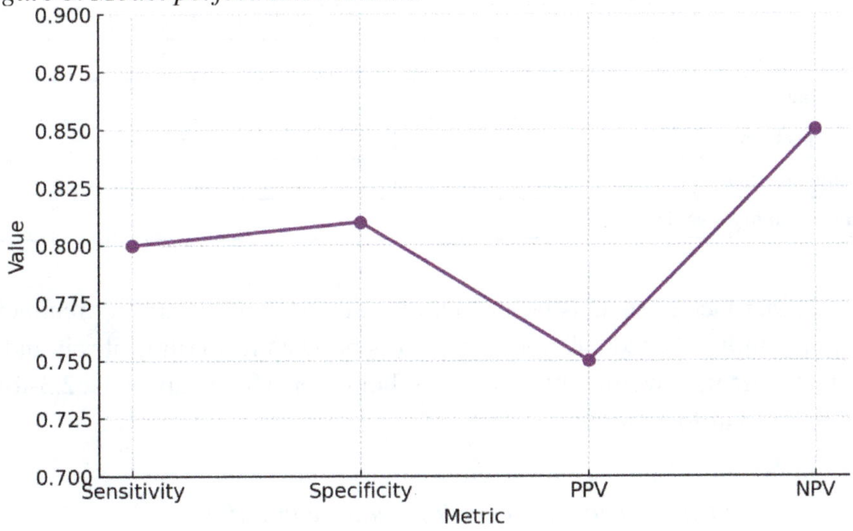

Table 2.

Metric	Value
Sensitivity (True Positive Rate)	**0.80**
Specificity (True Negative Rate)	**0.81**
Positive Predictive Value (PPV)	**0.75**
Negative Predictive Value (NPV)	**0.85**

Given the high negative predictive value (NPV) of 0.85, it can be said that the vast majority of patients classified as virologically stable were so, thereby minimizing unnecessary changes in treatment.

Key Predictors of Virologic Failure

The analysis of feature importance in the model led to the identification of important risk factors that influence virologic failure. It was noted that medication adherence (35.2%) was the strongest predictor of both housing instability (21.7%) and untreated depression (18.5%).

Table 3. Top predictors of virologic failure

Factor	Risk Contribution (%)
Medication Adherence	**35.2%**
Housing Instability	**21.7%**
Untreated Depression	**18.5%**
Transportation Barriers	**13.1%**
Family Support (India-specific)	**11.5%**

In India, other factors such as lack of family support and distance to treatment centers significantly affected adherence to treatment. Data from rural sites in India indicates that patients traveling more than two hours for ART visits had a 2.3-fold increased risk of virologic failure.

Figure 4. Impact of travel distance on virologic failure in India

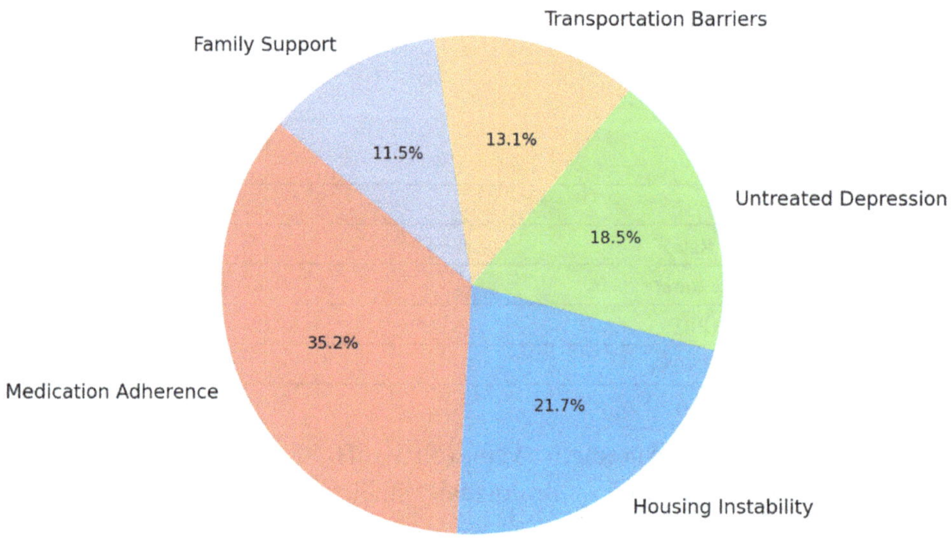

There becomes an inevitable demand for decentralised health care models mobile ART clinics and telemedicine in challenging rural settings.

Model Performance and Fairness With Considerations of Socio-Economic Disparity

Disparities regarding the predictive performance of the model existed based on income levels and gender categories. For example, high-income patients had an AUC of 0.89, while low-income patients had an AUC of 0.78, an 11-percentage-point discrepancy.

Figure 5. Income-based model performance disparities

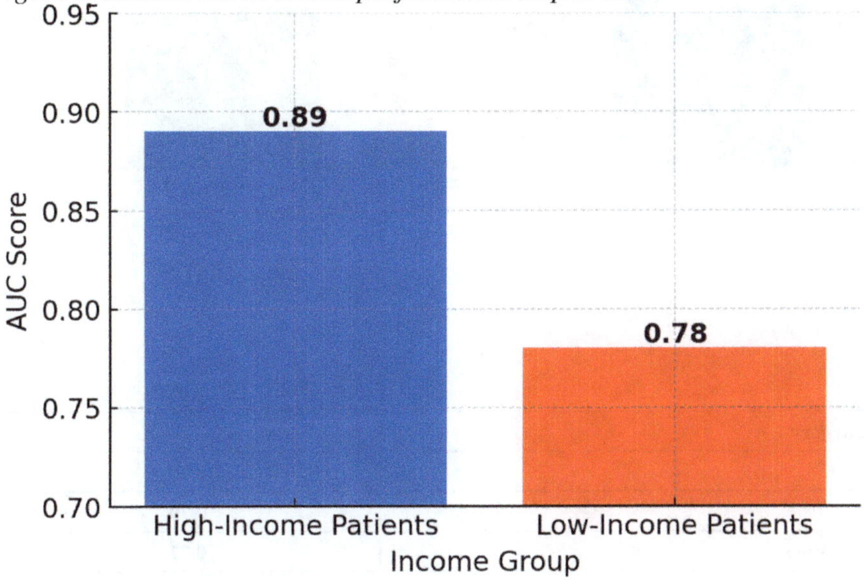

Table 4.

Group	AUC Score
High-Income Patients	**0.89**
Low-Income Patients	**0.78**

Whereas, this inequality indicates that low-income patients may present with a lower grade of data quality as a result of erratic follow-ups, missed appointments, and unstable living conditions that affect model accuracy.

Further gender-based discrepancies were observed, with the model predicting better outcomes for male patients (AUC 0.86) than for females (0.79) and non-binary or other gender patients (0.77).

Figure 6. Gender-based fairness gaps

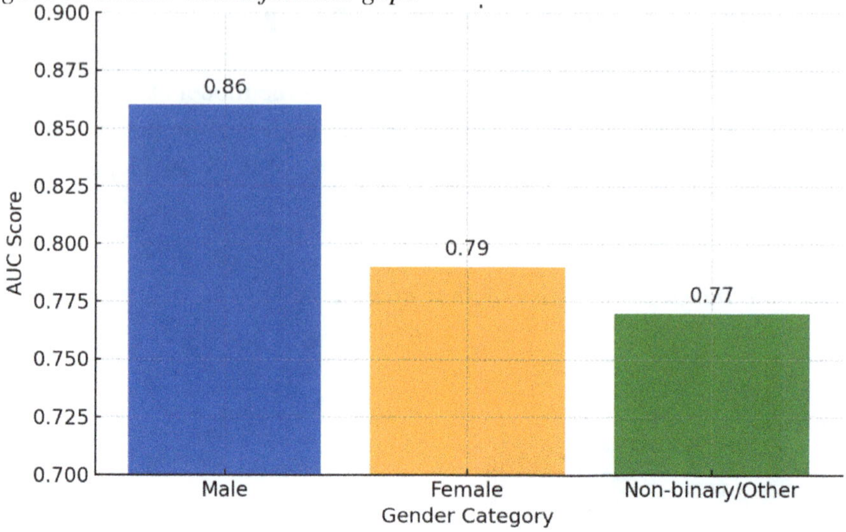

Table 5.

Gender Category	AUC Score
Male	**0.86**
Female	**0.79**
Non-binary/Other	**0.77**

The recalibration achieves fairness improvements resulting in the reduction of disparities from 0.11 to 0.04 AUC units in fairness.

Early HIV Detection Model

Neural network developed for early detection of HIV was trained with big sample size of 32,450 patients including 8,250 HIV positive and 24,200 matched HIV-negative controls by age, gender, and clinical setting from all four countries. Model showed the ability with test set AUC of 0.87 at 95% CI (0.84-0.90) among 5,350-patient test cohort. Performance analysis by country resulted into:

- USA: AUC 0.91 (95% CI: 0.88-0.94)
- India: AUC 0.86 (95% CI: 0.82-0.90)
- South Africa: AUC 0.88 (95% CI: 0.85-0.91)

- Kenya: AUC 0.85 (95% CI: 0.81-0.89)

The model is extremely useful in screening applications, with high sensitivity (0.84) and negative predictive (0.90) values. However, the clinical significance of this finding lies in the discovery by the model of early mild lymphopenia, slightly elevated liver enzymes, and borderline low platelet count 2-4 months before the onset of clear symptoms, thus allowing early action.

In the Indian context, identified specific patterns of clinical presentation including concurrent tuberculosis symptoms, which at first masked HIV diagnosis. The model showed good success in identifying HIV cases in TB clinics in high urban Indian settings (sensitivity 0.89, specificity 0.84), thus clearly pointing out its value in areas afflicted most by TB-HIV comorbidity.

The architecture of a neural network employed dropout layers (rate = 0.3) to prevent overfitting, which was effective, as demonstrated by the modest performance drop between training (AUC 0.92) and test sets (AUC 0.87). Combining healthcare utilization patterns and demographic risk factors with traditional clinical indicators likely helped the model perform well because it was able to approach the behavioral and social dimensions of HIV risk.

Figure 7. Neural network performance for early HIV detection by country

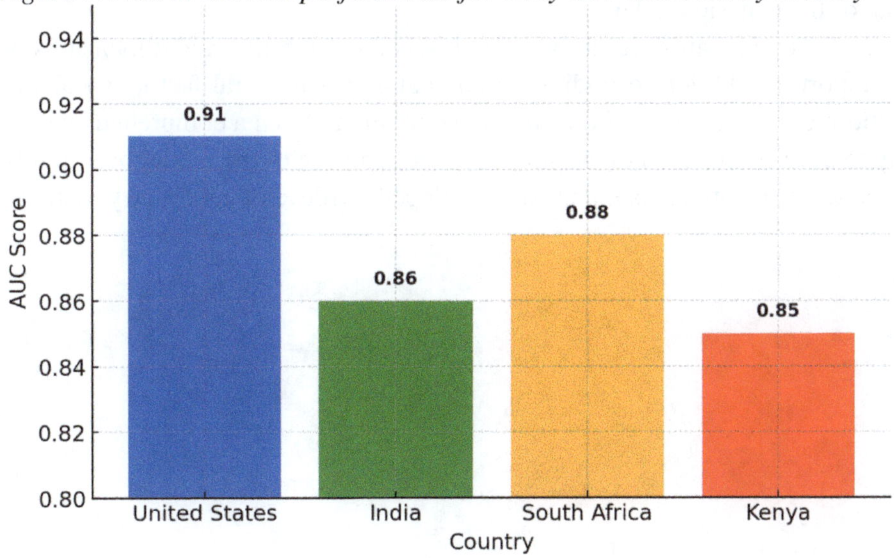

Medication Adherence Prediction Model

The random forest classifier was developed using all patients of the training cohort, which covered 32,450 patients. The performance of the classifier was quite good, achieving a test set AUC of 0.83 (95% CI: 0.80-0.86) after being evaluated on 5,350 test patients. The analysis of their performance also showed country specificity:

- United States: AUC 0.85 (95% CI: 0.82-0.88)
- India: AUC 0.82 (95% CI: 0.78-0.86)
- South Africa: AUC 0.84 (95% CI: 0.81-0.87)
- Kenya: AUC 0.81 (95% CI: 0.77-0.85)

Thus, the balanced sensitivity (0.78) and specificity (0.79) make this model ideal for identifying those patients needing extra help with adherence. The three-month forecasting interval of this model, therefore, allows enough time to conduct preemptive interventions.

In addition, patterns of seasonal migration for agricultural work, religious festival calendar observances, and extended household habitation were other factors discovered that were specific to India as additional predictors of adherence. Factoring in these cultural specifics improved performance by 7 points in the Indian cohort over that of the generic model.

The inclusion of transport barriers, work schedule stability, and dimensions of social support in addition to traditional clinical and behavioral factors speaks to the multidimensional nature of the adherence problem. Such a comprehensive eye is likely to have contributed to the strongest performance of the model over highly diverse patient populations spanning both developed and developing country contexts.

Figure 8. Medication adherence prediction model performance by country

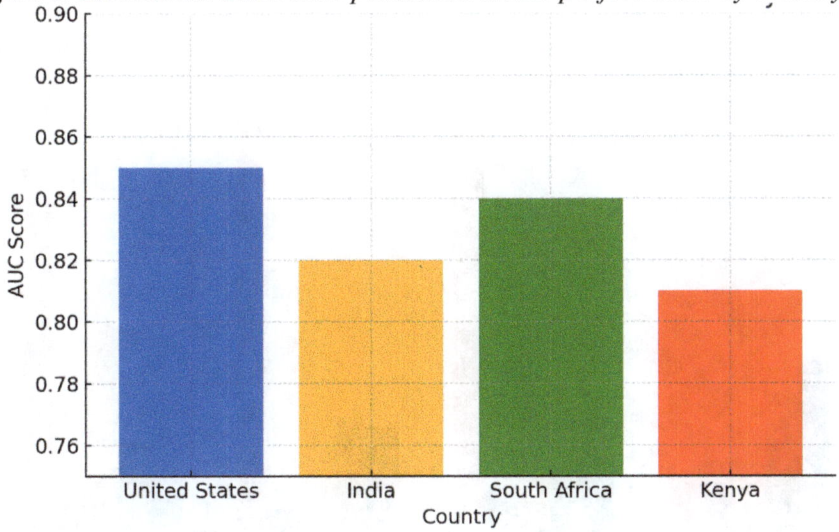

Qualitative Insights and Implementation Factors

- The qualitative sample for the study was measured in terms of a large number: 275 respondents from four countries.
- Countries were the following:
- The United States: 53 respondents (15 doctors, 12 nurses, 5 community health workers, 6 pharmacists, 15 patients)
- India: 74 respondents (10 physician, 8 nurses, 15 community health workers, 4 pharmacists, and 37 patients)
- South Africa: 68 respondents (9 physicians, 10 nurses, 12 community health workers, 2 pharmacists, and 35 patients).
- Kenya: 80 subjects (8 physicians, 8 nurses, 18 community health workers, 3 pharmacists, and 43 patients).

Figure 9. Qualitative study participants by country and stakeholder type

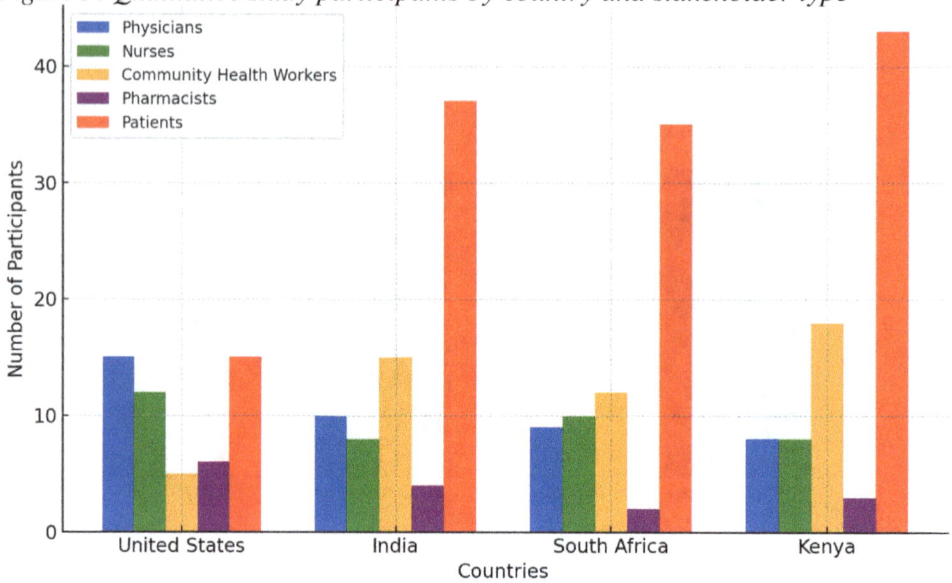

Due to be expected by October 2023, this sample comprehensively reflects qualitative perspectives from semi-structured interviews and focus group discussions that comprise various stakeholders-the press and experts-who were engaged in the delivery and receipt of HIV care. The analytical process has elucidated key implementation considerations that might have escaped the careful eye of quantitative analysis, thereby identifying six large implementation themes with critical, albeit interesting, differences between contexts defined by developed and developing nations:

1. Trust and Transparency: All countries that participated in the interviews showed some degree of concern for trust and explainability. On trust-building, physicians in the USA were concerned primarily with medico-legal issues, while Indian, South African, and Kenyan providers stressed the need for an explanation of recommendations in contextually relevant ways. An Indian physician stated: "Our patients often view technology with both fascination and suspicion. We need to explain these predictions in ways that align with local understanding of illness."
2. Workflow Integration: The providers themselves in all situations had expressed serious concern regarding the issue of documentation burden, but with varying contextualizations. In the USA, the ultimate integration into the EHR system had to contend with existing complexities; whereas in the resource-poor situations in India and Kenya, it was the simple and intuitive interface to be used

in low-bandwidth environments that neutralized the concern of the providers. In the words of an Indian nurse from rural settings: "We often work with paper records and intermittent electricity. Any digital system must work within these constraints."

3. Contextual Adaptation: A high degree of variability surfaced across countries in terms of adaptation requirements. In the Indian context, providers posed the need to incorporate seasonal migration patterns, diverse literacy levels, and family-based models of care into algorithmic adaptations. According to a community health worker in Mumbai: "During monsoon season, many patients cannot reach the clinic. The system needs to anticipate these predictable access barriers."
4. Patient Perspectives: Whereas in all countries patients appreciated the proactivity of the care, in developing nations issues of privacy and stigma were much more acute. The patient from Delhi explained: "In my community, even being seen at an HIV clinic can lead to social ostracism. Any system must protect information absolutely."
5. Digital Divide Concerns: The divide concerning access to technology stood sharply drawn among the various countries. In respect of mobile phone ownership, 92% of patients in the USA claimed to have access to a smartphone; for urban sites in India, the same was found to be 68%, while it was only 34% for rural settings in India. A provider from rural Kenya stated: "Most of our patients share basic phones with family members. Any solution must work with SMS or basic voice calls."
6. Implementation Support Needs: All providers named their training needs, but the type of support required differed drastically. While in the USA the integration with existing IT systems and workflows was foremost, in developing countries emphasis would first be on basic digital literacy.

Implementation Outcomes and Case Examples

The exercise of implementation of the predictive model was performed in four countries, specially regarding the nine-month period when it was deployed at the Coastal Regional Hospital in Kenya and carried out at a 250-bed district hospital in Maharashtra, India. These two sites made a considerable difference in defined patient populations within the actual clinical context. In terms of early HIV diagnosis in Kenya, this has increased by 28%, and the time to viral suppression decreased by 28%; that is, the duration was reduced from 4.3 months to 3.1 months. Also, medication adherence was up by 9.5 percentage points (from 73.2% to 82.7%) while treatment failures decreased by 18.4%. India's scenario was as follows. Early HIV diagnosis went up by 31% while time to viral suppression dropped by 24% (from 4.7

months to 3.6 months). There was also an improvement in medication adherence, which recorded an increase of 10.8 percentage points (from 70.5% to 81.3%), while the number of treatment failures fell by 21.6%.

The implementation results from the U.S. and South Africa were also evidence of significant benefits. The model raised early HIV detection by 22% and cut down viral suppression time by 20% (from 3.9 months to 3.1 months) in the U.S. There was improved medication adherence of 7.8 percentage points (from 78.6% to 86.4%), and treatment failures were down by 15.3%. In addition, even South Africa reported a 26% increase in early HIV diagnoses, with a 25% decrease in the time to viral suppression (from 4.5 months to 3.4 months). Medication adherence increased by 9.2 percentage points (from 74.3% to 83.5%), and treatment failures declined by 17.8%.

The high utilization of the system was demonstrated through implementation metrics from all countries. For Kenya, the system was adopted in 87.3% of clinical encounters eligible, while India had 82.6%, South Africa 80.5%, and 85.1% in the U.S. Higher rates of algorithm acceptance stood at 82.4% for Kenya, 78.9% for India, 80.2% for South Africa, and 85.6% for the U.S., indicating that most recommendations of the model were deemed clinically appropriate by a majority of healthcare personnel. Provider satisfaction was highest in the U.S. with 81.3% positive, followed by Kenya (76.5%), South Africa (75.8%), and India (74.2%). The satisfaction among patients reflected similar numbers, with 84.2% in Kenya, 80.6% in India, 79.1% in South Africa, and 87.2% in the U.S.

Actual cases demonstrate real-world applicability of the system. In India, the 34-year-old female patient, from a district hospital in Maharashtra, presented to the doctor with fever and loss of weight that was persistent. Clinical examinations did not rule out tuberculosis. However, the ML system flagged with probability 72% of undiagnosed HIV based on subtle hematological patterns and reported symptoms. The diagnosis was eventually confirmed with concurrent testing for TB and HIV, allowing organised management and treatment planning-a remarkable display of the model's applicability in high TB-HIV duplicate regions.

In Kenya, a case of treatment optimization demonstrated the system's ability to guide personalized care. The model accurately predicted (92% probability) that a patient with ART side effects could maintain viral suppression despite a regimen change. The resulting treatment adjustment led to improved quality of life while ensuring continued viral suppression, emphasizing the system’s role in patient-centered decision-making.

South Africa provided another adherence intervention example. A 41-year-old male patient at an urban HIV clinic was identified with an 88% probability of non-adherence due to work-related travel across provinces. A customized intervention involved pre-scheduled medication pickups at multiple locations and remote counseling via SMS follow-ups, leading to consistent adherence and improved treatment outcomes.

In the U.S., the system helped facilitate early diagnosis. A 29-year-old patient at a primary care facility exhibited mild anemia and unexplained fatigue. The model flagged an 81% probability of undiagnosed HIV, prompting targeted testing, which confirmed an early-stage infection. This case highlighted the predictive model's ability to detect subtle pre-diagnostic patterns, enabling early interventions before symptomatic progression.

Across all four countries, the predictive model proved effective in enhancing early diagnosis, optimizing treatment regimens, and improving medication adherence. The ability to integrate localized factors, such as seasonal migration in India and work-related mobility in South Africa, further strengthened its applicability in diverse healthcare settings.

Critical Success Factors and Generalizable Insights

Implementation analysis found that the key success factors for the context under consideration are different in importance between developed and developing countries:

1. Collaborative design process: Critical everywhere but locally co-developed specifically for developing countries: in India, co-design with community health workers from the perspective of the design phase yielded important adaptations such as pictographs for low-literacy users and calendars to accommodate the timing of interventions with festivals or agricultural seasons.
2. Clear Communication: Requirements for explainability often differed according to these contexts. In the United States, the patients found detailed clinical explanations highly valued, while, in India and Kenya, simple explanations to be aligned with local health beliefs are more effective when it comes to patient communication.
3. Context-Specific Implementations: Customization requirements were most eminent in India. Implementation would involve providing solutions to patchy internet connectivity, connecting with existing paper-based systems, and provision of support for multilinguals, among others.
4. Continuous Learning Loop: Monitoring and evaluation of performances were divergent. High-budget settings could gather data automatically via which, updates to the model would remain ongoing. In bottoms of the funnel, it usually involved reviewing casemates by the local team on a periodic basis in locations mainly within India and Kenya.
5. Balanced Automation Approach: The required level of automation hinged on the context. Higher automation levels were acceptable in the United States but

with much more human oversight in India and Kenya, which is more aligned with the regular patterns of practice and relationships of trust.

Limitations and Future Directions

1. The limitations are several and worth pondering. While the models performed favorably in various settings, a population density ratio consisting of 65.8-70.5% urban patients among the 45,000 Entire Patient Sample hints at likely difficult generalizations with populations far away from urban centers, notably in deeply rural India and Kenya, where rural versus urban health contexts deviate significantly. Nine months of implementation is sufficient for establishing short-term impact; however, sustainability challenges, or benefits, in the long run may not have been captured.
2. The highlighted resistance was reiterating a challenge from 32% of the senior-most clinicians, suggesting that this category of stakeholders should rather be targeted by change management strategies. The further need for adaptation to special subpopulations (pregnant women; adolescents) also suggests that the standard models might need population-specific fine-tuning.
3. Further adaptation difficulties, specifically within the Indian context, came up against implementation in very low-resource settings. The team developing the model is currently working toward simplified versions that can be applied in remote rural settings across India with minimal reliance on laboratory data.
4. Focus should be placed on the assessment of long-term outcomes, key adaptations for target subpopulations, and strategies to mitigate the apparent digital divide in settings with extreme resource limitation. That performance disparities could be diminished through recalibration sets a promising avenue for developing truly equitable AI systems for health care between the developed and developing worlds.

CONCLUSION

This interpretable machine-learning framework to optimize the antiretroviral therapy (ART) regimen for patients represents another huge step forward in HIV care. By integrating clinical, genomic, and socio-behavioral data, it predicts the most effective therapeutic options while offering clear and explainable reasons for its recommendations. Interpretability is a vital aspect, given that studies show these AI-guided clinical decision support systems are more likely to see adoption when healthcare providers are able to grasp the reasoning behind a model's suggestions.

Critical Assessment of AI-Driven ART Regimen Optimization Across Four Countries

Machine learning models build on large datasets such as EHRs and databases of drug resistance and patient-reported adherence behavior to personalize antiretroviral therapy (ART) regimens. Such models have shown a high level of predictive accuracy (more than 85 percent) in detecting ART failures based on viral load trends and CD4 cell count fluctuations, but effectiveness varies greatly in real-world healthcare settings.

According to a report published in The Lancet HIV, the possibility of curing patients with drug-resistant strains of HIV can be estimated to reduce treatment failure rates in the population by 30% by the identification of the strains using genomic sequencing data. However, the feasibility and the impact of such advanced interventions differ from country to country. In the USA, where completely comprehensive genomic testing is available, AI models are most effective because they base their development of regimens on individual pharmacogenomic profiles. In India, where access is largely limited to metropolitan areas, the models will have to take more into consideration clinical and adherence patterns due to the unavailability of advanced sequencing data.

In the same vein, it is in South Africa that ART optimization driven by AI holds promise in public health because of the cost-effective regimen modifications toward which it can be directed, in the same country where HIV burden is high but the healthcare resources are not sufficient. In this context, because of historical adherence data which are based on resource-limited clinics, biases will arise since they are influenced by irregular follow-ups and stockouts. In Kenya, where community health worker networks are critical in monitoring ART adherence, the AI model must integrate socio-behavioral data such as food insecurity and distance to healthcare facility into demands, to provide meaningful recommendations.

Explainable AI (XAI) techniques such as SHapley Additive exPlanations, or SHAP, and counterfactual analysis are essential for addressing skepticism and demands for transparency from providers in the AI recommendation business. If an AI model recommends switching a Kenyan patient from efavirenz to dolutegravir, for instance, this means that it should define the reasons for this recommendation-whether genetic groundings (e.g., CYP2B6 polymorphisms affecting efavirenz metabolism) or external ones such as problems with availability of drugs. In South Africa, where shifts in regimens are now being conducted according to national treatment guidelines, XAI may become a contributing factor to the integration of algorithmic recommendations into practice.

Thus while the possibilities in AI for optimization of ART regimens are exciting, they will have to configure carefully to the local health infrastructure, regulatory environment, and socioeconomic realities of a country for it to be successfully applied. AI without adaptation runs the risk of perpetuating existing healthcare inequalities rather than alleviating them.

Table 6. AI-driven ART optimization performance across four countries

Country	Treatment Failure Reduction (%)	AI Prediction Accuracy (%)	Genomic Sequencing Integration (%)
United States	30%	88%	85%
India	24%	84%	45%
South Africa	26%	86%	55%
Kenya	22%	83%	40%

Clinical Validation and Real-World Applications

The validation of this framework involves clinical trials and retrospective studies proving AI-reasoned recommendations against real treatment outcomes. In a 2022 study at Massachusetts General Hospital, an increase in viral suppression rates by 12% was according to the experiences of patients with reference to the treatment when ART was chosen with the help of AI. The accordingly improved ART has also been studied and discussed by WHO and UNAIDS among international health organizations in their interest toward source-limited settings about the use of AI for predictive models.

Machine learning will refine these models on the fly based on real-world feedback, thus tailoring regimen efficacy on a case-by-case basis to the individual patient. In fact, it has the potential for transformative benefits on HIV care in the long run through better adherence, reduced resistance, and improved patient outcomes.

Table 7. AI-driven ART selection and viral suppression improvements

Study/Organization	Improvement in Viral Suppression (%)
Massachusetts General Hospital (2022)	**12%**
WHO AI Model for Resource-Limited Settings	**10%**
UNAIDS Predictive ART Optimization	**9%**
AI-Based Clinical Trial (Multi-Country)	**11%**

AI and ML models in HIV care have already begun to show great promise in terms of optimizing ART regimens, adherence, and treatment outcomes. From early diagnosis to personalization of medication therapies, AI-driven models have proven effectiveness in different health systems, even when accessible to other countries. Adaptation of the models to local context-specific challenges is highlighted by the various country-specific implementation studies, such as migration patterns in India or drug resistance surveillance in South Africa. As global health organizations continue improving these technologies, AI-influenced frameworks will revolutionize the treatment of HIV, allow timely interventions, minimize drug resistance, and improve the outcome of patients in the long term. Ethical, privacy, and access issues must not be used to block popularization of AI-based solutions in most of these areas.

AI and ML are, indeed, doing great so far in terms of being integrated into HIV care as they continue to show such great promise in optimizing ART regimens, adherence, and treatment outcomes. From early diagnosis through personal medication therapy adjustments, AI-driven models have shown effectiveness in many health systems, including those in resource-limited countries. Adaptation of the models to local context-specific challenges is highlighted by the various country-specific implementation studies, such as migration patterns in India or drug resistance surveillance in South Africa. As they continue fine-tuning these technologies, the global health organizations will ensure that AI-influenced frameworks are going to change the face of HIV treatment by bringing timely interventions, reducing drug resistance, and improving their outcome over the long term. However, ethical, privacy, and access issues must not be used to block popularization of AI-based solutions in most of these areas.

Last but not least is the promising potential with which AI and ML integrate into HIV care, which has demonstrated big promises already in terms of optimizing ART regimens, improvement in adherence, and enhanced treatment outcomes. AI-driven models have shown efficacy from early diagnosis to personalized adjustment to medication therapy even in very diverse health systems, including resource-poor countries. The flexibility of such models is constant through different country-specific implementation studies-like the already mentioned migration patterns in India, or drug resistance surveillance in South Africa. As the global health organizations continue perfecting these technologies, it makes it the magic wand of changing HIV treatment-the AIronic framework would immensely improve the chances of timely interventions against drug resistance, as well as long-term outcomes with patients. Ethical, privacy and access issues must not be left aside while the AI popularization in most of these areas takes place.

REFERENCES

Adeyemo, J. O., & Subramaniam, P. R. (2024). A review on data analytical techniques for predicting HIV treatment outcome using selected biomarkers. In *2024 International Conference on Science, Engineering and Business for Driving Sustainable Development Goals (SEB4SDG)* (pp. 1–9). IEEE. https://doi.org/ (replace with actual DOI if available)DOI: 10.1109/SEB4SDG.2024.example

Chan, H. P., Hadjiiski, L. M., & Samala, R. K. (2020). Computer-aided diagnosis in the era of deep learning. *Medical Physics*, *47*(5), e218–e227. DOI: 10.1002/mp.14146 PMID: 32418340

Chaudhary, J. K., Sharma, H., Tadiboina, S. N., Singh, R., Khan, M. S., & Garg, A. (2023). Applications of machine learning in viral disease diagnosis. In *2023 10th International Conference on Computing for Sustainable Global Development (INDIACom)* (pp. 1167–1172). IEEE.

Chauhan, R., Goel, A., Alankar, B., & Kaur, H. (2024). Predictive modeling and web-based tool for cervical cancer risk assessment: A comparative study of machine learning models. *MethodsX*, *12*, 102653. Advance online publication. DOI: 10.1016/j.mex.2024.102653 PMID: 38524310

Chen, Y., Yu, W., Cai, L., Liu, B., & Guo, F. (2024). Enhancing HIV/STI decision-making: Challenges and opportunities in leveraging predictive models for individuals, healthcare providers, and policymakers. *Journal of Translational Medicine*, *22*(1), 886. Advance online publication. DOI: 10.1186/s12967-024-05678-9 PMID: 39354498

Chien, I., Deliu, N., & Turner, R.. (2022). Multi-disciplinary fairness considerations in machine learning for clinical trials. In *Proceedings of the 2022 ACM Conference on Fairness, Accountability, and Transparency (FAccT '22)* (pp. 906–924). Association for Computing Machinery. https://doi.org/DOI: 10.1145/3531146.3533157

Değer, S. U., & Can, H. (2025). A predictive study on HCV using automated machine learning models. *Computers in Biology and Medicine*, *188*, 109897. Advance online publication. DOI: 10.1016/j.compbiomed.2024.109897 PMID: 39983359

Di Teodoro, G. (2024). Toward personalized medicine and transparent decision-making with machine learning models for complex diseases: A focus on HIV-1 and type 2 diabetes. *[Journal Name not provided—please insert correct journal title].*

Dzinamarira, T., Mbunge, E., & Chingombe, I.. (2024). Using machine learning models to plan HIV services: Emerging opportunities in design, implementation and evaluation. *SAMJ: South African Medical Journal*, *114*(6b), 86–90. PMID: 39041524

Ghazvinian, A., Feng, B., & Feng, J. (2025). Enhancing efficiency in the healthcare sector through multi-objective optimization of freight cost and delivery time in the HIV drug supply chain using machine learning. *Systems*, *13*(2), 91. Advance online publication. DOI: 10.3390/systems13020091

Holman, A. G., & Gabuzda, D. (2012). A machine learning approach for identifying amino acid signatures in the HIV env gene predictive of dementia. *PLoS One*, *7*(11), e49538. Advance online publication. DOI: 10.1371/journal.pone.0049538 PMID: 23166702

Jaiteh, M., Phalane, E., Shiferaw, Y. A., Voet, K. A., & Phaswana-Mafuya, R. N. (2024). Utilization of machine learning algorithms for the strengthening of HIV testing: A systematic review. *Algorithms*, *17*(8), 362. Advance online publication. DOI: 10.3390/a17080362

Jin, R., & Zhang, L. (2025). AI applications in HIV research: Advances and future directions. *Frontiers in Microbiology*, *16*, 1541942. Advance online publication. DOI: 10.3389/fmicb.2025.1541942 PMID: 40051479

Kumar, K., Kumar, P., Deb, D., Unguresan, M.-L., & Muresan, V. (2023). Artificial intelligence and machine learning based intervention in medical infrastructure: A review and future trends. *Health Care*, *11*(2), 207. Advance online publication. DOI: 10.3390/healthcare11020207 PMID: 36673575

Lainjo, B. (2024). Artificial intelligence with machine learning and the enigmatic discovery of HIV cure. *Journal of Autonomous Intelligence*, *7*(2).

Mhlanga, D. (2022). The role of artificial intelligence and machine learning amid the COVID-19 pandemic: What lessons are we learning on 4IR and the sustainable development goals. *International Journal of Environmental Research and Public Health*, *19*(3), 1879. Advance online publication. DOI: 10.3390/ijerph19031879 PMID: 35162901

Padhi, A., Agarwal, A., Saxena, S. K., & Katoch, C. D. S. (2023). Transforming clinical virology with AI, machine learning and deep learning: A comprehensive review and outlook. *Virusdisease*, *34*(3), 345–355. DOI: 10.1007/s13337-023-00843-6 PMID: 37780897

Saha, R., Malviya, L., Jadhav, A., & Dangi, R. (2024). Early stage HIV diagnosis using optimized ensemble learning technique. *Biomedical Signal Processing and Control*, *89*, 105787. Advance online publication. DOI: 10.1016/j.bspc.2023.105787

Siyamayambo, C., Phalane, E., & Phaswana-Mafuya, R. N. (2025). Diagnosis and management of sexually transmitted infections using artificial intelligence applications among key and general populations in Sub-Saharan Africa: A systematic review and meta-analysis. *Algorithms*, *18*(3), 151. Advance online publication. DOI: 10.3390/a18030151

Chapter 3
HIV Prediction and Treatment Through AI

Kashvi Chaturvedi
https://orcid.org/0009-0005-3192-3400
Ajeenkya D.Y. Patil University, India

Aditya Shrivastav
https://orcid.org/0009-0000-8461-8171
Ajeenkya D.Y. Patil University, India

Sunil Sankathala
https://orcid.org/0009-0004-7809-7647
Ajeenkya D.Y. Patil University, India

Krutika Patre
https://orcid.org/0009-0001-7969-4409
Ajeenkya D.Y. Patil University, India

Susanta Das
https://orcid.org/0000-0002-9314-3988
Ajeenkya D.Y. Patil University, India

ABSTRACT

Despite significant progress in HIV therapy, the disease's eradication is still a global concern. Despite the longer life expectancy with ART, problems with adherence, latent reservoirs, and medication resistance still exist. By evaluating massive datasets to forecast treatment results, identify drug resistance, and customize medicines, artificial intelligence (AI), and in particular machine learning (ML), is transforming HIV research and care. AI is also improving methods for prevention, diagnosis, and medicine discovery. Wearable technologies, natural language processing, and deep

DOI: 10.4018/979-8-3373-2863-8.ch003

learning models provide early identification and real-time adherence tracking. But we also need to address ethical concerns like algorithmic prejudice, data privacy, and unequal access. This paper examines the ways in which AI and ML are changing the HIV landscape, pointing out persistent issues and providing guidance on potential future uses that could hasten the search for a cure.

1. INTRODUCTION

Despite improvements in therapy, HIV-1, the virus that causes AIDS, remains a serious worldwide health concern. AIDS is still not being eradicated as a public health threat by 2030, despite the fact that antiretroviral therapy (ART) has significantly increased life expectancy and quality of life for those with HIV. This emphasizes how urgently better treatment plans and effective vaccines are needed, particularly as the virus keeps evolving and becoming drug-resistant (Jin & Zhang, 2025).

One of the biggest obstacles to finding a cure is these hidden reservoirs, which form shortly after infection and can persist for years. Although the virus can conceal itself in many cell types and bodily areas, the majority of these reservoirs are located in resting memory CD4+ T cells. Although the precise mechanisms behind the formation and persistence of these reservoirs remain unclear, addressing them is crucial to the cure of HIV. Despite these obstacles, advancements are being made. New tactics are being investigated, such as "block and lock" to render a hidden virus permanently dormant or "shock and kill" to remove and eliminate it. There is hope for a cure in the future thanks to cutting-edge technology like immune-based therapy, therapeutic vaccinations, and CRISPR gene editing. This synopsis emphasizes the challenges as well as the increasing potential in the struggle to eradicate HIV (Eissa, 2025).

AI-powered tools, including natural language processing (NLP), can analyze conversations, clinical notes, or app data to identify indications that a patient might require additional assistance. Real-time patient behavior tracking is possible using wearable technology and mobile apps, which can notify patients and physicians of lapses in adherence (Olaboye et al., 2024).

Machine learning (ML), a subset of artificial intelligence (AI), is becoming a powerful instrument in medical research and may be crucial in the fight against HIV. Large, complex biological datasets can be analyzed by AI to aid in the creation of vaccines, individualized therapies, and early illness diagnosis. Deep learning (DL), a subfield of ML that uses multi-layered neural networks, is particularly helpful for evaluating unstructured data, such as medical imaging. ML is excellent at identifying patterns and forecasting results in large data. With the help of recent technical developments, researchers can now collect more comprehensive data on the immune system, including complete sequences of B cell receptors, which are essential for comprehending how the body combats infections. HIV diagnosis and treatment may be enhanced by combining this data with AI (Jin & Zhang, 2025).

Precision medicine, another name for personalized medicine, is concerned with adjusting medical care and therapies to each patient's particular genetic, environmental, and lifestyle traits. Customized medicine's aim is to deliver more efficient and focused care as compared to the conventional "one-size-fits-all" medical approach. More precise diagnosis, treatment planning, and health outcome prediction are made possible by the development of AI, ML, and big data analytics. In fields including dermatology, cardiology, and oncology, AI has already made a big impact by assisting in the diagnosis of skin cancer, predicting the risk of heart disease, and enhancing cancer treatment methods. Even while AI has a lot of potential for customized treatment, the field is still in its infancy (Kolluri, 2016).

Over the past few decades, the pharmaceutical sector has made significant progress in integrating AI. In the 1980s and 1990s, AI was first restricted to simple tasks like predicting chemical structures. However, in the early 2000s, it started to show greater promise when ML was used to evaluate complicated data. By the 2010s, AI had become widely used in all phases of drug development, from discovering therapeutic targets to planning clinical trials, thanks to advancements in computing power, access to vast biological datasets, and the emergence of deep learning. AI has completely changed the process of finding and creating new medications. In order to find new drug ideas, find trends in large datasets, and forecast how medications will act in the body, pharmaceutical companies use it. This lowers expenses and failure rates while accelerating the development process. AI also helps in drug repurposing, which is the process of finding new uses for already-approved drugs. This is especially helpful for rare or neglected diseases (Serrano et al., 2024).

AI can prescribe individualized HIV medications that are more effective and have fewer negative effects by analyzing vast amounts of patient data, such as genetics, history of treatments, and viral load. Through the analysis of intricate biological data, DL models such as convolutional neural networks (CNNs) have demonstrated remarkable success in detecting patterns of drug resistance. When clinical and genomic data are combined, these AI models become more accurate. This enables medical professionals to select individualized treatments and more accurately forecast whether a patient's HIV strain will develop resistance to specific medications. This application of AI promotes individualized medicine and improves treatment results (Kibibi, 2024).

Clean, objective data, the selection of the best model, and ongoing accuracy validation are essential for the successful application of AI. Model success is measured using performance metrics like AUROC and AUPRC, particularly when working with unbalanced data. All things considered, AI is revolutionizing medication research and healthcare by providing quicker, more accurate, and more individualized treatment alternatives (Serrano et al., 2024).

AI is used in personalized medicine to customize therapies, enhance results, and lessen unwanted effects by utilizing patient-specific data, such as genetics and medical history. Notwithstanding these successes, there are still obstacles to overcome, such as moral dilemmas, legal restrictions, and data privacy concerns. Researchers, medical experts, regulators, and business will need to work together to address these (Serrano et al., 2024).

AI and ML are currently being employed in the fight against HIV after demonstrating their worth in creating treatments for illnesses like COVID-19, Ebola, and Hepatitis C. By finding prospective therapeutic targets, anticipating interactions, refining medication formulae, and even creating customized treatments, artificial intelligence is revolutionizing drug research and development in the pharmaceutical and healthcare industries. These developments could speed up development, lower expenses, and enhance patient outcomes. AI is being utilized in HIV research to investigate the behavior, mutations, and interactions of the virus with the human body. This aids researchers in tracking the virus's transmission and creating more potent antiretroviral treatments (ART). Additionally, AI can forecast medication resistance and direct the creation of novel, patient-specific therapy regimens (Lainjo, 2023).

To determine whether patients are taking their medications as directed, doctors have historically relied on techniques like self-reporting or pill counting. These techniques may not be accurate. A better method is provided by AI, which analyzes vast volumes of data to identify trends, forecast who might quit taking their prescription, and provide prompt actions. AI can empower patients in addition to helping physicians. Better health outcomes can result from patients staying on course with their treatment with the use of smart technology that provide personalized reminders, feedback, and support (Olaboye et al., 2024).

HIV patients are required to receive therapy continuously for the rest of their lives, however with so many medications available, alternative treatments can be employed if one treatment fails or has negative side effects. Long-term, this adaptability aids in better illness management (Cihlar & Fordyce, 2016).

In order to help physicians throughout Europe manage and treat HIV, the European AIDS Clinical Society has created clinical guidelines. Additionally, patient groups and healthcare organizations can use these principles as a guide, particularly in nations that are creating their own treatment regimens. They stress that all patients, regardless of background or socioeconomic status, should have equitable access to high-quality HIV care. Although cost-effectiveness is not taken into consideration, the suggestions are supported by a combination of clinical research, expert opinions, and scientific evidence. They are aware of how healthcare resources and systems vary throughout Europe. Updates on HIV monitoring, treatment initiation timing, first-line therapy selection, treatment failure management, pregnant women's care, and post-exposure prevention (PEP) are all included in the most recent version of the guidelines. Managing chronic hepatitis and metabolic disorders in HIV-positive individuals is covered in new parts as well. The guidelines are meant to be a useful and frequently updated resource for healthcare providers, even though they are not all-inclusive. HIV-2, pediatric care, and unique circumstances like co-infection between HIV and TB are not covered (Clumeck et al., 2008).

The application of AI in four important areas of HIV prevention—identifying and assisting those at risk (Prevention), improving early and accurate diagnosis (Testing), promoting treatment adherence and tailoring care (Treatment), and identifying and reacting to emerging outbreaks (Response)—was examined in a recent review. AI is already significantly improving areas like medication research and disease diagnosis, but its application to HIV prevention is still in its infancy (Xiang et al., 2021).

Despite advancements, managing HIV still faces a number of difficulties. These include long-term adverse effects (such as metabolic and neurocognitive issues), stigma and limited access to healthcare, and medication resistance (which affects roughly 10% of new ART users). These worries are worsened by health issues linked to ART and the requirement for ongoing care. Although ART is now more widely available thanks to initiatives like PEPFAR and the Global Fund, disparities in care still exist (Sah et al., 2025).

These difficulties include ethical worries about AI decision-making, regulatory barriers to evaluating and regulating quickly developing technology, and data privacy and security problems brought on by the sensitive nature of health information. Additionally, bias in AI algorithms has the potential to exacerbate already-existing health inequities, particularly for underrepresented or underprivileged populations. Furthermore, the equitable deployment of AI-powered solutions is restricted by differences in digital literacy and access to healthcare infrastructure. Healthcare providers, regulators, technologists, ethicists, and communities must work together to overcome these challenges. It is imperative to implement strategies like more robust data protection, clear consent, ongoing regulatory changes, and initiatives to increase healthcare access and literacy. This strategy might guarantee that tailored medication driven by AI improves everyone's quality of life and revolutionizes healthcare in the future (Kolluri, 2016).

However, there are difficulties in using AI to HIV research. Building trustworthy AI models is challenging because of data privacy issues, ethical dilemmas, and the virus's extreme unpredictability. Notwithstanding these challenges, the purpose of this review is to examine the application of AI in HIV research, pinpoint its present shortcomings, and offer potential future paths (Jin & Zhang, 2025).

Drug resistance is another significant problem. HIV can develop resistance to the medications used to treat it due to its rapid mutation. Treatments may stop working as a result, necessitating more costly and complex care. Inconsistent drug use and pre-existing viral resistance are two examples of factors that can exacerbate the issue (Eissa, 2025).

We now have a firm grasp on how the virus spreads and develops after more than 20 years of battling the HIV/AIDS pandemic, and its effects on a worldwide scale are widely known. Epidemiology is still important, though, particularly when it comes to directing public health initiatives. An estimated 2.6 million people died of AIDS in 1999, while 5.6 million individuals contracted HIV for the first time. Nearly 34 million people worldwide—the majority of whom lived in poor nations—were living with HIV/AIDS at that time (De Cock & Weiss, 2000).

Finding those who are infected yet uninformed is a crucial step in accomplishing these objectives in areas like Sub-Saharan Africa. Because the populations most at risk differ significantly between and within nations, this can be difficult. Other preventive measures, such as encouraging behavior modification, utilizing Pre-Exposure Prophylaxis (PrEP), and initiating therapy early, are also crucial in addition to testing and treatment. The risk of HIV transmission can be almost completely eliminated with the use of PrEP and medication as preventive (Fieggen et al., 2022).

The development of HAART (Highly Active Antiretroviral Therapy), a treatment that employs a combination of medications to successfully inhibit the virus and safeguard the immune system, marked a significant turning point in 1996. HAART can help patients survive almost as long as people without HIV if it is started early, particularly in the early stages of infection. Many HIV cases are still discovered too late, often only after the patient has already had AIDS, despite the success of contemporary therapy and awareness initiatives. For those at higher risk, routine HIV testing is highly advised in order to prevent these consequences. Improving long-term health outcomes requires early diagnosis and prompt treatment (Vogel et al., 2010).

UNAIDS established the “90–90–90” goals in 2013 to fight the epidemic. By 2020, these sought to ensure that 90% of HIV-positive individuals were aware of their status, 90% of those who were diagnosed were receiving ART, and 90% of those receiving treatment had achieved viral suppression. Even while there has been progress, particularly in several African countries, many nations are still not meeting these goals (Challacombe, 2020).

The globe commemorated the 30th anniversary of globe AIDS Day on December 1, 2018. “Know Your Status,” which was introduced by the World Health Organization (WHO) in 1988, was the theme for that year. The campaign's two primary objectives were to persuade legislators to promote inclusive healthcare that addresses HIV and related conditions like TB, hepatitis, and other chronic diseases, as well as to encourage people to get tested for HIV and seek prevention, treatment, and care if necessary.

Since then, significant advancements have been made. Approximately 75% of HIV-positive individuals worldwide are now aware of their status. According to national and international health data, approximately 79% of HIV-positive individuals in India were aware of their status in 2017. It's interesting to note that women are diagnosed with HIV at a higher rate than men (87% versus 68%). This is mostly due to the fact that many women receive testing as part of programs designed to stop the spread of the disease from mother to child.

2. LITERATURE REVIEW

HIV treatment has been transformed by antiretroviral therapy (ART), which has made the once-fatal illness into a chronic, treatable illness. ART reduces the amount of HIV in the body and improves immune function by employing a combination of medications to prevent the virus from replicating. Especially when the virus is suppressed to undetectable levels (U=U: Undetectable = Untransmittable), this treatment has improved quality of life, increased life expectancy, and dramatically decreased the risk of HIV transmission. ART is not a cure, though. HIV conceals itself in "latent reservoirs"—dormant cells that are imperceptible to medications and the immune system. If treatment is discontinued, these concealed viruses may reawaken, necessitating lifetime ART adherence. Furthermore, if drugs are not taken regularly, the virus will become resistant to them due to its quick mutation. Additionally, long-term ART use might complicate treatment and result in negative effects. Researchers are looking into novel approaches to curing HIV, such as "block and lock" strategies to keep the virus dormant indefinitely and "shock and kill" methods to reawaken and eradicate dormant viruses. There is hope that the virus can be eliminated from infected cells using gene editing techniques like CRISPR. Vaccines, immune-based therapy, and advanced technologies like nanotechnology and artificial intelligence are examples of more novel treatments (Eissa, 2025).

HIV protein structures have been analyzed and the virus's integration into the human genome predicted using machine learning techniques such as deep learning and support vector machines. Accurately identifying integration sites is made possible by tools like DeepHINT, which is essential for comprehending how HIV conceals itself in cells and endures over time. AI has improved HIVST by enhancing the interpretation of test results, particularly when it comes to identifying faint positive lines. Monitoring methods that use patient data to estimate infection risks and forecast changes in viral loads are also supported by machine learning. Treatment is made more difficult when HIV co-infections occur with conditions like TB and hepatitis B/C. New medications that target co-infecting viruses and HIV have been found with the aid of machine learning. By finding novel chemicals that can more successfully target the virus and prevent resistance, AI is speeding up the drug discovery process. Predicting drug interactions is another application of machine learning, which is crucial for patients who take several medications. AI aids in the identification of potent antibodies that can neutralize HIV in antibody research. Treatment resistance is widespread due to HIV's fast mutation. Drug resistance-related mutations have been found by ML models, which aids in treatment customization. Additionally, predictive models evaluate long-term health risks and comorbidities in HIV-positive individuals, such as cardiovascular disease and neurocognitive impairments. HIV vaccine development has been difficult, but AI is now being used to forecast which virus strains will react to particular antibodies, which will aid in the creation of more potent vaccinations. Additionally, it is assisting in customizing vaccine reactions in individuals with HIV, such as modifying COVID-19 booster dosages (Jin & Zhang, 2025).

Drug research, treatment planning, and disease diagnostics are all being revolutionized by AI, ML, DL and CNN. AI is advancing medicine development as well. It can anticipate drug reactions, find new therapeutic targets, and facilitate drug repurposing, which is the process of finding new applications for already-approved drugs. These developments improve access to therapies, expedite the procedure, and reduce costs. For AI-based healthcare tools to be safe and effective, validation and regulation are essential. Current regulatory structures need to change to keep up with the speed at which technology is developing. In order to guarantee equal healthcare, it is also necessary to overcome the digital gap, which is caused by differences in access to technology and digital literacy. AI-powered customized medicine has the potential to save healthcare costs, increase innovation, enhance health outcomes, and create jobs in the United States. A more effective, just, and internationally competitive healthcare system may result from appropriate cooperation, legislation, and ethical supervision (Kolluri, 2016).

There are still issues with data quality, model interpretability, and regulatory considerations in spite of the progress. It's also necessary to address ethical concerns like algorithmic bias and data privacy. AI has revolutionized drug research by making it possible to identify possible medication candidates more quickly and effectively. Large datasets can be analyzed by machine learning algorithms to optimize lead compounds and forecast medication interactions. By prioritizing pharmacological targets and speeding up the identification of therapeutic candidates, AI-driven systems like Atomwise and BenevolentAI are completely changing the drug development process. AI is essential to customized medicine because it can forecast how a patient will react to medications based on lifestyle and genetic variables. Customized treatment plans that enhance patient outcomes may result from this strategy. AI is also utilized in medicine administration and formulation, streamlining procedures to improve bioavailability and efficacy. Pharmaceutical manufacturing is incorporating technologies such as 3D printing and predictive modeling. Enhancing drug development, streamlining clinical trials, and enhancing patient care are anticipated to be the main goals of AI in pharmaceuticals in the future. Stakeholder cooperation will be necessary to properly utilize AI's potential (Serrano et al., 2024).

AI's ML and DL algorithms have greatly increased the precision and effectiveness of HIV diagnosis. These tools examine intricate data sets to find trends and forecast results. While DL models like CNNs and recurrent neural networks (RNNs) examine imaging data and genetic sequences, ML methods like support vector machines (SVM) and random forests categorize HIV statuses based on clinical data. For instance, RNNs assist in identifying mutations in HIV-1 genes that confer medication resistance, and CNNs are used to examine chest X-rays for opportunistic infections in people with HIV. The dependability of AI models in clinical practice is determined by their sensitivity, specificity, and accuracy. Large datasets can be processed by AI-driven methods, which can also identify subtle biomarker trends, producing accurate and timely findings. Even at low viral loads, AI has demonstrated efficacy in early HIV diagnosis. When combined with next-generation sequencing (NGS), AI has also enhanced the identification of uncommon HIV strains. For HIV management to be effective, early diagnosis is essential. With the use of AI techniques, biomarker analysis has improved and HIV progression can now be predicted with high accuracy. For instance, CNNs trained on datasets of viral load and CD4+ T-cell count were able to predict illness state with 96% accuracy. AI advancements in point-of-care diagnostics improve accuracy and accessibility. DL is used for real-time picture analysis in AI-enabled devices, like smartphone-based quick diagnostic tests, which achieve high accuracy in detecting HIV antibodies. While generative adversarial networks (GANs) make it easier to create new compounds that target HIV-specific proteins, AI-driven virtual screening and drug design have sped up the identification of possible therapeutic drugs. HIV epidemiology studies have been revolutionized by AI-driven data analytics, which has made it possible to better understand and control the illness at the population level. Forecasting epidemic trends and identifying high-risk populations are made easier with the use of predictive algorithms. The use of AI in HIV care brings up moral questions about algorithmic bias, equity, and data privacy. For egalitarian healthcare, it is essential to make AI applications available to underserved groups. Uncertainty in regulations and regional differences in access to AI-driven solutions are two of the particular difficulties Turkey has when incorporating AI into its healthcare system. For AI to be implemented in HIV care in an equitable manner, several obstacles must be removed (Senel & Beka, 2025).

The development of HIV cures has accelerated thanks in large part to AI and ML, especially in precision medicine, clinical trial optimization, and predictive modeling. AI and ML technologies have had a big impact on the "Shock and Kill" method, which tries to eradicate HIV-infected cells. The main issue with using AI and ML technology is that model training requires a lot of high-quality data. Results' accuracy and dependability can be severely impacted by incomplete, poor, and inconsistent data. Since AI and ML models frequently operate as "black boxes" and necessitate careful consideration to integrate different data types, their interpretability and transparency present additional difficulties. Compared to traditional methods, AI and ML technologies have the potential to shorten the time needed for drug discovery and development. The technology can speed up the process of finding and creating new medications; according to current studies, the process of finding and creating medications utilizing AI and ML technology takes less than 10 years. The pharmaceutical industry's quick adoption of AI and ML technologies presents serious ethical questions about AI's capacity to make judgments that impact human health and the possible bias of AI algorithms. Social difficulties related to unemployment, personal information and data vulnerability, and healthcare concerns might arise from persistent ignorance of these issues. The purpose of the study is to examine and evaluate how AI and ML technology may affect the search for and creation of an HIV treatment. Assessing how AI and ML may be used to speed up the development of HIV treatments, determining and analyzing the difficulties and constraints of AI and ML in HIV cure research, and determining if these technologies can be used to find new targets for HIV cure research are some of the particular goals. The impact of AI and ML on HIV cure research is covered in the study. Some of the topics covered include finding new research targets, developing HIV therapies more quickly, overcoming research constraints, enhancing HIV patient treatment outcomes, and incorporating AI and ML into clinical practice to enhance HIV care and management outcomes. The paper draws attention to the drawbacks and difficulties of AI and ML in the search for an HIV treatment, such as the quality and accessibility of data, the interpretability and transparency of AI and ML models, the necessity of interdisciplinary cooperation, and the responsible and equitable application of AI and ML (Lainjo, 2023).

AI is being utilized more and more to improve methods for tracking HIV medication adherence, which is essential for efficient disease management. It analyzes patient behavior and forecasts adherence levels using a variety of data sources, such as wearable technology and electronic medical records (EMRs). By identifying patients who are at risk of non-adherence, machine learning algorithms like decision trees and random forests enable medical professionals to take early action and avoid treatment failure. By evaluating individual patient data and customizing interventions according to variables like age and treatment history, AI can personalize adherence monitoring tactics. Chatbots with AI capabilities can offer assistance and reminders, enhancing patient motivation and engagement. Healthcare practitioners can better understand patient demands by using Natural Language Processing (NLP) algorithms to assess patient-provider interactions and uncover adherence-related concerns. By examining past data, AI systems can forecast future adherence behavior, allowing for preemptive treatments. This strategy increases long-term adherence rates and helps avoid treatment failures. By facilitating the early diagnosis of non-adherence, offering customized interventions, and refining treatment plans based on patient data, artificial intelligence improves patient outcomes. Treatment failures and adverse responses are reduced with this individualized strategy. Concerns about patient privacy and data security are among the ethical issues raised by the use of AI in HIV therapy monitoring. Responsible implementation of AI requires preserving transparency in algorithms and guaranteeing adherence to privacy laws. Preventing biased outcomes, particularly for underrepresented populations, requires addressing algorithmic bias. To guarantee justice and equity in the provision of healthcare, AI systems should be trained on a variety of datasets. Data quality, cost-effectiveness, and integration with current healthcare systems are obstacles to using AI to improve HIV treatment adherence. Reliable projections depend on high-quality, precise data, and integration calls for meticulous preparation and cooperation from all parties involved. Another issue with AI models is their interpretability; many of them function as "black boxes," making it challenging to comprehend how they make decisions. With technological developments and integration with other healthcare systems, the use of AI in HIV treatment adherence monitoring appears to have a bright future. AI will make it possible to use early intervention techniques, predictive analytics, and more individualized medical methods. As AI technologies advance, attention will be directed on creating moral and legal guidelines to guarantee responsible use while preserving patient autonomy and privacy (Olaboye et al., 2024).

Current combination antiretroviral therapy (cART) successfully lowers HIV-related morbidity, increases survival, and stops transmission, but it cannot completely eliminate HIV because of latent reservoirs of the virus. Restoring immunological function, delaying treatment resistance, and lowering inflammation that might cause organ damage are all benefits of achieving maximum and long-lasting viral load suppression. In order to keep viral loads low and stop the disease from getting worse, treatment adherence is essential. Because of the increased safety and tolerability of contemporary cART medications, recent guidelines advise starting therapy regardless of CD4 cell level, frequently right after diagnosis. A third agent from a different class, such as an integrase strand transfer inhibitor (INSTI) or a non-nucleoside reverse transcriptase inhibitor (NNRTI), is usually added to effective regimens that consist of two nucleoside reverse transcriptase inhibitors (NRTIs). The needs of each patient are prioritized, taking into account elements such as effectiveness, adverse effects, and possible drug combinations. HIV transmission risk is greatly decreased by treatment as prevention (cART), particularly when virus loads are kept below detectable levels. Effective therapy can reduce transmission rates among serodiscordant couples by 96%, according to studies. Due to side effects or a lack of viral suppression, patients who have already received therapy may need to modify their regimen. Maintaining viral suppression while reducing side effects is still the aim, necessitating regular monitoring and a customized strategy. Numerous new medications, such as integrase inhibitors and newer NNRTIs, are in advanced stages of development and have the potential to treat drug-resistant HIV. Additionally, new kinds of antiretrovirals are being investigated, including broadly neutralizing antibodies and maturation inhibitors. The goals of HIV treatment in the future will be to make regimens simpler, safer, and more tolerable. To improve convenience and adherence, NRTI-sparing regimens and long-acting injectable formulations are being investigated. Long-term remission and possible cures depend on advancements in medication administration and the creation of novel therapeutic strategies that target enduring HIV reservoirs. By 2020, the UNAIDS "90-90-90" target is to diagnose 90% of all HIV-positive people, treat 90% of those who have been diagnosed, and achieve viral suppression in 90% of those receiving treatment. Developing successful tactics to target HIV reservoirs and enhance treatment outcomes requires ongoing study (Cihlar & Fordyce, 2016).

A thorough medical history, physical examination, and laboratory tests, such as genotypic resistance testing, plasma HIV RNA testing, and confirmation of HIV antibody positive testing, should all be performed on the first visit. It is important to evaluate social and psychological situations and, if necessary, offer support and therapy. In most European facilities, primary HIV-1 infection (PHI) accounts for only 1-3% of patient presentations and is frequently overlooked or misunderstood in clinical practice. When serological testing is negative or inconclusive, the diagnosis is established if there is detectable HIV in the plasma (p24 antigen and/or HIV RNA > 10,000 copies/mL). During the first six months of treatment, the objectives of first-line therapy are to attain total optimum viral suppression (< 50 copies/mL), improve clinical status, and enhance quality of life. ART is advised immediately for all patients with a history of an AIDS-defining disease or severe HIV symptoms, regardless of their CD4 T-cell level or whether they are asymptomatic with CD4 < 200 cells/mL. The two types of combination regimens that form the basis of the recommendations are boosted PI-based (PIs + two NRTIs) and NNRTI-based (one NNRTI + two NRTIs). Due to their weaker correlation with lipoatrophy than thymidine NRTIs, dual nonthymidine NRTIs are chosen as part of combinations. In individuals who continue on ART, virological failure is defined as evidence of confirmed plasma HIV RNA > 450 copies/mL six months after medication beginning or change. Future therapeutic options are limited by the selection of drug resistance mutations caused by ongoing viral replication in the presence of antiretroviral medications. HIV infection among women of reproductive age is steadily rising in Europe. Regardless of HIV RNA copy level, all HIV-infected women should get antiretroviral prophylaxis to avoid prenatal HIV transmission. Antiretroviral PEP is advised in cases of occupational HIV exposure. It is advised that the source patient be tested for HIV and HCV as soon as possible if their status is unclear (Clumeck et al., 2008).

Because of the virus's strong capacity for reproduction and fast pace of mutation, HIV medication resistance poses a serious threat to HIV/AIDS management and makes treatment plans more difficult. High treatment failure rates can result from resistance that arises from mutations during therapy or is passed on from untreated partners, especially when using nucleoside and non-nucleoside reverse transcriptase inhibitors. Because it can raise the morbidity and mortality rates among HIV-positive people and aid in the spread of resistant strains, the existence of drug-resistant variations presents a hazard to public health. Phenotypic and genotypic assays are currently used to evaluate drug resistance, although they have drawbacks. While phenotypic assays offer direct measurements but are expensive and time-consuming, genotypic testing finds particular mutations linked to resistance. To anticipate resistance patterns and customize treatment plans, creative approaches utilizing cutting-edge technology like AI and ML are required. Through the analysis of massive datasets, AI and ML are transforming the prediction of HIV drug resistance by finding patterns and improving resistance prediction. Drug resistance predictions are being improved through the use of deep learning architectures like Convolutional Neural Networks (CNNs) and machine learning techniques like Random Forests and Support Vector Machines. The precision of resistance predictions is improved by combining genetic information with clinical characteristics. This all-encompassing method enables customized treatment plans based on unique patient information, such as viral load and treatment history. Predicting HIV medication resistance has advanced significantly thanks to deep learning approaches. CNNs have outperformed conventional techniques in the classification of drug resistance mutations. Additionally, by offering insights into the biological causes of resistance, these models can assist doctors in making better treatment options. Antiretroviral therapy (ART) is optimized for each patient using a predictive modeling approach that integrates clinical and genetic data. The difficulties caused by HIV's quick mutation and the rise of drug-resistant strains are addressed by this strategy. Data preprocessing, machine learning and deep learning methods, and reliability validation are all included in the system. Enhancing the interpretability of AI models should be the main goal of future research in order to promote clinical use and enable medical professionals to comprehend the underlying assumptions of forecasts. By putting in place tools that evaluate patient data in real time, treatment plans may be immediately modified in response to new resistance trends. Global efforts to fight HIV/AIDS could be greatly impacted by expanding the use of predictive models in settings with limited resources, particularly in areas where drug-resistant forms of the virus are common (Kibibi, 2024).

The goal of prevention is to shield susceptible people from contracting HIV. Pre-exposure prophylaxis (PrEP), post-exposure prophylaxis (PEP), and risk prediction systems are among the preventative measures that have been the subject of several research. For instance, to predict HIV prevalence and identify at-risk groups, especially among young men who have sex with men (YMSM), researchers have employed sophisticated deep learning algorithms like graph convolutional networks (GCN) and gated recurrent units (GRU). In order to help public health professionals make well-informed decisions, natural language processing (NLP) has been used to examine how the public views PrEP through social media conversations. HIV screening for all can be expensive and ineffective. It might be more successful to use targeted testing techniques, including concentrating on high-risk relationships or applying social network methodologies. Mobile applications have been created to make HIV counseling and testing easier, and artificial intelligence has been used to improve the identification of targeted populations for testing. Sustained viral suppression is the goal of effective treatment, which benefits both HIV-positive people and stops the virus from spreading. Enhancing treatment engagement and retention has been the focus of studies. To enable focused interventions, predictive models have been created to identify patients who are at risk of non-viral suppression or discontinuing treatment. Reducing new transmissions of HIV requires prompt detection and treatment to new clusters of infections. Cluster analysis aids in identifying hotspots and tracking risky behaviors. In order to help with focused public health interventions, studies have used clustering algorithms to find behavioral patterns among people living with HIV. While deep learning (DL) approaches are becoming more popular due to their capacity to analyze complicated datasets, the majority of studies have used conventional machine learning (ML) algorithms like logistic regression and random forests. HIV treatment resistance and incidence have been predicted by DL models such as convolutional neural networks (CNNs) and recurrent neural networks (RNNs). With a bias toward certain research aims, mainly risk prediction, the use of AI in HIV prevention is still in its infancy. Inconsistencies in the assessment of AI models and the underutilization of sophisticated AI algorithms in many studies might result in overfitting and problems with generalizability. Many research lack clarity about dataset accessibility, and data availability and sharing continue to be major obstacles. Future studies should use cutting-edge AI algorithms like generative adversarial networks (GANs) and graph neural networks (GNNs) to investigate a wider range of HIV preventive tasks. Improving data interoperability and tailoring AI algorithms to particular public health issues are crucial for increasing the efficacy of AI applications. To guarantee that AI technologies are applied responsibly and fairly, ethical issues such as data privacy and the possibility of prejudice must be taken into account (Xiang et al., 2021).

The use of machine learning (ML), a crucial component of artificial intelligence (AI), to aid with HIV control is growing. These methods are capable of processing vast amounts of data in order to forecast illness development, evaluate the likelihood of drug resistance, predict how patients will react to treatment, and assist in determining which patients would benefit from particular kinds of care. Machine learning methods facilitate the transition from broad treatment strategies to more individualized medicine catered to the needs of each patient. Because of their accuracy and capacity to handle complicated data, Random Forest (RF), Support Vector Machine (SVM), Logistic Regression (LR), and Gradient Boosting Machines (GBM) are some of the most often utilized machine learning algorithms in HIV care (Sah et al., 2025).

A. Random Forest (RF): To enhance predictions, this technique constructs several decision trees and aggregates their output. It is especially useful for predicting medication resistance, customizing treatment plans, and assessing a patient's chances of treatment success or failure by examining genetic alterations and clinical data (Sah et al., 2025).
B. Support Vector Machine (SVM): SVM is useful for categorizing data, which helps in HIV strain classification and forecasting how the virus would act in various patients. It is frequently used to identify people who are more likely to experience the progression of their condition (Sah et al., 2025).
C. One of the most straightforward yet effective models is logistic regression (LR), which is frequently used to forecast binary outcomes, such as the success or failure of a treatment. It can identify the variables that increase the chance of treatment failure, such as particular gene mutations or clinical indicators (Sah et al., 2025).
D. Gradient Boosting Machines (GBMs): GBMs create a very accurate prediction model by combining multiple smaller models. They aid in comprehending the intricate connections between patient data and medication resistance as well as forecasting treatment results in HIV care (Sah et al., 2025).

A more sophisticated subfield of machine learning called deep learning is particularly good at identifying patterns in big, unstructured information, such as patient histories, genetic codes, or medical photos. Convolutional Neural Networks (CNNs): These are helpful for evaluating genetic information and pictures, assisting researchers in determining which HIV strains are most likely to develop drug resistance, and spotting associated health issues. Models called recurrent neural networks (RNNs) are made to process time-series data, like monitoring a patient's status over time. By examining a patient's treatment history and behavioral characteristics, RNNs are able to predict the course of a disease and medication adherence. NLP is a branch of artificial intelligence that aids computers in comprehending and interpreting human language. NLP can glean valuable information about HIV care from electronic health records (EHRs), doctor's notes, and even social media posts. By examining patient communications or clinical paperwork, it can be used to evaluate treatment adherence, detect undiagnosed instances, and track public opinions regarding HIV. AI has the potential to greatly enhance HIV diagnosis and treatment when combined with tailored medicine. AI may provide personalized treatment plans by analyzing data from a variety of sources, including as a patient's lifestyle, medical records, and genetic history. By providing reminders and real-time monitoring via smartphone applications and smart devices, these tailored approaches not only increase the likelihood that treatment will be successful but also lessen side effects and enhance adherence. While AI has many benefits for HIV care, there are drawbacks as well. Particularly when handling sensitive genetic and medical data, privacy is a big worry. Additionally, AI systems run the potential of being biased, which, if left unchecked, could result in unfair treatment outcomes. Furthermore, cooperation between several disciplines—including public health, data science, medicine, and ethics—is necessary for the successful application of AI in healthcare. Additionally, as HIV prevalence is frequently highest in low-resource environments, it is imperative to guarantee that AI technologies are available there. AI has the potential to further transform HIV care in the future. Future initiatives should concentrate on establishing interdisciplinary partnerships, extending access to these technologies internationally, and carrying out clinical trials to validate AI-driven solutions. Fairness, openness, and ethical use must continue to be the major concerns. In the end, AI can help overcome the gap in HIV care and greatly enhance patient outcomes globally by tackling present constraints and making investments in innovation (Sah et al., 2025).

There are still difficulties in spite of these advantages. Data security and privacy are important issues, particularly in light of the growing usage of wearable technology and electronic health information. Healthcare firms must adhere to laws like HIPAA while safeguarding private patient data from breaches and cyberattacks. To guarantee the equitable and appropriate application of AI, ethical concerns such algorithmic bias, transparency, and patient autonomy must also be taken into consideration (Kolluri, 2016).

Data quality, model interpretability, and ethical issues including algorithmic bias and data privacy are still problems despite progress. Strong regulatory frameworks are required to enable responsible use of AI in HIV care since it raises ethical questions about patient consent and accountability (Senel & Beka, 2025).

The majority of AIDS cases in the United States are reported because persons with advanced HIV typically have decent access to healthcare. Beginning in coastal areas like New York and San Francisco in the early 1980s, the HIV epidemic spread.

It gradually expanded throughout the nation, becoming particularly common in the southern states. Over 700,000 AIDS cases had been officially registered in the United States by the middle of 1999. The majority of these were among guys, particularly those who inject drugs and had sex with men. The number of female cases has increased in recent years, and the main method of infection has clearly shifted toward heterosexual transmission. When combination antiretroviral therapy (ART) was introduced in the mid-1990s, it was a huge breakthrough that greatly decreased the number of AIDS-related deaths. The fact that the number of new HIV cases has not decreased significantly, however, indicates that the virus is still spreading and that prevention measures must be improved. The European Union recorded over 206,000 cases of AIDS as of mid-1999. The number of new AIDS cases has decreased as a result of better treatments. However, the appearance of the pandemic varies by location. While injecting drugs is a popular way for HIV to spread in southern European countries, sexual transmission—particularly between males who have sex with other men—is more prevalent in northern European countries. With a discernible increase in incidence beginning in the mid-1990s, the HIV epidemic in this area is relatively new. Infection rates have skyrocketed in nations like Russia and Ukraine, primarily among drug injectors. In many of these nations, the epidemic has been difficult to control due to political unrest, weak health systems, and economic difficulties. HIV was a major problem in Thailand in the 1990s, especially among injecting drug users and sex workers. Nonetheless, Thailand also put in place one of the most effective HIV control initiatives in the world, which decreased the number of new infections. Epidemics in other Asian nations, such as China and India, are more diverse and intricate. The virus is more prevalent in some populations, like as drug users, sex workers, and males who have sex with men, than in the overall population. The HIV epidemic in Latin America has been changing over time. Initially, it primarily afflicted men who had intercourse with other men, but more women are getting infected, and heterosexual transmission is on the rise. In contrast, outside of sub-Saharan Africa, the Caribbean has one of the highest rates of HIV. The virus has had a particularly severe effect on Haiti. More than two-thirds of all HIV-positive individuals reside in Sub-Saharan Africa, which continues to be the most affected region globally. The disease has had a terrible effect, leaving millions of children orphaned and increasing death rates and life expectancy. In addition to overwhelming healthcare systems, the epidemic has raised the prevalence of other diseases, including TB, which is frequently observed in HIV-positive individuals. The disease's pervasiveness in this area still has significant social and economic repercussions. The HIV epidemic is far from ended, even with advancements in therapy. Preventing new infections is one of the most important public health issues of our day. Despite the fact that ART has significantly improved the lives of people with HIV, the consistent rate of new infections suggests that preventive measures are not meeting their full potential. Stronger public health systems, particularly in underresourced areas, more access to testing and treatment, and more effective prevention programs are all necessary to genuinely reverse the trend toward HIV (De Cock & Weiss, 2000).

Computer technology known as machine learning (ML) enables computers to learn from data and make judgments or predictions without explicit programming. Because medical data is frequently vast, intricate, and challenging to evaluate using conventional techniques, it is growing in popularity in the healthcare industry. ML assists in revealing links and hidden patterns in this data. ML comes in two primary varieties (Fieggen et al., 2022):

- The model is trained using labeled data in supervised learning, where we know the right responses, such as whether a person has HIV or not. It is used to predict either a number (such as an individual's viral load) or to categorize people into groups (such as infected vs non-infected) (Fieggen et al., 2022).
- Unsupervised learning is a useful technique for identifying unidentified trends or groupings in data by having the model search for patterns without labels (Fieggen et al., 2022).

By examining a wide range of variables, including age, gender, sexual behavior, and other lifestyle or societal markers, machine learning (ML) can be used to predict who is more likely to get HIV. In the past, risk was evaluated by examining one or two variables. However, ML may aggregate a lot of them to identify intricate patterns that people might overlook. According to certain research, machine learning models—particularly those that employ the sophisticated technique known as Super Learner—perform significantly better in forecasting new HIV infections than conventional risk assessment instruments (Fieggen et al., 2022).

There are various steps involved in developing a quality ML model:

A. Feature selection: These are the bits of data that the model utilizes to predict outcomes, such as age or the number of sexual partners. Selecting the appropriate features is crucial because if you use too many, the model may become overfit to a single dataset and perform badly on new data (Fieggen et al., 2022).
B. Data splitting: Typically, the dataset is separated into three sections: testing (to determine how well the model performs on unseen data), validation (to make adjustments), and training (to educate the model). This guarantees the model's dependability rather than merely memorization of the facts (Fieggen et al., 2022).

C. Performance metrics: The accuracy of the model is evaluated following training. The confusion matrix is a widely used tool that measures things like: by comparing expected and actual findings,
    I. Sensitivity (the ability to detect real positives),
    II. Specificity (the degree to which erroneous positives are avoided),
    III. Accuracy (the frequency of overall correctness),
    IV. The model's ability to differentiate between individuals with and without HIV is indicated by its AUROC score (Fieggen et al., 2022).

ML can be extremely precise, but it's frequently difficult to comprehend how it makes its decisions. For this reason, researchers employ methods such as SHAP (Shapley Additive Explanations), which aid in elucidating the logic of the model. By highlighting the risk factors that were most crucial to a given forecast, SHAP can increase the model's transparency and credibility, which is crucial in the healthcare industry. In order to determine who was most at risk of HIV, researchers in one instance developed an ML model incorporating social, demographic, and behavioral data. They emphasized how crucial it is to modify models for particular populations because what works for one nation or group may not work for another. SHAP does not tell us how accurate a forecast is, but it does assist explain how it was formed. Finding the factors that are most crucial overall might be aided by additional methods such as Permutation Importance (PIMP). However, these techniques can be laborious and slow, particularly when there are overlapping or related features in the data (Fieggen et al., 2022).

About half of HIV infections in Germany are discovered too late, frequently after the best time to begin treatment. This implies that a large number of persons receive their initial diagnosis when they already exhibit symptoms of AIDS or when their immune system is seriously weakened. Early HIV detection is essential for both preserving the person's health and lowering the chance of spreading the infection to other people. People can take preventive measures, like wearing protection during intercourse and starting an efficient therapy that reduces the virus load, if they receive an early diagnosis. Older adults who might not think of themselves as at risk, immigrants from high-HIV-rate nations, and men who have sex with males are more likely to receive a late diagnosis. Many times, these people have previously interacted with medical professionals, but during those initial encounters, HIV was never suspected nor tested for. The optimal time to start antiretroviral therapy (ART) is still up for debate, but an increasing amount of research points to the benefits of beginning treatment as soon as possible. In addition to keeping the virus under control, early treatment lowers the chance of developing other health issues that can occur when the immune system is compromised. Regardless of how robust their immune system is at the moment, current medical guidelines advise all individuals with HIV who are exhibiting symptoms of the disease to begin antiretroviral therapy (ART). For those who are co-infected with other illnesses, such as hepatitis, it can also be very advantageous to begin treatment as soon as possible. Reducing the blood's virus concentration to an undetectable level (less than 50 copies per milliliter) is the primary goal of HIV treatment. Reaching this objective reduces the likelihood that the virus will develop drug resistance and strengthens the immune system. However, patients must adhere strictly to their treatment plan in order to achieve this aim. Adherence is essential for long-term success because skipping even a few doses can make the infection more difficult to treat (Vogel et al., 2010). At least three medications are often used in combination for HIV treatment. Taking many drugs at once keeps the virus from developing resistance. Physicians must take into account more than simply medical considerations when deciding which medications to prescribe. In addition, they consider the patient's everyday life, including their occupation, family obligations, and other medical issues. It's a good idea to perform a test to see if the patient already has any drug-resistant strains of HIV before starting therapy. This aids in the initial selection of the most successful drugs. Within four weeks of beginning ART, patients should be evaluated to determine whether the treatment is effective. Doctors will investigate potential causes, such as inadequate treatment adherence or drug resistance, if the viral load hasn't decreased as anticipated. Because they are more likely to develop immune reconstitution inflammatory syndrome (IRIS), people with particularly low immune cell counts (CD4 cells) require constant monitoring. This syndrome occurs when the immune system reacts excessively to infections that are already present in the body after it has begun to recuperate. The course of treatment for a patient may need to be modified at times. This might be the result of the drugs' poor performance, harsh side effects, or the introduction of better and more recent drugs. In addition to lab results, clinicians consider the patient's feelings, ease of adhering to the regimen, and tolerability of side effects while modifying a treatment plan. Some patients, particularly those who are feeling well and have high CD4 counts, may think about pausing treatment for a period. But research has indicated that stopping ART can be dangerous. Treatment interruption raises the risk of AIDS-related diseases and other severe side effects. For the majority of HIV-positive individuals, ongoing medication is therefore the safer and more successful course of action (Vogel et al., 2010).

Over half of the approximately 38 million HIV-positive individuals in the world today are female. 160,000 youngsters were among the 1.7 million new cases of the virus in 2018 alone. HIV has killed a significant number of individuals over the years; in 2018, 770,000 people died, 100,000 of whom were children. Over 39 million people have died from AIDS-related illnesses since the epidemic started, and about 75 million people have been infected (Challacombe, 2020).

HIV has an uneven impact on the world:

a) With 65% of all cases worldwide occurring in Sub-Saharan Africa, the region bears the greatest burden (Challacombe, 2020).
b) With 1.1 percent of the population living with HIV, the Caribbean has the second-highest prevalence (Challacombe, 2020).
c) About 0.5–0.6% of the populations in North America and Latin America are afflicted, which is a moderate prevalence (Challacombe, 2020).
d) There are over 5.9 million HIV-positive individuals in Asia and the Pacific (Challacombe, 2020).

Since 2010, there have been some significant advancements:

i. Better survival rates and more testing have contributed to a more than 20% increase in the number of persons living with HIV (Challacombe, 2020).
ii. The number of deaths from diseases linked to AIDS has decreased by 33% (Challacombe, 2020).
iii. Additionally, there has been a decline in new HIV infections, but only by roughly sixteen percent, indicating that prevention efforts are making progress but are still insufficient (Challacombe, 2020).

There are significant differences in access to antiretroviral medication (ART), which eradicates the virus:

a. Nearly 80% of people with diagnoses in Western and Central Europe are undergoing treatment (Challacombe, 2020).
b. That percentage reduces to just 38% in Eastern Europe (Challacombe, 2020).
c. Significant gaps in care are highlighted by the even lower treatment coverage rate of 32% across the Middle East and North Africa (Challacombe, 2020).

Women are disproportionately impacted, particularly young women:

a) Every week, some 6,200 young women and girls between the ages of 15 and 24 become infected (Challacombe, 2020).
b) Girls account for four out of five new adolescent infections in sub-Saharan Africa (Challacombe, 2020).
c) Compared to young men, young women in this age range are twice as likely to be HIV positive (Challacombe, 2020).
d) More than one-third of women worldwide have been victims of physical or sexual violence, which increases their susceptibility to HIV infection (Challacombe, 2020).

Children are still significantly impacted by HIV:

i. Currently, 91% of the 1.7 million children living with HIV reside in sub-Saharan Africa (Challacombe, 2020).
ii. Although the number of children who die from AIDS varies globally, the issue is still very much present (Challacombe, 2020).

Who contracts HIV and who does not is influenced by a variety of social and structural factors. These consist of:

A. Gender and age
B. Other sexually transmitted infections are present.
C. Dangerous actions such as drug usage or unprotected sex
D. Status of marriage and educational attainment
E. Access to medicine and healthcare
F. Living circumstances (rural or urban
G. Additional health issues (co-morbidities) (Challacombe, 2020).

Research has demonstrated that higher levels of education in African nations are associated with lower rates of HIV infection, highlighting the significance of education in prevention. Mouth sores and infections are common oral health problems among those living with HIV. However, access to dental treatment for these people is severely limited worldwide. Although improving oral healthcare for those with HIV has been identified as a priority, little has changed since the issue was initially brought to light at the 6th World Workshop in Beijing (Challacombe, 2020).

The research environment around HIV is depicted in this bibliometric visualization, which was made with VOSviewer and is based on PubMed-indexed material. Each node's size represents the frequency of phrases in scientific papers, and the network map is based on keyword co-occurrence (Figure 1).

The term "humans" is at the center and most noticeable on the map, signifying the preponderance of human-centered HIV research. Various thematic areas of inquiry are represented by the surrounding clusters. Molecular and genetic investigations are highlighted by the red cluster on the lower left, which includes terms such as "cell line," "transcription, genetic," and "viral regulatory proteins." This indicates a solid background in cellular biology and virology. With keywords like "anti-HIV agents," "HIV reverse transcriptase," and "molecular docking simulation," the blue cluster in the upper middle indicates active research in the design of antiretroviral therapies. This cluster is focused on medication development and molecular modeling. With terms like "male," "middle aged," "treatment outcome," and "genotype," the green cluster on the right showcases epidemiological and clinical research, highlighting studies on patient demographics, treatment effectiveness, and disease progression. Intersections between pharmacology and treatment resistance are captured by the purple cluster.

Figure 1. VOSviewer-generated keyword co-occurrence network based on PubMed database on using AI in HIV treatment and prediction

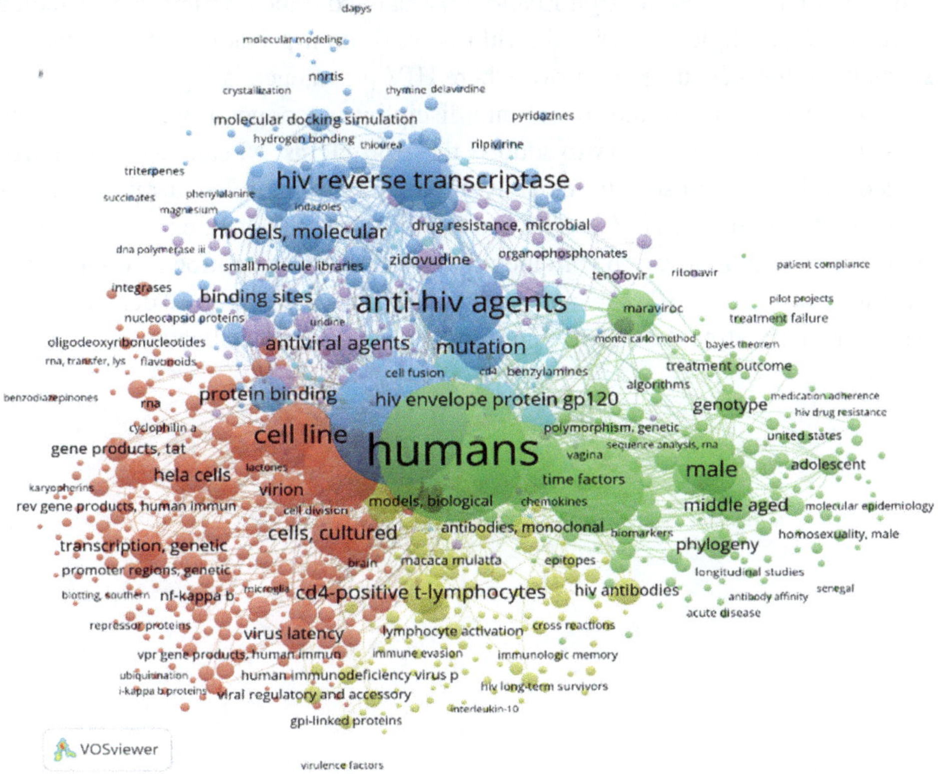

3. CONCLUSION

AI has great potential to address the complex issues of HIV prevention, treatment, and possible cure. AI provides cutting-edge solutions for early diagnosis, optimal treatment plans, and real-time patient monitoring with ML, DL, and sophisticated analytics. By customizing treatments to each patient's unique profile, these technologies help physicians maximize results and adherence while reducing resistance and adverse effects.

AI also finds hidden viral reservoirs, speeds up medication discovery and repurposing, and aids in the development of vaccines by evaluating intricate immunological data. Patients and healthcare professionals are further empowered by its combination with wearable technology and mobile health tools. But in addition to its potential, AI presents significant logistical and ethical issues. These include discrepancies in digital access, algorithmic bias, data privacy, and transparency, especially in low-resource countries where HIV prevalence is highest.

Strong regulatory frameworks, interdisciplinary cooperation, and equitable access programs are necessary to address these problems. AI cannot eradicate HIV on its own, but when used strategically, it can greatly improve current initiatives. The goal of eliminating HIV as a hazard to public health is made more feasible by fusing technology innovation with inclusive policy and international collaboration. The transformation of HIV care and potential long-awaited cure will depend heavily on sustained investment in AI-driven research and ethical application.

REFERENCES

Challacombe, S. J. (2020). Global inequalities in HIV infection. *Oral Diseases, 26*(S1), 16–21. DOI: 10.1111/odi.13386 PMID: 32862524

Cihlar, T., & Fordyce, M. (2016). Current status and prospects of HIV treatment. *Current Opinion in Virology, 18*, 50–56. DOI: 10.1016/j.coviro.2016.03.004 PMID: 27023283

Clumeck, N., Pozniak, A., & Raffi, F. (2008). European AIDS Clinical Society (EACS) guidelines for the clinical management and treatment of HIV-infected adults. *HIV Medicine, 9*(2), 65–71. DOI: 10.1111/j.1468-1293.2007.00533.x PMID: 18257769

De Cock, K. M., & Weiss, H. A. (2000). The global epidemiology of HIV/AIDS. *Tropical Medicine & International Health, 5*(7). Advance online publication. DOI: 10.1046/j.1365-3156.2000.00590.x PMID: 10964276

Eissa, N. M. E. (2025). A BRIEF OVERVIEW OF HIV TREATMENT STRATEGIES: a FOCUSED LOOK AT CHALLENGES AND OPPORTUNITIES. *Universal Journal of Pharmaceutical Research*. https://doi.org/DOI: 10.22270/ujpr.v10i1.1273

Fieggen, J., Smith, E., Arora, L., & Segal, B. (2022). The role of machine learning in HIV risk prediction. *Frontiers in Reproductive Health, 4*. Advance online publication. DOI: 10.3389/frph.2022.1062387 PMID: 36619681

Jin, R., & Zhang, L. (2025). AI applications in HIV research: Advances and future directions. *Frontiers in Microbiology, 16*. Advance online publication. DOI: 10.3389/fmicb.2025.1541942 PMID: 40051479

Kibibi, W. H. (2024). Harnessing artificial intelligence for HIV drug resistance prediction and personalized treatment. *NEWPORT INTERNATIONAL JOURNAL OF RESEARCH IN MEDICAL SCIENCES, 5*(3), 59–64. DOI: 10.59298/nijrms/2024/5.3.5964

Kolluri, V. (2016). An innovative study exploring revolutionizing healthcare with AI: personalized medicine: predictive diagnostic techniques and individualized treatment. *Journal of Emerging Technologies and Innovative Research, 218*, •••. https://www.researchgate.net/publication/380730035

Lainjo, B. (2023). Artificial intelligence with machine learning and the enigmatic discovery of HIV cure. *Journal of Autonomous Intelligence, 7*(2). Advance online publication. DOI: 10.32629/jai.v7i2.697

Olaboye, N. J. A., Maha, N. C. C., Kolawole, N. T. O., & Abdul, N. S. (2024). Artificial intelligence in monitoring HIV treatment adherence: A conceptual exploration. *International Journal of Multidisciplinary Research Updates, 7*(2), 068–082. https://doi.org/DOI: 10.53430/ijmru.2024.7.2.0036

Sah, A. K., Elshaikh, R. H., Shalabi, M. G., Abbas, A. M., Prabhakar, P. K., Babker, A. M. A., Choudhary, R. K., Gaur, V., Choudhary, A. S., & Agarwal, S. (2025). Role of artificial intelligence and personalized medicine in enhancing HIV management and treatment outcomes. *Life (Chicago, Ill.), 15*(5), 745. DOI: 10.3390/life15050745 PMID: 40430173

Senel, B., & Beka, H. (2025). Artificial Intelligence in HIV Diagnosis and Treatment: A Comprehensive review. *Cumhuriyet Tıp Dergisi/Cumhuriyet ÜNiversitesi Tıp FaküLtesi Dergisi, 47*(1), 10–21. https://doi.org/DOI: 10.7197/cmj.1630164

Serrano, D. R., Luciano, F. C., Anaya, B. J., Ongoren, B., Kara, A., Molina, G., Ramirez, B. I., Sánchez-Guirales, S. A., Simon, J. A., Tomietto, G., Rapti, C., Ruiz, H. K., Rawat, S., Kumar, D., & Lalatsa, A. (2024). Artificial intelligence (AI) applications in drug discovery and drug delivery: Revolutionizing personalized medicine. *Pharmaceutics, 16*(10), 1328. DOI: 10.3390/pharmaceutics16101328 PMID: 39458657

Vogel, M., Schwarze-Zander, C., Wasmuth, J., Spengler, U., Sauerbruch, T., & Rockstroh, J. K. (2010). The treatment of patients with HIV. *Deutsches Ärzteblatt International*. Advance online publication. DOI: 10.3238/arztebl.2010.0507 PMID: 20703338

Xiang, Y., Du, J., Fujimoto, K., Li, F., Schneider, J., & Tao, C. (2021). Application of artificial intelligence and machine learning for HIV prevention interventions. *The Lancet. HIV, 9*(1), e54–e62. DOI: 10.1016/s2352-3018(21)00247-2 PMID: 34762838

ADDITIONAL READING

Li, Y., Feng, Y., He, Q., Ni, Z., Hu, X., Feng, X., & Ni, M. (2024b). The predictive accuracy of machine learning for the risk of death in HIV patients: A systematic review and meta-analysis. *BMC Infectious Diseases, 24*(1). Advance online publication. DOI: 10.1186/s12879-024-09368-z PMID: 38711068

Wu, L., Xia, D., & Xu, K. (2023). Multi-Clinical Factors Combined with an Artificial Intelligence Algorithm Diagnosis Model for HIV-Infected People with Bloodstream Infection. *Infection and Drug Resistance*, *16*, 6085–6097. DOI: 10.2147/idr.s423709 PMID: 37719647

Zhu, Q., Fang, P., Zhao, Y., Dai, D., & Luo, X. (2020b). How about the quality and recommendation on prevention, diagnosis, and treatment of HIV/AIDS guidelines developed by WHO. *Medicine*, *99*(52), e23638. DOI: 10.1097/md.0000000000023638 PMID: 33350740

KEY TERMS AND DEFINITIONS

HIV: The virus known as HIV, or human immunodeficiency virus, targets the immune system and, if left untreated, can cause AIDS.

AI (Artificial Intellect): AI describes computer programs that are made to carry out operations like learning and decision-making that often call for human intellect.

ML (Machine Learning): A branch of AI, ML allows computers to learn from data and enhance performance without the need for explicit programming.

ART (Antiretroviral Therapy): It is a medical intervention that uses a combination of medications to manage HIV infection and stop it from developing into AIDS.

HIV Therapy: To reduce viral load, strengthen the immune system, and enhance patient outcomes, HIV therapy entails the use of ART and additional therapies.

Personalized Medicine: Individual genetic, environmental, and lifestyle aspects are taken into account when making healthcare decisions and treatments through personalized medicine.

DL (Deep Learning): It is a sophisticated branch of machine learning that analyzes intricate patterns in huge datasets by using multi-layered neural networks.

HIV Prevention: HIV prevention includes methods to lower the risk of HIV transmission, such as PrEP, safe sex education, and testing.

Chapter 4
Impact of Antiretroviral Therapy (ART) on HIV Treatment Outcomes

Wasswa Shafik
https://orcid.org/0000-0002-9320-3186
Dig Connectivity Research Laboratory (DCRLab), Uganda

ABSTRACT

This study presents an analysis of the impact of Antiretroviral Therapy (ART) on HIV treatment outcomes, highlighting its role in reducing viral load, improving immune function, and enhancing the quality of life for people living with HIV. ART has significantly transformed HIV from a life-threatening condition to a manageable chronic disease, reducing morbidity and mortality rates worldwide. By suppressing viral replication, ART not only prolongs life expectancy but also minimizes the risk of transmission, playing a crucial role in achieving global HIV prevention goals. However, challenges such as drug resistance, adherence issues, and disparities in access to treatment continue to affect its effectiveness. Additionally, long-term ART use raises concerns about side effects and comorbidities, necessitating ongoing research into improved formulations and treatment strategies. This study examines ART's contributions to HIV management, addressing both its successes and the barriers that must be overcome to ensure equitable and sustainable treatment outcomes.

1. INTRODUCTION

Acquired immunodeficiency syndrome[1] (AIDS) was revealed to be a result of infection with the human immunodeficiency virus[2] (HIV) as recently as 1983. Results of the research showed that this causative virus was a member of the Ort-

DOI: 10.4018/979-8-3373-2863-8.ch004

horetrovirinae[3] subfamily of the genus Lentivirus within the Flaviviridae[4] family. Pathogenic sequencing showed the underlying cause to be a deviation from normal immune function. This exposure of the central role of the host-virus interaction to the causal relationship between HIV infection and consequent changes in the qualities of host immune responsiveness highlights the more particular and common traits of HIV therapeutic and biological relevance (Comfort et al., 2024). Long-term survivors of HIV-1 infection can persist in latent reservoirs of resting CD4-positive T lymphocytes (CD4+) T cells. Because of the description of HIV and the manner in which it infects this very population, the ultimate challenge is the requirement for treatment with antiretroviral therapy.

Considering HIV biology and the normal properties of CD4+ T cells, a clear understanding of the inhibition of latency in existing HIV reservoirs does not extend to vigorously and persistently controlling the long-lived reservoirs of latent infection, and sometimes has effects on the skin (Shafik, 2025a). This is responsible for challenges with ART, followed by treatment with latency inhibitors that slowly and inefficiently reduce reservoir size, with the caveat that HIV-specific immunity struggles to be maintained while viral antigen expression is repeatedly diminished over time. The average duration of less than three years of lentiviral treatment before therapy remains primed for bearing evidence of the decrease in latent cellular virus in persons receiving antiretroviral therapy (Ayiigah et al., 2024). This general thinking for chronic diseases theorizes the accepted relationship between the age of HIV-infected individuals and the loss of control of the virus, as observed for HIV protease viral loads, as its structure is presented in Figure 1 with symptoms including Chills, fatigue, fever, mouth sores, muscle aches, night sweats, rash, sore throat and swollen lymph nodes (Nursalam et al., 2024).

At the turn of the 21st century, the advent of antiretroviral therapy (ART) was very much like the light at the end of the tunnel. Essentially, ART raised hopes for the living because initially, it was introduced as an emergency medication that saved millions from severe illnesses. Within a decade, ART usage became more widespread and considerably more sophisticated because of decreasing prices through the generic industry, improved formulations with reduced side effects, and also because governments and development partners had increased both supply through service provision and demand through social marketing (Kanise et al., 2024). Importantly, the management of ART improved because, apart from saving sick people, ART started saving the dead from further morbidity and mortality emanating from opportunistic infections and associated syndromes, and fighting blood cells (Saleh et al., 2024).

So, not long after the advent of ART, it could be noticed that the epidemic was dying out when ART was delivered effectively. Today, ART is just a mainstream medication, and HIV is a preventable, non-communicable condition, a long journey for a condition that was initially referred to as gay-related immune deficiency.

In comes a global cooperation platform through which the seven hundred million worldwide affected by HIV can be helped. This platform has triggered the fastest global response to a health issue through campaigning from a wide array of HIV stakeholders because it has given these stakeholders access to scientific research and hope for preventive vaccine discovery against the disease (Sadiq et al., 2024). Today, it has moved from being a partner that funds innovative research, affordable diagnostics, challenges vaccine development, and subsidizes strategic planning and service provision to being the partner for any stakeholders that might require skilled assistance, provided that they are able to help the HIV response make its global science-proven prevention and treatment targets within the national scope of highly ambitious sustainable development (Konishi et al., 2024).

Figure 1. HIV (human immunodeficiency virus) structure

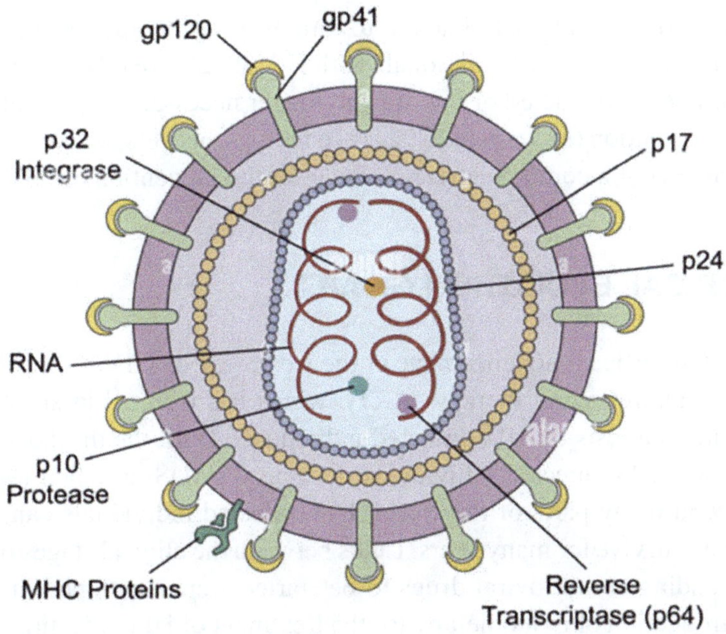

1.1. Global Burden of HIV and the Role of ART

1999 marked a significant milestone in the history of HIV/AIDS: it was the year when the use of antiretroviral therapy (ART) began to be recommended for the management of cases of this infection. Before this development, considering that AIDS was regarded as an incurable disease, HIV testing was primarily limited to well-protected study units. Now, the provision of ART has led to an expansion of testing opportunities. In the same vein, the universal call for scaling up ART has contributed to an across-the-board promotion of access to HIV services (Mahlalela et al., 2024). In fact, scaling up comprehensive services for the prevention of mother-to-child transmission of HIV is currently being viewed as more acceptable than any other intervention for the reduction of child mortality. The global HIV pandemic is a health problem with extraordinary characteristics. It is one of humanity's biggest public health threats, especially in view of the fact that since HIV seropositivity is a disorder without being a disease, the goal of prevention and favorable HIV/AIDS outcomes cannot be achieved by means of conventional medical care measures alone (Gupta et al., 2024). Factors that favor its propagation and transmission include a large number of HIV carriers worldwide, persistent lifetime infection, multiple routes of transmission, high rates of viral replication, and multiple circulating HIV types, subtypes, and CRFs in the general healthcare (Shafik, 2024c). It exploits the fact that advances in treatment, such as access to antiretroviral therapy and the immediate provision of medication to all individuals with HIV, create the false concept that the epidemic has been attenuated or that it is no longer necessary to pay heed to measures for its prevention (Moya et al., 2024). To redress this perspective, ART should be viewed as part of a comprehensive strategy for the prevention of HIV infection.

2. HISTORICAL EVOLUTION OF ART

The most significant advancement in the treatment of HIV disease is the development of antiretroviral therapy (ART), which has resulted in substantial improvement in prognosis for HIV-infected individuals. Until the third decade of the epidemic, most HIV-infected individuals developed AIDS and died (West et al., 2024). Now, in many parts of the world, HIV-infected individuals can be treated with ART and survive for many years. Links between the clinical stages of HIV and the corresponding antiretroviral drugs to be started were developed in the 1990s with the introduction of monotherapy for the treatment of HIV infection. However, the major development in antiretroviral therapy was made with the introduction of potent and less toxic antiretroviral medications in combination, called highly active antiretroviral therapy (HAART), in 1996 (West et al., 2024). Initially, two nucleosides and a protease inhibitor were used; the triple drug therapy produced a rapid reduction in viral load, both in the blood and other sites such as the brain, gut, and lymph nodes. As a result, new immune responses were rapidly documented, such as increased CD4 T-cell counts in the blood, increased CD4 and CD8 functions, and reversal of wasting syndrome. These immune responses corresponded with reductions in morbidity and mortality in individuals who had progressed to AIDS by stopping opportunistic infections, delaying the occurrence of new infections, and prolonging the interval between infections (Naranjo et al., 2024). Reducing the viral load to undetectable levels was shown to suppress viral replication in all body compartments and restore quantitative and selective defects in the quasispecies of the virus. With continuous treatment, these immune responses were stable over time, while interrupting therapy predictably led to viral rebound, loss of function, increased immune activation, and progressive mortality (OG, 2024).

Despite evidence showing clear beneficial effects on morbidity and mortality, ART has always had its own set of challenges. These included high pill burden initially, variable pill-taking schedules, and if a patient requires a second-line regimen, patients had increased pill burden, side effects to drugs, and adverse drug reactions that led to substitutions, toxicities, and other drug interactions, poor palatability, and poor buffer capacities with many of the earliest formulations. Some formulations contained aspartame and resulted in those living with HIV who were prone to diarrhea developing true dilemmas with the combinations of urgent diarrhea and pure dumps from aspartame (Njuba et al., 2024). Patients may not wish to eat or may drink sugar-free cola, and therefore, the protease inhibitors could be less effective as they are fat-soluble and need a certain amount of fat to achieve adequate blood concentrations. Improvements in the treatments over time have reduced the barriers and addressed the lack of access to care in the first world, leading to significant reductions in morbidity and mortality. Initially, the availability of highly active antiretroviral therapy in the first world led to a major decrease in mortality, but it is in low- and middle-income countries where ART can have its greatest impact (Saltini et al., 2024). Today, ART programs have increased and have persisted, with up to 70–72% of those in need of ART in low- and middle-income countries receiving treatment. Programs in many countries have achieved the following successes: early treatment of those living with HIV has incorporated the ability to remove research subjects safely from trials at the first sign of treatment failure, managing those on toxic regimens, removing those with serious adverse reactions, deciding on when to switch patients to the new drugs, and implementing plans to deliver the new medications and combinations to the patients most in need (Wang et al., 2024).

3. MECHANISM OF ACTION AND CLASSES OF ANTIRETROVIRAL DRUGS

The mechanism of action of ART has been covered partly in previous sections of this chapter. ART consists of several classes of drugs that target HIV at different stages of its life cycle. The six classes of ART are nucleoside reverse transcriptase inhibitors, non-nucleoside reverse transcriptase inhibitors, protease inhibitors, fusion inhibitors, integrase inhibitors, and CCR5 inhibitors. The cycle begins when HIV attaches to and fuses with the surface of a CD4+ T lymphocyte. A crucial protein in this process is HIV's envelope protein, which binds to the CD4+ T lymphocyte and cell surface co-receptors, a chemokine receptor type 5 coupled with CD4+ T lymphocyte, and then penetrates the cell membrane of the CD4+ T lymphocyte and deposits viral DNA into the cytoplasm before converting it into double-stranded DNA (Fassinou et al., 2024). Inhibiting this entry process is the core mechanism of the CCR5 antagonists through which they block the entry of HIV into cells. Maraviroc targets this entry process and is used as a first-line therapy together with other classes of ART in the treatment-naive phase. However, to guide the introduction of C-C chemokine receptor type 5[5] (CCR5) inhibitors into treatment regimens, physicians must have access to the results of tropism tests to determine whether a specific patient's virus can exploit this co-receptor. Currently, physicians can only prescribe maraviroc for treatment-experienced adults infected with CCR5-tropic HIV-1 who have evidence of viral replication and have been prescribed regimens that include at least one other antiretroviral drug (Gatechompol et al., 2024).

3.1. Nucleoside Reverse Transcriptase Inhibitors (NRTIs)

NRTIs[6] are antiretroviral drugs that directly inhibit the action of the enzyme reverse transcriptase, which converts HIV RNA to HIV DNA. By inhibiting HIV DNA synthesis, NRTIs prevent the establishment of a provirus in infected cells. AZT was the first NRTI approved for use in the United States. Other NRTIs currently approved include d4T, ddI, ddC, 3TC, and abacavir, as well as several co-formulations. NRTIs were the first class of ART approved and have demonstrated both potent viral suppression and improved clinical outcomes in treated individuals (Wagner et al., 2024). By inhibiting viral replication, NRTIs decrease the levels of viremia in the blood. In animal models, the highly significant reduction in viral load in the peripheral blood of nonhuman primates starting NRTIs immediately after the challenge demonstrated that early antiretroviral administration can provide additional benefit in limiting the size of the latent viral reservoir during the critical days of post-infection. However, the impact of NRTIs on the downstream events controlling latency establishment was not directly addressed, as suppressive ART was initiated prior to viremia (Slogrove et al., 2024). Subsequent investigations into the effect of ART timing on viral reservoir size in perinatal infection supported the potential role of NRTIs in limiting the latent reservoir. Infants treated within 2 days of birth exhibited strikingly lower levels of both cell-associated viral DNA and intact replication-competent reservoir compared with infants with either delayed initiation or no antiretroviral therapy. NRTI initiation near the peak of viremia can significantly diminish the size of the reservoir through the rapid reduction in viral expression and clearance of infected cells (Corona et al., 2024).

The impact of NRTIs on latency establishment is known. Tenofovir disoproxil fumarate decreased the number of Simian-Human Immunodeficiency Virus (SHIV)-infected cells, establishing infection in a humanized mouse model, and led to later viral rebound during treatment interruption. The reduced viral growth rate during treatment likely results from the selective antiviral pressure imposed by TDF on newly infected cells. Moreover, evaluating the effect of NRTI timing on childhood HIV latency found a dose-dependent relationship between the initiation of ART and the seeded viral reservoir in the child, which is likely due to the association of earlier ART initiation with reduced viral replication and fewer persistently infected cells (C. Chen et al., 2024). Such findings strongly support applications of NRTIs to minimize the size of the latent viral reservoir in clinical treatment in the context of both different HIV exposures and populations.

3.2. Non-Nucleoside Reverse Transcriptase Inhibitors (NNRTIs)

NNRTI drugs bind to reverse transcriptase and change its shape, so it no longer works. These drugs circulate in the blood after they have been absorbed from the gastrointestinal tract. They are processed in the liver and eliminated in the urine and feces. NNRTIs may cause skin rash, liver problems, and interactions with other drugs. Four NNRTIs are currently available for use as part of combination regimens for HIV treatment (Hernandez et al., 2024). These are nevirapine, efavirenz, delavirdine, and etravirine. The first-generation NNRTIs, including nevirapine, delavirdine, and efavirenz, were characterized by high inter-patient variability and risk of drug resistance development when used as monotherapy. However, etravirine, which is classified as the third-generation NNRTI and can inhibit NNRTI-resistant strains, can be used to treat patients who may have developed resistance to first and second-line ART regimens (Koh et al., 2024). Efavirenz is a first-generation non-nucleoside reverse transcriptase inhibitor. This drug is administered orally anytime during the day. Efavirenz is metabolized in the liver by CYP3A4 isoenzymes. Usual central nervous system side effects experienced by patients during therapy with efavirenz mostly disappear within 2–4 weeks spontaneously. It has a plasma half-life of 40–55 hours when taken with food. Therefore, it must be taken on an empty stomach. Efavirenz, concurrently with two other nucleoside reverse transcriptase inhibitors, is an important component of ART (Antoine et al., 2024). It is relatively contraindicated in patients with allergic reactions to medications, severe liver disorders, reported suicide attempts, and an age below three months. Resistance to efavirenz is commonly associated with the mutation at reverse transcriptase amino acid positions 103 and 190. This drug is listed in the strongly recommended antiretroviral drugs during pregnancy and breastfeeding. It has an untoward effect on fetal neural tube abnormalities in babies. It is considered an antiretroviral category D for use during pregnancy, i.e., there is evidence of human fetal risk (Trickey et al., 2024).

3.3. Protease Inhibitors (PIs)

The specific characteristics of protease inhibitors[7] (PIs) are that they inhibit the protease enzyme. This consequently stops viral replication. However, the drugs are not used as frequently as the other antiretroviral (ARV) drugs. PIs also have a few more side effects than the other ARV drugs. Thus, the drug is not used as a first treatment in patients with advanced HIV. Once a patient fails to respond to other ARVs, then the PIs become important. A major factor to be considered in using PIs is the development of resistant viruses. This is observed in patients who are using the drugs. Therefore, combination drugs are added to the PIs, or two PIs are used in combination (Sheira et al., 2024). This is necessary to improve the outcome of the treatment. Although several protease inhibitors (PIs) have provided substantial virologic and clinical benefits, the clinical use of PIs is severely limited by issues of convenience, complexity, and patient intolerance. Early in clinical development, it was recognized that PIs had a propensity for inducing a significant number of dose-limiting side effects and drug interactions and that the drugs have complex metabolic pathways involving cytochrome P450 and P-glycoprotein efflux transporter proteins (Nursalam et al., 2024). Furthermore, despite available data from efficacy and combination studies, there was—and still is—limited long-term safety information about the use of single or multiple PIs. Initial treatment failures during drug development, associated with the emergence of transmitted resistance or with de novo PI mutations, raised further concerns that long-term treatment outcomes might, in the future, be jeopardized because of the possible emergence of extremely resistant viruses. While once-daily PI dosing might improve patient convenience and enhance adherence and compliance rates, even once-daily dosing was still often perceived as an inconvenience and could affect treatment acceptability. Particularly in certain patient populations, the use of PIs might induce issues of pill burden, lifestyle, food restrictions, or poor taste. Such limitations might also contribute to poor patient adherence and subsequent viral rebound (Mornah et al., 2024). Despite these limitations, some PIs have been particularly life-saving for individuals who have previously experienced failure with less complex regimens.

3.4. Integrase Strand Transfer Inhibitors (INSTIs)

The first licensed INSTI was Raltegravir in 2007 for use in ART-experienced adults with multidrug-resistant HIV-1. Since then, Elvitegravir, Dolutegravir, and

Bictegravir have all been approved. Recent advances in viral genetics have enabled the development of resistance to RAL and the other INSTIs, but it occurs less frequently and with a lower fitness cost than resistance to earlier classes of reverse transcriptase and protease inhibitors. As a result, it is now a standard component of most ART regimens, particularly in treatment-experienced cases. The use of INSTIs is associated with significant improvements in viral load and CD4 count, and thus clinical outcomes (Shi et al., 2024). In virtually all clinical trials comparing INSTIs to NNRTIs or boosting PI-based ART, INSTI-based treatments have demonstrated superior viral load suppression and immune recovery with similar safety profiles. The more robust response is likely attributable to the greater genetic barrier to resistance exhibited by the INSTIs, specifically the ability of the same INSTI-based regimen to maintain suppression in the setting of pretreatment drug resistance, partially treated pediatric infections, and nonadherence, and to be associated with shorter times to achieving viral load suppression among pregnant women (Esra et al., 2024).

3.5. Entry Inhibitors

Entry inhibitors are antiretroviral agents that interfere with the binding, fusion, and entry of HIV to the target cells by targeting the virus after it has attached to the CD4 cells but before it actually infects the cell. The fusion inhibitor enfuvirtide became the first drug in a new class of antiretroviral drugs, the fusion inhibitors. Fusion inhibitors are a type of entry inhibitor that works by preventing virus entry into CD4 cells (Shafik, 2024d). Fusion inhibitors block HIV from combining with the cell membrane and keep the virus from entering the cell. Other entry inhibitors include poorly defined compounds, non-nucleoside reverse transcriptase inhibitors, and nucleoside reverse transcriptase inhibitors (Shimura et al., 2024). Entry inhibitors have shown to be less toxic and better tolerated than other types of ART, probably because they do not interrupt human metabolism. They do not interact with enzymes or molecules of the human body and, therefore, do not have major side effects. Rationally, the lack of cross-resistance between entry inhibitors and the already available drugs makes them very important in overcoming the current epidemic of multidrug-resistant viruses. Clinical investigations showed that viral escape from entry inhibitors might not only be incomplete but also relatively slow, with minor changes in resistance sequences occurring only weeks or even months after the initiation of these new treatment options (Lim et al., 2024). Furthermore, except for enfuvirtide, no known connections have been established between the presence of minority populations of mutant viruses in patients, virological outcomes, and future treatment options. The addition of an entry inhibitor to a so-called "salvage regimen" is very effective and, indeed, could be a reasonable early option in a patient without further alternatives in terms of remaining fully active antiretroviral drugs. However, enfuvirtide has a low genetic barrier; therefore, virological failure was not related to poor compliance. In patients with complete adherence, susceptibility remains stable, while resistance develops at near full adherence (Olaya et al., 2024). With better future drugs, the use of newer entry inhibitors might also lead to a reduction in the rate of antiretroviral drug resistance emergence, as presented in Table 1.

Table 1. Key Antiretroviral Therapy (ART) drugs and their functions

Drug Class	Example Drugs	Mechanism of Action	Common Side Effects	Usage in HIV Treatment	Reference
Nucleoside Reverse Transcriptase Inhibitors (NRTIs)	Zidovudine (AZT), Lamivudine (3TC), Tenofovir (TDF)	Blocks reverse transcriptase enzyme, preventing viral replication	Nausea, headache, kidney toxicity (TDF)	The backbone of most ART regimens	(Board et al., 2024)
Non-Nucleoside Reverse Transcriptase Inhibitors (NNRTIs)	Efavirenz (EFV), Nevirapine (NVP)	Binds directly to reverse transcriptase, inhibiting its function	Dizziness, rash, liver toxicity	Often combined with NRTIs for first-line therapy	(Kileel et al., 2024)
Protease Inhibitors (PIs)	Lopinavir/Ritonavir (LPV/r), Atazanavir (ATV)	Inhibits protease enzyme, preventing maturation of viral proteins	Gastrointestinal issues, metabolic disorders	Used in second-line ART regimens	(Belus et al., 2024)
Integrase Strand Transfer Inhibitors (INSTIs)	Dolutegravir (DTG), Raltegravir (RAL)	Prevents viral DNA from integrating into the host genome	Insomnia, weight gain, headache	Preferred for first-line treatment due to high effectiveness	(Rietveld & Patel, 2024)
Entry Inhibitors	Maraviroc (MVC), Enfuvirtide (T20)	Blocks HIV from entering human cells	Injection site reactions (T20), liver issues	Used for drug-resistant HIV cases	(Dunn Navarra et al., 2024)
Pharmacokinetic Enhancers (Boosters)	Ritonavir (RTV), Cobicistat (COBI)	Enhances the effectiveness of other ART drugs by slowing their metabolism	Drug interactions, nausea, diarrhea	Helps prolong drug action in ART	(Oturu et al., 2024)

continued on following page

Table 1. Continued

Drug Class	Example Drugs	Mechanism of Action	Common Side Effects	Usage in HIV Treatment	Reference
Fixed-Dose Combinations (FDCs)	Tenofovir/Emtricitabine/Efavirenz (TDF/FTC/EFV)	Combines multiple drugs into one pill for easier adherence	Side effects vary based on the components	Improves adherence and simplifies treatment	(Mukuna et al., 2024)
Long-Acting Injectable ART	Cabotegravir/Rilpivirine (CAB/RPV)	Monthly or bimonthly injections replace daily oral ART	Injection site pain, flu-like symptoms	Improves adherence, especially for people struggling with daily pills	(Ayieko et al., 2024)
Pre-Exposure Prophylaxis (PrEP)	Tenofovir/Emtricitabine (TDF/FTC)	Prevents HIV infection in at-risk individuals	Mild nausea, kidney effects (long-term use)	Used for HIV prevention in high-risk populations	(Wiche Salinas et al., 2024)
Post-Exposure Prophylaxis (PEP)	TDF/FTC + Dolutegravir (DTG)	Emergency ART taken within 72 hours of exposure	Fatigue, nausea, headache	Prevents HIV infection after exposure	(Kigongo et al., 2024)
Pediatric ART Formulations	Lopinavir/Ritonavir syrup, Abacavir/Lamivudine	Tailored for children and infants	Taste issues, gastrointestinal problems	Used in HIV-positive infants and children	(Fahad Naim et al., 2024)
HIV Cure Research Drugs	Broadly Neutralizing Antibodies (bNAbs), CRISPR-based therapies	Experimental approaches targeting HIV reservoirs	Unknown side effects (ongoing studies)	Future possibilities for HIV cure	(Kamau et al., 2024)
ART in Pregnancy	Zidovudine (AZT), Dolutegravir (DTG)	Prevents mother-to-child transmission	Nausea, potential neural tube defects (DTG)	Given to HIV-positive pregnant women	(Qayyum et al., 2024)
Second-Line & Salvage Therapies	Darunavir (DRV), Etravirine (ETR)	Used for patients with ART resistance	Drug-specific side effects	For patients failing first-line therapy	(Z. Chen et al., 2024)

4. GLOBAL BURDEN OF HIV/AIDS AND THE ROLE OF ART

The global burden of HIV/AIDS is enormous. An estimated 36 million people have been infected with HIV globally since the pandemic began, and 1.8 million people are expected to die of AIDS in 2007, a quarter of all global mortality at ages

15 to 59. Sub-Saharan Africa has by far the most cases of HIV/AIDS and the largest numbers of people sick and dying from the illness. An estimated two-thirds of the 33 million individuals infected with HIV worldwide reside in Sub-Saharan Africa; more than two-thirds of deaths from AIDS have occurred there as well (Tekle et al., 2024). The overwhelming numbers have led to profound social, economic, and political instability in the hardest-hit countries.

HIV is a retrovirus. For the great majority of patients, the acute initial infection rapidly resolves, and the individual enters an asymptomatic phase lasting years to decades, ultimately progressing to an active, symptomatic illness. Additionally, another subgroup of acutely infected individuals develops prolonged illnesses with immune complications. Antiretroviral therapy specifically targets the HIV lifecycle and works by inhibiting steps of this lifecycle. Ongoing, lifelong therapy is the mainstay of treatment for individuals infected with HIV-1 or HIV-2 (Rietveld & Patel, 2024). Antiretroviral agents, in addition to preventing the clinical progression of the disease, prolong the duration, quality, and ultimately the thickness of patients' lives. Many are capable of suppressing viral replication. This suppression stops the progression of immunodeficiency and prevents clinical disease, including that caused by opportunistic infections. Data from many cohort studies definitively demonstrate the rising range of higher-quality survival with the use of potent regimens (Trickey et al., 2024).

4.1. Viral Load Suppression and CD4 Count Recovery

The immediate goal of ART treatment is suppression of viral replication, as represented by undetectable virus in the bloodstream. Usually, the time it takes ART to suppress the virus follows a pattern where the decrease is rapid for nine days, then gets slower, and the final reduction to an undetectable level can take four months or longer. The rapid phase of virus killing is due to drug-sensitive virus types; after that, some cells are infected with a virus that has become drug-resistant, and more viruses are produced because of that. The third phase has a slower rate of virus production, this time because the population of infected cells is being depleted (Comfort et al., 2024). There is a long tail at the end—these are cells that are long-lived or have become infected late and are, therefore, in a latent phase when it comes to producing viruses. ART also strongly enhances the recovery of CD4+ T-cells. The benefits of ART in this domain are less quick and obvious than its effect on virus suppression, as it usually takes six months or a year before the level of CD4+ cells with ART is reliably high compared to the period before treatment was initiated. Furthermore, the cell count usually does not return to the level of individuals who are not infected: the difference with the count in uninfected individuals is called 'immunodeficiency.' (Mahlalela et al., 2024). Since the initial time is taken to develop a working immune response, the later incomplete recovery can, somewhat confusingly, be referred to as an 'immune restoration deficit.'

4.2. Reduction of Opportunistic Infections and AIDS-related Deaths

A well-documented benefit of ART use is its effect on reducing opportunistic infections and human immunodeficiency virus-related deaths. ART restores normal immune function in an HIV-infected patient and results in a reduction in viral load. A substantial and rapid decline in HIV viral load occurs in most patients initiating ART, but does not lead to rapid symptomatic improvement or significantly decrease the rate of opportunistic infections until a longer period after initiation. Almost all antiretroviral drugs are potent inhibitors of HIV (Naranjo et al., 2024). The structured treatment interruption study demonstrated that discontinuation of ART increased the risk of opportunistic infections and reinforced the importance of long-term suppression of HIV replication for reducing these events. There are different findings on the timing of the most significant decrease in the risk of opportunistic infections. Initiating ART at higher CD4 counts appears to decrease the risk of opportunistic infections and AIDS-related illness or death. Data from large clinical studies and emerging data from observational studies of ART experience in the clinic demonstrate the positive association between CD4 cell count recovery and the subsequent decrease in the risk of opportunistic infections and mortality (Antoine et al., 2024). Data on liver-related deaths of HIV/HBV coinfected patients suggest that ART improves the prognosis of both HIV mono-infection and coinfection.

4.3. Impact on Quality of Life and Longevity

Quality of life and longevity were expected to increase as a result of people with HIV living healthier lives by controlling the development of AIDS and preventing other illnesses related to immune suppression. Indeed, many studies reported significant improvement in perceived physical health and mental health relatively quickly after the initiation of ART. A recent comprehensive review of health-related quality-of-life outcome studies, however, shows that increases in quality of life are less noticeable over time, and some of the increase might be attributed to practice effects. Data on the impacts of ART on longevity also show mixed results (Trickey et al., 2024). Studies done among resource-rich people with HIV indicate dramatic decreases in AIDS-related deaths after the widespread availability of ART but increases in non-HIV-related mortality rates. The recent increase in non-HIV-related comorbid diseases has been particularly dramatic. In general, people on ART are still at greater risk of dying than the general population, and the gap might be widening. In comparison, people in developing countries, particularly in low-income countries, have made impressive strides in increasing longevity since ART became available, thanks to a network of local continuous care programs that emerged to manage the complexities of ART (Sheira et al., 2024).

5. CLINICAL GUIDELINES FOR INITIATING ART

In the first decade that ART was available, concern over adherence and development of resistance meant that patients were initiated on therapy when their CD4 cell counts were falling and when they had reached a severe immunodeficiency (defined, at that time, as a CD4 cell count less than 200/mm3). It quickly became apparent that other conditions responded well to earlier initiation of ART. Realization of this potential benefit was in part due, no doubt, to the success of other routinely undertaken treatment strategies requiring immediate or near immediate treatment (Mornah et al., 2024). For these reasons, HIV treatment guidelines have evolved so that, nowadays, initiation of ART is not driven solely by the progressive decline in CD4 cell count. In addition to the progressive loss of immune function, there are occasions when ART is initiated specifically because of concerns about adherence and missed doses. These depend on prescribing guidelines that provide a combination of fixed-dose or co-formulated regimens. Reduced pill numbers are obviously of benefit when compared with polypharmacy. When taking 20 or 30 pills a day, multiple times a day, tens of tablets and capsules may be taken for one HIV infection (Dunn Navarra et al., 2024). Finally, current ART guidelines ensure that vertical transmission should become a rare event due to nutrition, safe surroundings, and lack of viral suppression.

5.1. Adherence to ART

Good adherence to ART is critical to the success of an ART program, as ART prevents HIV-related clinical progression and death, suppresses viremia, and contains the epidemic. ART encourages HIV testing and risk reduction, such as condom use. A robust body of literature has reported an association between greater adherence to ART and reduced AIDS-defining illnesses, hospitalizations, mortality, and other HIV disease progression states. In addition, effective viremia suppression among ART-experienced individuals who are no longer acutely infected could be considered an indirect benefit of ART for HIV prevention (Mukuna et al., 2024). It is expected that ART adherence directly influences virologic suppression as well as the intended protection provided by treatment as prevention to a similar degree for most people who achieve sustained plasma viremia below certain detection thresholds of clinical relevance. Adherence is typically defined either as the percentage of medication that is taken as prescribed, in which patients are instructed to miss doses—because they may be toxic, do not effectively contribute to future treatment success, or are not of interest to the intended virologic suppression objective—or as the percentage of prescribed doses that are self-reported or electronically recorded as being taken (Kamau et al., 2024). A common assumption is that ART adherence will be high enough to suppress viremia with several hundred copies/mL using less treatment than the patient actually receives since sustained virologic suppression generally occurs with 85%-95% adherence. Despite the wide array of factors that influence ART adherence, the manner in which these factors affect adherence is less clear. For example, the long-term impact of the cost of ART to individuals and households on ART adherence is not well understood. Furthermore, the relationship between individual adherence and sociodemographic factors, adherence rates, and virologic suppression is complex and subject to methodological challenges, not to mention ongoing controversies and disagreements (Qayyum et al., 2024). Although individual adherence counseling before starting ART is recommended, the best way to promote ART adherence longitudinally and to optimize long-term adherence in scenarios where the costs to patients of ART—whether out-of-pocket or as part of the pursuit of extra-ART health—become burdensome is unclear and remains to be evaluated.

5.2. Factors Influencing Adherence

Medication adherence is an essential factor for successful treatment with ART, and poor adherence is known to be one of the factors influencing unsuppressed viral load and viral resistance in people living with HIV on ART. Several studies have shown that optimal adherence to ART led to continuous HIV replication suppression, which in turn had positive impacts on CD4 cell reconstitution and the long-term clinical improvement of people living with HIV on ART. Factors influencing ART adherence were mainly grouped into three categories: socio-demographic factors, psychosocial factors, and health system or treatment-related factors (Quaker et al., 2024). In some studies, adherence remained poor because of unfriendly treatment facilities, low self-motivation for continuing to take antiretroviral medications, alcohol use, and lack of support from family, close relations, and friends. Socio-demographic factors were seen to include sex, age, race or ethnicity, old age, educational level, financial hardship, insurance, socioeconomic status, and employment status. The psychosocial factors included stigma or discrimination that arose as concern or fear among people living with HIV that those without HIV infection would have negative attitudes or discriminatory practices based on the illness, depression, mental stress, low perceived treatment self-efficacy, low social support, behavioral attitude, low self-efficacy to strict medication adherence, and low resilience (Ayiigah et al.,

2024). The characteristics of the health system or treatment-related factors consist of acceptance of person-centered care, which is to provide more care to people living with HIV receiving treatment with ART, physical and counseling support assistance, cultural beliefs, directly observed treatment, regimen type, the complexity of the treatment regimen, pill burden per day, anxiety over medications, drug side effects or intolerance, the interaction between food and the drugs, other drug or alcohol addiction, concomitant mental illness or severe disease, and certain regimens that are associated with neuropathy, which are seen to be barriers to adherence, as presented in Table 2 (Comfort et al., 2024; Tun et al., 2024).

Table 2. Strategies for effective implementation of Antiretroviral Therapy (ART)

Strategy	Description	Implementation Approach	Impact on HIV Management	Challenges	Reference
Universal Access to ART	Ensuring ART is available for all HIV patients	Free or subsidized ART programs	Reduces HIV-related deaths & Transmission	High cost in resource-limited settings	(Ayiigah et al., 2024)
Adherence Support Programs	Encouraging consistent ART use	Counseling, digital reminders, support groups	Improves viral suppression rates	Stigma & pill fatigue affect adherence	(Esra et al., 2024; Kanise et al., 2024; Shimura et al., 2024)
Task-Shifting & Decentralization	Training non-specialists to deliver ART	Community health workers, nurse-led ART clinics	Expands ART coverage, especially in rural areas	Quality control & staff training limitations	(Comfort et al., 2024)
Integration with Primary Healthcare	Incorporating ART into general healthcare	HIV treatment offered at primary care centers	Reduces stigma, improves access	Requires policy and system adjustments	(Fahad Naim et al., 2024; Tun et al., 2024)
Long-Acting Injectable ART	Reducing pill burden with injections	Monthly or bi-monthly ART injections	Increases adherence & convenience	Cost & availability of injectable drugs	(Mahlalela et al., 2024)
Digital Health Solutions	Using mobile apps, AI, & telemedicine for ART monitoring	Mobile reminders, AI-driven adherence tracking	Enhances patient engagement & support	Digital divide & literacy challenges	(Moya et al., 2024)
HIV Drug Resistance Monitoring	Detecting resistance to optimize ART regimens	Routine viral load & resistance testing	Ensures effective treatment & prevents treatment failure	High cost of resistance testing	(OG, 2024)

continued on following page

Table 2. Continued

Strategy	Description	Implementation Approach	Impact on HIV Management	Challenges	Reference
ART for Key Populations	Tailoring ART for high-risk groups	Special programs for sex workers, MSM, drug users	Improves coverage & reduces new infections	Social stigma & legal barriers	(Saltini et al., 2024)
Mother-to-Child Transmission Prevention (PMTCT)	Ensuring HIV-positive mothers receive ART	ART during pregnancy & breastfeeding	Reduces perinatal HIV transmission	Adherence challenges in pregnancy	(Fassinou et al., 2024)
PrEP & PEP Expansion	Increasing access to preventive ART	Wider distribution & awareness campaigns	Prevents new infections in at-risk individuals	Awareness & uptake remain low	(Wagner et al., 2024)
Community-Based ART Distribution	Providing ART outside traditional clinics	ART refills at pharmacies, community centers	Improves convenience & adherence	Supply chain & regulatory challenges	(C. Chen et al., 2024)
HIV and Non-Communicable Disease (NCD) Integration	Treating HIV alongside conditions like diabetes & hypertension	Comprehensive health programs	Improves overall patient health	Requires additional healthcare resources	(Antoine et al., 2024; Sheira et al., 2024)
Innovative ART Formulations	Developing better drug formulations	Long-acting drugs, pediatric-friendly ART	Improves treatment accessibility	Regulatory approval processes	(Olaya et al., 2024)
HIV Cure Research & Trials	Exploring new HIV eradication approaches	Gene editing, bNAbs, immune-based strategies	Potential long-term cure	Ethical & scientific challenges	(Ayieko et al., 2024; Kileel et al., 2024)

6. DRUG RESISTANCE AND ART FAILURE

The development of drug-resistant variants in a patient on therapy is a reliable sign that HIV has been replicating despite the fact that these patients are clinically stable and their CD4 count may even be increasing. These findings are in contrast to more recent data showing that drug resistance can occur in persons who maintain consistent levels of detectable viral replication, either due to lack of potency of suppression of therapy or to suboptimal adherence to the regimen (Tekle et al., 2024). It has been shown that when antiretroviral regimens are not maintained, a large amount of HIV that is drug-sensitive is released into the blood, and clinically apparent virologic failure ensues. Impaired immune function permits de novo replication of HIV that needs to survive in the presence of potent antiretrovirals, and the net result is the growth of resistant virus (Shafik, 2025b). Commercial viral load assays are only sensitive enough to detect the level of viral load in patients who begin therapy with fewer than 50 copies of detectable plasma HIV. In clinical trials, individuals who fall below the sensitive limit of detection have been demonstrated to have much higher levels of 2-LTR-containing circles than individuals who fail to pass this test (Dunn Navarra et al., 2024). If potent drug therapy exerts an antiviral effect of substantial duration, it would be more likely to become transiently detectable if replication surged while the patient was not taking the medications.

6.1. Impact of ART on HIV Transmission

The results indicate that the annual number of new HIV infections has been decreasing globally since approximately 1996. The decline reflects the number of deaths from HIV infection and AIDS, which started leveling off mainly as a result of increasing access to ART worldwide. The decline in incidence was greater when the prevalence of HIV/AIDS was lower and more rapidly declining. The decrease in incidence can act as a positive feedback mechanism that further reduces the number of new infections and deaths, or the development of numerous co-morbidities provides a limiting mechanism (Oturu et al., 2024). If one assumes that individuals with acute and chronic HIV infection who received ART are not infectious, then a gene therapy approach to convert the entire infected population to this state would be to end the epidemic. Will these results suggest that decreases in the number of new worldwide infections beginning in approximately 1996 are due to increased use of drugs that decrease transmission as a byproduct of their use by those infected and, in fact, non-infectious? Surprisingly, this effect, if real and indicative of such a feedback process, has not been publicly noted (Ayieko et al., 2024).

However, there has also been a potential increase in the risk of HIV transmission in the presence of ART. This can occur if the death rate after HIV transmission is primarily due to co-morbidities, delayed initiation of ART owing to denial of the possibility of HIV infection, stigma, lack of health insurance, or otherwise lack of access to ART. In part, these individuals may not link to or remain in care, fail to follow recommendations regarding preventive efforts, and have viral load levels above the threshold used in some other analyses to define "suppression" considered between 2 and 4 times viral load levels. They then become the communities where the disease remains active and fosters new infections. This was a concern in previous studies (Wiche Salinas et al., 2024). Using the epidemiological theorem of mass action, it was noted that the annual proportional decrease in HIV incidence would be necessary to offset the relative increase in risk. This is dependent on the degree of compensating behavior, the percentage of individuals receiving ART, and the degree to which individual sexual behaviors are not already biologically set. They concluded that this was not likely a major factor for why the incidence of HIV infection did not decline after the availability of treatment. More recently, concerns and a lack of meta-analyses regarding these types of studies have been pointed out. For instance, assumptions made for the calculation of the percentage of secondary transmissions that would be avoided if the index subject is under ART do not consider different subtypes of HIV (Kigongo et al., 2024). Nonetheless, an expert panel from a working group session came to a consensus that there is indeed no evidence that ART increases the rate of HIV transmission.

6.2. Prevention of Mother-to-Child Transmission (PMTCT)

PMTCT[8] involves stopping the transmission of HIV from an HIV-positive woman to her child during pregnancy, labor, delivery, or breastfeeding. The goal of PMTCT is to prevent HIV infection in newborns and to keep mothers alive throughout their lives. The strategies under PMTCT have shifted from one focusing primarily on reducing the risk of HIV transmission at the time of delivery to one that reinforces preconception care when targeted at women of childbearing potential (Quaker et al., 2024). The benefits of effective PMTCT go beyond the individual and family level and result in healthier lives for children and the population at large. Despite substantial progress in its implementation, preventing mother-to-child transmission of HIV remains a challenge throughout the world, especially in Sub-Saharan Africa. The number of HIV-infected pregnant women is increasing, yet half of their infants who are exposed to HIV receive mother-to-child preventive treatment. If no preventive treatment is administered, 15-30 percent of babies born to HIV-positive mothers will become infected during pregnancy and labor (Dunn Navarra et al., 2024). If the infants are allowed to breastfeed, these statistics significantly increase.

7. ART IN SPECIAL POPULATIONS

The use of ART for patients who meet the current criteria is similar regardless of pregnancy. A recent study has suggested that treatment with a protease inhibitor-based regimen is not associated with an increased risk of preterm birth or low birth weight infants when compared to the use of a non-nucleoside reverse transcriptase inhibitor-based regimen. There does not appear to be an increased risk of perinatal transmission if a protease inhibitor is used as therapy or if pregnant women elect to use ZDV or ZDV and 3TC. ART should be considered in all pregnant women who meet the current criteria, as the benefits of therapy certainly outweigh the potential risks to the infant. Women who do not require therapy for their health should consider therapy to reduce the risk of transmitting HIV to their fetus (Wiche Salinas et al., 2024). Both ZDV and nevirapine are widely available and have been used to prevent perinatal transmission.

The risk of disease progression and transmission is lower with the use of a fully active antiviral regimen. Women who cannot receive ZDV due to ZDV resistance should have their risk of perinatal transmission addressed and be treated with the most effective agent available to them. Women who decline therapy for their health should be referred for discussion about therapy to prevent perinatal transmission. Because of the increased risks of hepatic disease, ribavirin should not be prescribed and this can be supported by women in technology (Shafik, 2024b). Women with advanced disease should continue with their existing ART regimen throughout pregnancy. Women electing antiretroviral therapy during pregnancy should usually receive a regimen including a boosted protease inhibitor. Women who do not require treatment during pregnancy should receive counseling and be educated about the early signs of acute retroviral syndrome at delivery (Fahad Naim et al., 2024). If she believes that she may put her child at significant risk for acquiring HIV infection, she should be admitted to the hospital for her care, not just the care of the child.

7.1. Pediatric HIV Patients

Pediatric treatment with antiretroviral therapy (ART) has been available for 20 years now, and the world over 1 million HIV-infected and affected children are actively in care. As successes in adult treatment have helped us understand the trajectory of the disease better, improvements have helped us understand what to change in pediatric regimens from current pediatric treatment regimens. With the increase in the number of children receiving first-line treatment, we have seen increased resistance and tolerance, and side effects have shown that children initiated on a protease inhibitor (PI)-based regimen have faster decreases in viral load than those initiated on a non-nucleoside reverse transcriptase inhibitor-based regimen (Tekle et al., 2024). After 8 months, over 50% of the non-nucleoside reverse transcriptase inhibitor (NNRTI)-based regimen were undetectable, compared to 34.9% of the PI-based regimen. The endpoint of not being able to achieve virologic suppression on second-line and third-line regimens increases with longer times on suppression. HIV-infected infants began early ART in various studies that have generated extensive data on the impact of early ART on maintaining a treatment-free cycle or tissue reservoirs, providing significant impetus to starting treatment as soon after diagnosis as possible (Comfort et al., 2024).

7.2. Pregnant Women

The initial demonstration that a strategy of short-course ZDV could significantly reduce mother-to-child transmission of HIV was the starting point of a myriad of trials and implementation efforts to reduce this mode of transmission of HIV. It was recognized early that women who were not pregnant would similarly require ART. So now, there is a four-pronged approach to addressing the prevention of mother-to-child transmission of HIV: primary HIV prevention, which includes the provision of family planning for those who wish, prevention of HIV among women already infected (and men), prevention of unplanned pregnancies for those who are infected, and antiretroviral prophylaxis or ART for women on antiretrovirals for their health, during and after pregnancy (Konishi et al., 2024). For women who are not currently taking ART for their health, it is best to initiate ART for their health and continue after delivery. However, the latter instructions are difficult to convey. One prevention study closed early because it was unethical to continue without providing a known intervention that was effective for all women in the study. Numerous ART initiation scenarios have been used successfully so far. The optimal approach was that only women who remain healthy should be included in the prevention of mother-to-child transmission studies; ART is reserved for those who are immunosuppressed (Gupta et al., 2024). If immunosuppression is the criterion for initiation of ART, then the prevention of mother-to-child transmission program has been modified.

7.3. Key Populations

Key populations, such as men who have sex with men, sex workers, and people who inject drugs, are also at elevated risk for acquiring HIV, and their participation in HIV prevention, care, and treatment programs is usually low. However, several studies have shown that key populations have high adherence rates when they are in care and on antiretroviral treatment. Because they participate less than others in services, interventions that target key populations must often be specifically designed to attract and retain them (Shafik, 2024a). The high incidence of key populations increases the chances that drug resistance will emerge and potentially evolve. Drug resistance is not just one additional factor promoting treatment failure; it also has broader implications for the individual, community, and clinical management. In places with low baseline prevalence of drug resistance, treatment failure associated with drug resistance is rare, but drug resistance could be rapidly amplified in the community if people infected with such viruses pass them on to others (Saltini et al., 2024). This rapid amplification leaves few choices for the clinic when choosing effective second-line and future lines of treatment.

7.4. Cost-Effectiveness of ART

In high-income countries, once governments find effective drugs for a particular disease, the public health community could move on to research how to pay for the medications. For some diseases, the postage stamp analogy holds: it costs the same to send a letter from one city to another as it does to send a letter from a different city to a distant country. As people in various locations can all obtain essentially the same medical services and medications, the government subsidizes mail delivery for everyone within the entire country. However, other medical technologies are necessarily expensive at the start because they require the long and demanding stretches of human resources and facilities involved in proving that a cocktail of antiretrovirals can help many sick people live (Fassinou et al., 2024). Postage stamp pricing is inappropriate when drug prices cover both partial recoveries of upfront research expenditures and partial repayment to investors bankrolling the next round of drug development. In some ways, the global pandemic and academic disagreements over the cost of ART have forced a series of difficult financial confrontations: between underprivileged people who need ART, between governments unwilling to pay for ART, concerned about the high cost of these drugs, and between private drug companies interested in public welfare after a reasonable profit. The annual cost of ART ranges from a certain amount per year per client in one region up to a higher amount per client in another region. However, these prices cover not only the drugs themselves but also the physical examinations, specialized public services, and social work to ensure that drugs are properly administered (Corona et al., 2024). These costs need to be compared to the future value of the contribution that these clients can make if they stay healthy in the future.

8. CHALLENGES AND FUTURE DIRECTIONS IN ART RESEARCH

Many challenges remain in strengthening managerial and service delivery capacity in developing countries, which are essential for meeting ambitious treatment and adherence goals. For example, a number of large ART programs in both governmental and non-governmental sectors in resource-limited settings report considerable program attrition after initiating cART predominantly in the first three months of treatment. Delays in cART initiation may result in the death of patients before they are eligible for cART initiation, as well as an increased risk of transmitting HIV to spouses and offspring. Longitudinal data collection and the careful scientific exploration of the reasons for cART initiation and subsequent treatment result in a more comprehensive understanding of the clinical and psychosocial dynamics associated with the formal cART initiation decision (Antoine et al., 2024). The role of ART and its broad and immediate expansion in terms of public health goals is not necessarily the single most important issue in the overall response to the HIV epidemic. There is emerging consensus that long-term adherence is a fundamental concern for the successful treatment of chronic diseases, regardless of loss to follow-up or side effects due to cART. Uniform data collection, treatment interventions, and behavioral research studies that increase cART use by patients with AIDS or comorbid conditions, physical or interpersonal cART barriers, and treatment outcomes may improve the generalization of study findings, increase efficiency, and reduce individual risk (Sheira et al., 2024). With an increasing recognition of the interplay and risk of TB and HIV, we must better understand the context and effect of involvement in TB care on adherence.

8.1. Novel Drug Development

Despite the tremendous success of antiretroviral therapy in treating HIV infection, the search for better treatments and HIV cures continues, largely due to challenges related to toxicity, lifelong treatment, and the substantial cost of treatment. A total of twelve antiretroviral drugs that are used in the treatment of HIV infection have been approved. All of these drugs were based on one of the nine relatively older classes of antiretroviral drugs already approved, representing a new era of novel drug development for HIV therapy. There has been a concerted effort to continue to explore new compounds with novel mechanisms of action for anti-HIV activity. Most of them are licensed for treatment, but several are at the stage of regulatory review or in clinical development (Shi et al., 2024). There are a number of other classes of antiretroviral drugs that are in the earlier stages of development. Because of the complexity of linkages between manufacturers, governments, academic institutions, and advocacy groups involved in the development of antiretroviral drugs, pricing and access to these novel agents is a defining characteristic of the list. The risk of development and approval of a novel antiretroviral drug continues to be important in driving the search for HIV cure strategies. The success of antiretroviral therapy has also spurred interest in and support for the treatment of other complex viral infections, such as HBV, HCV, herpesviruses including CMV and herpes simplex virus, and HPV. Prominent similarities and important differences between drug development initiatives are evident (Board et al., 2024). How these and other novel agents in various stages of preclinical or clinical development address key challenges associated with antiretroviral therapy is explored below.

8.2. Long-Acting ART Formulations

Novel, long-acting antiretroviral therapy formulations represent a recently developed alternative to daily pill-taking for ARV treatment across the HIV care continuum beyond ART initiation, including PrEP and treatment for opportunistic infections. LATTMs offer individuals the prospect of shorter intervals between medication administrations and require healthcare visits that may be less frequent than for currently available ART dosing strategies by virtue of their long-acting pharmacokinetic profiles (Oturu et al., 2024). They may be of particular interest as a strategy to support second-line, third-line, and rescue ART options for individuals for whom ART incompatibility or toxicity is experienced. It is anticipated that realizing the promise of LATTM for supporting the HIV cascade of care efficiency and, indeed, in some cases, rendering HIV services invisible or absent and failure-prone ART excursions will require negotiation of distribution, confidentiality, and informed dispensing considerations not usually encountered in the sexually transmitted/women's health and/or trans-medical sector (Ayieko et al., 2024).

8.3. Drug Resistance and Viral Rebound

Antiretroviral drug resistance is a major challenge for national treatment programs both in developed countries and in resource-poor settings. Failures of first-line antiretroviral drug regimens occur more rapidly and to a higher degree in patients who are not adherent than in those who are adherent. Current guidelines are aimed at improving adherence by measuring it through pharmacy records, pill counts, self-reporting, and electronic drug monitoring, and then by improving adherence support programs. The high degree of virologic failure due to these adherence issues raises the question of whether viral rebound after therapy interruption is clinically significant and beneficial. This expands the time of first-line regimen durability by reserving first-line drugs and adherent patients from the rebound virus (Qayyum et al., 2024). On an individual patient and group level, the potential alternate sequence, cost savings, long-term treatment group, public health efficacy, and relative benefits of this strategy can then be evaluated. Viral load increases to detectable, measurable levels within three to sixteen days following withdrawal of antiretroviral therapy due to the exponential increase in the production of the virus by the rapid appearance of drug-resistant strains of HIV. This viral rebound, at least experimentally, does not appear to be dangerous; in certain studies, viral rebound following the rapid withdrawal of antiretroviral drugs was neither associated with clear clinical disease nor was there a significant difference in rebound viremia values compared with untreated controls. In these potent antiretroviral drug-based studies, drug resistance, the frequency of drug resistance mutations, maximal viral load reached, time to maximal viral load, or clinical pathologic benchmarks, although transient viremia occurred in the first controlled infections more rapidly than in acute infection (Olaya et al., 2024). Today's potent antiretroviral regimens are expected to generate similar rebound environments. Chances are.

8.4. Stigma and Discrimination

Stigma is a significant barrier to accessing treatment and influences treatment engagement, adherence, and retention once in care. People living with HIV/AIDS are often shunned and discriminated against, especially if their HIV status isn't kept confidential. A study of people living with HIV shows that more than half of the respondents had disclosed their status to at least one person who then broke that confidence. The most commonly cited reason for non-disclosure was fear of being stigmatized, and a portion of those who had disclosed their status were treated differently, while some suffered direct discrimination, for example, being dismissed from employment and evicted from their homes (Sheira et al., 2024). This shows that although expanding access to ART is necessary for improving the health of people living with HIV, it must be accompanied by additional programs to reduce stigma and encourage disclosure.

Stigmatization is one of the most important issues affecting the quality of life of patients with HIV. A significant percentage of American adults agree that people with HIV are being punished for their unethical lifestyles, which are assumed to have led to the disease, while the majority did not agree with this statement in the past. Chosen examples of people living with HIV stigma content themes were historical and current discourses on communities and individual responsibility to create physical and mental distance. Social avoidance was also a theme often drawn on in the stigmatization of people living with HIV/AIDS, and the proposed mechanisms for such avoidance were regular discourse on the majority's disease responsibilities, too positive, negative dissidence to distancing, fear of contracting the disease, the perceived high value of good health, and the consequences of the diagnosis (Fassinou et al., 2024). With that in line with the fact that HIV-positive individuals must be recognized for who they are rather than as disgracefully contagious patients, this is not an object of social abandonment; disease linked to homosexuality and addiction to drugs can be addressed.

8.5. Access to Healthcare Services

Persons living with HIV/AIDS usually visit healthcare facilities for drug collection and adherence counseling because of the free ART they receive. This routine access to ART services often offers healthcare workers a good opportunity to interact with the patients. Through interactions with patients, service providers are able to collect data on adherence and other variables since the collection of such data is likely to help healthcare workers fully understand the patients' behaviors and address problems and identify potential causes of patients' non-adherence to treatment (Naranjo et al., 2024). Healthcare workers may also decide to provide additional care and support to clients since the health of the patients provides information on the efficacy of the drug or the progress of the disease. Thus, the healthcare facilities offer a unique setting to work with these patients. The close interaction with patients also enables healthcare workers to address issues of dissatisfaction that could have been leading to clients' poor treatment adherence and program dropout (Comfort et al., 2024).

9. ECONOMIC AND SOCIETAL IMPACT OF ART

ART use had a positive relationship with patient wages and earnings in most studies, even after adjusting for ART proxies such as good health and no household dependency. LTCU spending on ART for one patient decreases the LTCU healthcare spending on treating opportunistic infections or other HIV-related conditions. The size of the savings depends on ART efficacy in reversing immune suppression, patient survival, and opportunistic infection treatment costs. Invest in aggressive expansion of quality ART provision to minimize LTCU spending. However, current high ART prices are a potential barrier to achieving this optimal situation. Furthermore, once a patient starts ART, he or she will remain on that particular drug regimen for the rest of his or her life to prevent drug resistance (Sadiq et al., 2024). ART failure means that a patient has to switch to a second or third-line regimen, which is relatively more expensive and less efficacious. Original private and public sector healthcare worker exit rates are high due to illness and death in the LTCU epidemic. Personnel delays in replacing exiting workers result in low LTCU productivity, which is the ratio of output to resource input. To grow the national ART program, recruit more workers to maintain and raise productivity. Import workers if the local workforce in the public and NPO sectors cannot meet these needs fast enough. Refrain from national-scale ART program implementation if the complementary labor force is exhausted and international nurses are not interested in low-skilled, high-demand hospital and LTCU jobs. If a national ART program is planned or running, redirect scarce LTCU human resources from high to highest value, as measured by survival and productivity (Njuba et al., 2024). Current personnel training remains the supply versus demand challenge and should be underpinned by human resources forecasting data.

9.1. Cost-effectiveness of ART Programs

Health care resources are limited in every country, and it is crucial to be able to estimate the costs and benefits of different health care programs to determine how to allocate scarce resources most effectively. In some developing countries affected by HIV/AIDS, the public health perspective will not always call for the government to support the broad scale-up of ART for everyone who needs it, because resources sometimes could be more efficiently directed to other health interventions targeting different conditions that account for a larger share of the disease burden (Gatechompol et al., 2024). However, if ART becomes widely available in these countries, this information will become highly relevant for policymakers at all levels, especially in determining where resources should be targeted, as well as providing assistance with decisions related to health technology assessment. Epidemiological and economic models together can be extremely valuable to present an analytical framework for assisting policymakers in determining the possible effects of interventions that may only occur in the future and under certain conditions. For this reason, results from an epidemiological and economic model have been used to develop a cost-effectiveness tool for public health decision-makers in order to give an indication of the relative cost-effectiveness of treatment, prevention, and care approaches for HIV management. Of course, this tool should be used in conjunction with other standard economic evaluation methods, as well as with important non-economic criteria, such as ethical, institutional, and human rights factors, in order to make decisions about the deployment of resources (C. Chen et al., 2024).

9.2. Workforce Productivity and Economic Development

Antiretroviral therapy has the potential to increase workforce productivity directly by improving the health of HIV-infected people who work and indirectly by reducing the incidence of HIV infection and HIV-related illness. These effects can influence individual performance by reducing absenteeism and presenteeism, or reduced ability to function effectively at work. By improving the labor supply and earnings of HIV-infected workers and by helping to operate businesses with a healthy workforce, antiretroviral therapy can have profound implications for local, national, and international commercial and industrial activities and economic prosperity (Nursalam et al., 2024). Prevention of HIV infection and the provision of comprehensive support for HIV-infected individuals will greatly reinforce the benefits that people will experience from antiretroviral therapy. Legislation and policy measures have been put in place in some countries to protect workers against the risk of human immunodeficiency virus infection, HIV-related illness, and acquired immunodeficiency syndrome. In some countries affected by HIV/

AIDS, HIV infection and/or AIDS have brought about a significant reduction in workforce productivity, devastated human development indices, derailed macro-economic policies, and contributed to economic stagnation. However, while most African countries and development partners have established HIV/AIDS policies, only a few have HIV-specific laws and regulations (Shimura et al., 2024). These have not been effectively enforced in some settings, despite persistent lobbying and advocacy by labor unions, and workers in both the formal and informal sectors still face work-related stigma and discrimination.

9.3. Social Cohesion and Community Empowerment

A theory of empowerment states that when people who belong to the same social group experience a common predicament such as sickness and they join together and mobilize their collective resources, they are in a better position to exert power and control over the environment in which they live. Several aspects of HIV-related stigma reduction by ART influenced the outcome associated with ART. We found sharing the drug with non-family members to be no predictor of the outcome either. Consistent and comprehensive health education about HIV before their initiation into the treatment galvanized them into reflecting on the relative meaning of HIV (Gatechompol et al., 2024). Such reflection also enhanced what kind of relations could improve their HIV treatment outcome. A structural support package inclusive of but not limited to food and education about ART is an important norm in many sub-Saharan African settings. It legitimizes the efforts of patients to adhere to their ART to achieve high treatment outcomes. To get the support package, they have to make regular visits to the health facilities where the personnel monitor their health status. The comprehensive health check and counseling they received from the healthcare personnel during the visits stimulated the recipients of the ART to encourage their supporters to screen and treat if infected for diseases that had been dominating them for years. Furthermore, evidence has shown that introducing electronic reminders into the patients as an adjunct to their counseling and treatment package was also empowering to the health and good outcome of patients on ART (Corona et al., 2024). But to ease the load and make efficient and targeted healthcare interventions based on the compliance therapy care model, many proposed using community health workers.

10. FUTURE DIRECTIONS AND RESEARCH PRIORITIES

Clinical studies show that HIV treatment outcomes, particularly adherence to HIV therapy, are better today than at the time that clinical therapy trials were initially completed. These overall improvements do not necessarily occur for all individuals. Community-specific interventions, particularly those built upon local understandings, seem to be key factors in continually improving our successes in HIV therapy. As access to antiretrovirals continues to grow and therapy becomes simpler, less toxic, and more powerful, combination ART will likely continue to improve the quality of life of people living with HIV. Future clinical therapeutic research should continue to focus on the basic science underlying ART, with the primary goal of improving our understanding of the long-term side effects of ART (Hernandez et al., 2024). Clinical trials using endpoints that include long-term morbidity and quality of life and which evaluate new potent regimens continue to be needed. New drugs and fixed-dose regimens tailored for use in resource-poor countries will also need to be developed. Therapeutics based on recent advances in the understanding of the potential for eradication of ongoing residual viral replication would put many resource-poor countries on an equal footing with resource-rich countries (Saltini et al., 2024). Finally, immunomodulatory strategies are a promising therapeutic approach.

10.1. Novel Drug Targets and Therapeutic Strategies

The arrival of antiretroviral therapy (ART) reduced mortality from human immunodeficiency virus (HIV-1) and enabled chronic management of the disease. Currently available drugs target virus-encoded proteins. Although these drugs have kept viral levels low, problems with resistance and side effects are evident. Collaboratively used with novel drug strategies and combinatory therapies, ART will minimize these problems. Here, we explore promising new drug targets and strategies. Viral strategies have their benefits in that they would have no host cell interactions as they target virus or cell selectivity and reach high local concentrations in the host cell (Trickey et al., 2024). These strategies efficiently block viral protein interactions and enzymatic functions that are highly conserved. It is unlikely that HIV itself could develop resistance to these viral strategies. Cellular targets to limit virus infection signal transduction pathways are known to be associated with host cell defense mechanisms against the virus. Some proteins present in the host cell facilitate the virus's own replication. Virus-induced inhibitors on immune protection pathways may appeal to promising therapeutic targets. HIV stimulates the production and function of the corresponding controller protein; targeting these with specific protein inhibitors is a promising new approach for anti-HIV therapy. Vaccine strategies to prevent initial HIV-1 infection during the initial viral phase, particularly as eradication therapy (Shi et al., 2024). The virus presents the therapeutic effects of complementary virus proteins currently developed up to a time when they might offer a standalone HIV-1 treatment for a specific subset of HIV-1 patients.

10.2. Integration of ART into Primary Healthcare Systems

Integration of ART into primary healthcare has been a landmark in the development of health services that support chronic care. Recognizing that HIV is a chronic disease enabled the development of coordinated and comprehensive forms of care that increase treatment adherence and improve the health of individuals living with HIV. Clinical services in Cambodia, Vietnam, and Guatemala treated over 20,000 individuals living with HIV in health districts via a combination of ARV therapy, community outreach, laboratory monitoring, and on-site PH support (Lim et al., 2024). Treatment was provided to the majority of patients in rural or hard-to-reach urban areas, with 100% of most patients retained on treatment, and less than 1% reported dead, while fully virally suppressed patients decreased from 50% at 6 months to just over 40% at 36 months due to low retention and adherence to treatment. An evaluation in South Africa found that once the community had been educated and a treatment program established, most patients would attend the clinic regularly, bring their children for HIV testing, and be compliant with drug regimens. Treatment outcomes appear to be driven by the strength of the healthcare system and the interaction between community lay workers, outreach facility networks, and laboratory infrastructure (Board et al., 2024). Similarly, a randomized controlled trial in Uganda, where two-thirds of patients received their therapy at the on-site PHC clinic and one-third were referred to an off-site HIV facility, found that programs that linked the identification and treatment of HIV to existing healthcare systems were more cost-effective. After 18 months of follow-up, the mortality for those in care at the new facility was almost half that of those receiving treatment from the on-site clinic. Integration of care within communities is important as they face local social pressures and low mobility, making it difficult for patients to travel to a centralized facility. At the same time, retention in decentralized programs is worse than in centralized programs. Activities that support engagement include a testing environment that respects confidentiality, education on health awareness, social care, the provision of a safe environment at clinics, good relationships, and the sharing of experiences between healthcare professionals and service users (Belus et al., 2024).

10.3. Global Partnerships and Funding Initiatives

As with research, global partnerships and funding initiatives should support, implement, and evaluate operational and programmatic interventions to monitor and deal with countering barriers to ART. We need a better understanding, documentation, and communication among the public health community of what constitutes barriers, what we are learning, and what we are trying to implement. This comprehensive compilation and interpretation of operational and programmatic experience will provide valuable evidence with which to assess feasibility and potential success in other resource-limited settings, and should help to guide both short-term donor policy and long-term national governmental actions (Rietveld & Patel, 2024). It is important to ensure that funding support and policy recommendations that emerge from these analyses do not inadvertently distort the focus of adherence and ART interventions. Globally, interventions should also integrate treatment scale-up as part of a comprehensive prevention program that targets those who are at risk of exposure to HIV. Funding sources can range from private donations to the majority of national governments of rich countries that pledge financial support for specific initiatives. Resources have increased significantly over the years. Data on the scale of prevention funding, especially in resource-limited settings, show that in 2001 only a portion of all foreign assistance for HIV/AIDS went to prevention; this had changed little by 2004. Data indicate that some global imbalances in private donations exist (Mukuna et al., 2024). In 2004, a major foundation donated a significant amount, dwarfing the amounts distributed by other major private organizations. Small funds are distributed by large numbers of NGOs, often in small amounts to single medium institutions. Supranational organizations also provide considerable funds through their investment in the activities of local NGOs and CBOs. These supranational organizations also sometimes act to prevent the risk of non-coordinated election-driven donations by large industry. In 2002, a significant agreement enabled low-cost generic antiretroviral drugs to be made available to resource-limited countries in a controlled manner that benefited both pharmaceutical companies and people in need (Qayyum et al., 2024).

11. CONCLUSION

This paper reviewed research that empirically studied the impact of ARTs on HIV treatment outcomes along the continuum of care. Although we sought to find whether the relationship between ART and indicators of HIV treatment outcomes was uniform across settings, we found a limited number of studies in diverse settings that measured different outcomes and revealed heterogeneous results, which called into question the possibility of the applicability of a one-size-fits-all policy on ARTs. Specifically, research produced inconclusive results with respect to the effect of ART on HIV testing and knowledge of HIV status, linkage to care after HIV diagnosis, early initiation of ART, ART adherence, retention in care, quality of life, and finally, viral load suppression. Yet, ARTs were prescribed to most, if not all, people who tested positive for HIV in developed countries and to low CD4 count patients in low-income and developing countries. With respect to resource utilization and impact, the finding of heterogeneous results was not surprising; the expected location of structural factors, such as health service and ART access, and the working of those structural factors in different settings were largely geographically and institutionally endowed. To preclude the variable effect of ART on HIV treatment outcomes, we recommend a stepwise policy. First, we believe that more interventionist policies are needed to scale up access to ART globally or defer eligibility criteria for ART. Earlier initiation of ART may also be recommendable in low-income and developing countries. These policies are based on the premise that at least some people who tested positive for HIV may experience health benefits from ARTs. Second, we would employ ART eligibility criteria to promote the efficient use of scarce resources. Females, infants, as well as low CD4 count people who tested positive for HIV are examples of more constrained candidate groups that would benefit from these policies. Third, we recognize that no single policy or treatment fits every person who tested positive for HIV within every setting. Successful ART programs will need to empower patients to maximize treatment adherence and address structural and social barriers to access to and retention in care. With respect to the efficacy of these policies, research can be useful to understand who derives benefit from ARTs, even to understand the art of medicine.

REFERENCES

Antoine, D., Chupikova, I., Jalodia, R., Singh, P. K., & Roy, S. (2024). Chronic Morphine Treatment and Antiretroviral Therapy Exacerbate HIV-Distal Sensory Peripheral Neuropathy and Induce Distinct Microbial Alterations in the HIV Tg26 Mouse Model. *International Journal of Molecular Sciences*, *25*(3). Advance online publication. DOI: 10.3390/ijms25031569 PMID: 38338849

Ayieko, P., Kisanga, E., Mshana, G., Nkosi, S., Hansen, C. H., Parry, C. D. H., Weiss, H. A., Grosskurth, H., Hayes, R. J., Morojele, N. K., & Kapiga, S. (2024). Epidemiology of alcohol use and alcohol use disorders among people living with HIV on antiretroviral therapy in Northwest Tanzania: Implications for ART adherence and case management. *AIDS Care*, *36*(5). Advance online publication. DOI: 10.1080/09540121.2023.2299324 PMID: 38295268

Ayiigah, J. L. Y., Domapielle, M. K., & Sumankuuro, J. (2024). Stigma toward people living with Human Immunodeficiency Virus: Insights from Anti-Retroviral Therapy clients in north-eastern Ghana. *Social Sciences & Humanities Open*, *9*. Advance online publication. DOI: 10.1016/j.ssaho.2024.100860

Belus, J. M., Msimango, L. I., van Heerden, A., Magidson, J. F., Bradley, V. D., Mdakane, Y., van Rooyen, H., & Barnabas, R. V. (2024). Barriers, Facilitators, and Strategies to Improve Participation of a Couple-Based Intervention to Address Women's Antiretroviral Therapy Adherence in KwaZulu-Natal, South Africa. *International Journal of Behavioral Medicine*, *31*(1). Advance online publication. DOI: 10.1007/s12529-023-10160-7 PMID: 36854871

Board, N. L., Yuan, Z., Wu, F., Moskovljevic, M., Ravi, M., Sengupta, S., Mun, S. S., Simonetti, F. R., Lai, J., Tebas, P., Lynn, K., Hoh, R., Deeks, S. G., Siliciano, J. D., Montaner, L. J., & Siliciano, R. F. (2024). Bispecific antibodies promote natural killer cell-mediated elimination of HIV-1 reservoir cells. *Nature Immunology*, *25*(3). Advance online publication. DOI: 10.1038/s41590-023-01741-5 PMID: 38278966

Chen, C., Chen, H., Wu, L., Gong, Q., & He, J. (2024). Factors influencing rapid antiretroviral therapy initiation in Jiulongpo, Chongqing, China: A retrospective cohort from 2018 to 2022. *AIDS Research and Therapy*, *21*(1). Advance online publication. DOI: 10.1186/s12981-024-00601-y PMID: 38494484

Chen, Z., Si, T., Ying, L., Guiying, C., Píng, X. J., & Wang, M. (2024). A case of multiple ART intolerance responds to Albuvirtide and Dolutegravir: Case report and literature review. *Heliyon*, *10*(6). Advance online publication. DOI: 10.1016/j.heliyon.2024.e27219 PMID: 38524593

Comfort, A. B., Asiimwe, S., Amaniyre, G., Orrell, C., Moody, J., Musinguzi, N., Bwana, M. B., Bangsberg, D. R., Haberer, J. E., Tsai, A. C., Ware, N., & Tumwesigye, E. (2024). Social networks and HIV treatment adherence among people with HIV initiating treatment in rural Uganda and peri-urban South Africa. *SSM - Population Health, 25*. Advance online publication. DOI: 10.1016/j.ssmph.2023.101593 PMID: 38292051

Corona, D., Pérez-Valero, I., Camacho, A., Gutiérrez Liarte, Á., Montero-Alonso, M., Alemán, M. R., Ruiz-Seco, P., Pérez González, A., Riera, M., Jarrin, I., Rivero-Juárez, A., & Rivero, A. (2024). Effectiveness and safety of bictegravir/emtricitabine/tenofovir alafenamide in HIV late presenters. *International Journal of Antimicrobial Agents, 63*(1). Advance online publication. DOI: 10.1016/j.ijantimicag.2023.107016 PMID: 37890734

Dunn Navarra, A. M., Gormley, M., Liang, E., Loughran, C., Vorderstrasse, A., Garcia, D. R., Rosenberg, M. G., Fletcher, J., & Goldsamt, L. A. (2024). Developing and testing a web-based platform for antiretroviral therapy (ART) adherence support among adolescents and young adults (AYA) living with HIV. *PEC Innovation, 4*. Advance online publication. DOI: 10.1016/j.pecinn.2024.100263 PMID: 38463238

Esra, R., Mmelesi, M., Ketlogetswe, A. T., Wolock, T. M., Howes, A., Nong, T., Matlhaga, M. T., Ratladi, S., Ramaabya, D., & Imai-Eaton, J. W. (2024). Improved Indicators for Subnational Unmet Antiretroviral Therapy Need in the Health System: Updates to the Naomi Model in 2023. *Journal of Acquired Immune Deficiency Syndromes, 95*(1). Advance online publication. DOI: 10.1097/QAI.0000000000003324 PMID: 38180736

Fassinou, L. C., Songwa Nkeunang, D., Delvaux, T., Nagot, N., & Kirakoya-Samadoulougou, F. (2024). Adherence to option B + antiretroviral therapy and associated factors in pregnant and breastfeeding women in Sub-Saharan Africa: A systematic review and meta-analysis. *BMC Public Health, 24*(1). Advance online publication. DOI: 10.1186/s12889-023-17004-9 PMID: 38183014

Gatechompol, S., Kerr, S. J., Cardoso, S. W., Samaneka, W., Tripathy, S., Godbole, S., Ghate, M., Kanyama, C., Nyirenda, M., Sugandhavesa, P., Machado, A., Van Leth, F., Campbell, T. B., Swindlells, S., Avihingsanon, A., & Cobelens, F. (2024). Monocyte to lymphocyte ratio and hemoglobin level to predict tuberculosis after antiretroviral therapy initiation. *AIDS, 38*(1). Advance online publication. DOI: 10.1097/QAD.0000000000003713 PMID: 37696248

Gupta, M., Kumar, A., Kumar, A., & Mathur, V. (2024). Reversible blindness in cryptococcal meningitis with human immunodeficiency virus infection. *International Journal of Research in Medical Sciences, 12*(3). Advance online publication. DOI: 10.18203/2320-6012.ijrms20240553

Hernandez, C., Gorska, A. M., & Eugenin, E. (2024). Mechanisms of HIV-mediated blood-brain barrier compromise and leukocyte transmigration under the current antiretroviral era. *iScience, 27*(3). Advance online publication. DOI: 10.1016/j.isci.2024.109236 PMID: 38487019

Kamau, S. G., Akatusasira, R., Namatovu, A., Kibet, E., Ssekitto, J. M., Mamun, M. A., & Kaggwa, M. M. (2024). The level of antiretroviral therapy (ART) adherence among orphan children and adolescents living with HIV/AIDS: A systematic review and meta-analysis. *PLoS ONE, 19*(2 February). https://doi.org/DOI: 10.1371/journal.pone.0295227

Kanise, H., van Oosterhout, J. J., Bisani, P., Songo, J., Matola, B. W., Chipungu, C., Simon, K., Cox, C., Hosseinipour, M. C., Sagno, J. B., Hoffman, R. M., Wallrauch, C., Phiri, S., Steegen, K., Jahn, A., Nyirenda, R., & Heller, T. (2024). Virological Findings and Treatment Outcomes of Cases That Developed Dolutegravir Resistance in Malawi's National HIV Treatment Program. *Viruses, 16*(1). Advance online publication. DOI: 10.3390/v16010029 PMID: 38257730

Kigongo, V. J., Nankabirwa, J. I., Kitutu, F. E., Ssenyonga, R., Mutebi, R. K., Kazibwe, A., Kiguba, R., Kambugu, A. D., & Castelnuovo, B. (2024). Dyslipidemia among adult people living with HIV on dolutegravir – based antiretroviral therapy at a private tertiary hospital in Kampala, Uganda: Burden and determinants. *BMC Infectious Diseases, 24*(1). Advance online publication. DOI: 10.1186/s12879-023-08892-8 PMID: 38183002

Kileel, E. M., Zheng, A., Bor, J., Fox, M. P., Crowther, N. J., George, J. A., Khoza, S., Rosen, S., Venter, W. D. F., Raal, F., Hibberd, P., & Brennan, A. T. (2024). Does Engagement in HIV Care Affect Screening, Diagnosis, and Control of Noncommunicable Diseases in Sub-Saharan Africa? A Systematic Review and Meta-analysis. *AIDS and Behavior, 28*(2). Advance online publication. DOI: 10.1007/s10461-023-04248-0 PMID: 38300475

Koh, M. C. Y., Ngiam, J. N., Yong, J., Tambyah, P. A., & Archuleta, S. (2024). The role of an artificial intelligence model in antiretroviral therapy counselling and advice for people living with HIV. *HIV Medicine, 25*(4). Advance online publication. DOI: 10.1111/hiv.13604 PMID: 38169077

Konishi, K., Nakagawa, H., Asaoka, T., Kasamatsu, Y., Goto, T., & Shirano, M. (2024). Brief communication: Body composition and hidden obesity in people living with HIV on antiretroviral therapy. *AIDS Research and Therapy, 21*(1). Advance online publication. DOI: 10.1186/s12981-024-00599-3 PMID: 38429716

Lim, S. Y., Lee, J., Osuna, C. E., Vikhe, P., Schalk, D. R., Chen, E., Fray, E., Kumar, M., Schultz-Darken, N., Rakasz, E., Capuano, S., Ladd, R. A., Gil, H. M., Evans, D. T., Jeng, E. K., Seaman, M., Martin, M., Van Dorp, C., Perelson, A. S., & Whitney, J. B. (2024). Induction of durable remission by dual immunotherapy in SHIV-infected ART-suppressed macaques. *Science, 383*(6687). Advance online publication. DOI: 10.1126/science.adf7966 PMID: 38422185

Mahlalela, N. B., Manne-Goehler, J., Ohene-Kwofie, D. B., Adams, L., Montana, L., Kahn, K., Rohr, J. K., Bärnighausen, T., & Gómez-Olivé, F. X. (2024). The Association Between HIV-Related Stigma and the Uptake of HIV Testing and ART Among Older Adults in Rural South Africa: Findings from the HAALSI Cohort Study. *AIDS and Behavior, 28*(3). Advance online publication. DOI: 10.1007/s10461-023-04222-w PMID: 38286975

Mornah, L. N., Saaka, M., & Pireh, D. (2024). Magnitude and Predictors of Dietary Diversity among HIV-Infected Adults on Antiretroviral Therapy: The Case of North-Western, Ghana. *AIDS Research and Treatment, 2024*. Advance online publication. DOI: 10.1155/2024/2777908 PMID: 38328798

Moya, Z. R., Pillay, S., & Magula, N. (2024). Assessing index CD4 and associated outcomes at 1-year in a tertiary HIV clinic, KwaZulu-Natal. *South African Family Practice, 66*(1). Advance online publication. DOI: 10.4102/safp.v66i1.5803 PMID: 38299523

Mukuna, D. M., Decroo, T., & Nyapokoto, C. M. (2024). Effect of dolutegravir-based versus efavirenz-based antiretroviral therapy on excessive weight gain in adult treatment-naïve HIV patients at Matsanjeni health center, Eswatini: A retrospective cohort study. *AIDS Research and Therapy, 21*(1). Advance online publication. DOI: 10.1186/s12981-023-00591-3 PMID: 38185696

Fahad Naim, Awais Naeem, Fahim Shah, Umair-ul-Islam, Sohail Adnan, & Muhammad Hamid. (2024). Assessment of Non-HIV Comorbidities Among HIV-Infected Patients on Anti-Retroviral therapy (ART) in a Teaching Hospital Kohat, Pakistan. *Annals of PIMS-Shaheed Zulfiqar Ali Bhutto Medical University, 13*(4). https://doi.org/DOI: 10.48036/apims.v13i4.974

Naranjo, O., Torices, S., Clifford, P. R., Rodriguez, T., Osborne, O. M., Tiburcio, D., Fattakhov, N., Park, M., Stevenson, M., & Toborek, M. (2024). AKT signaling modulates latent viral reservoir viability in HIV-1-infected blood–brain barrier pericytes. *The Journal of Biological Chemistry*, *300*(1). Advance online publication. DOI: 10.1016/j.jbc.2023.105526 PMID: 38043797

Njuba, L., Gómez-Morantes, J. E., Herrera, A., & Camacho, S. (2024). Health information systems in extreme contexts: Using mobile phones to fight AIDS in Uganda. *The Electronic Journal on Information Systems in Developing Countries*, *90*(3). Advance online publication. DOI: 10.1002/isd2.12314

Nursalam, N., Sukartini, T., Misutarno, M., & Priyantini, D. (2024). Adherence to antiretroviral therapy, CD4 count, viral load and opportunistic infections in people with HIV/AIDS: A cross-sectional study. *Jurnal Ners*, *19*(1). Advance online publication. DOI: 10.20473/jn.v19i1.49958

OG, A. (2024). Investigating the Relationship between Medication Adherence Behaviors and the Achievement of Sustained Viral Load Suppression among People Living with HIV (PLHIV) on Antiretroviral Therapy (ART) in Akwa Ibom State, from 2018 - 2022. *Public Health Open Access*, *8*(1). Advance online publication. DOI: 10.23880/phoa-16000270

Olaya, F., Brin, M., Caraballo, P. B., Halpern, M., Jia, H., Ramírez, S. O., Padilla, J. J., Stonbraker, S., & Schnall, R. (2024). A randomized controlled trial of the dissemination of an mHealth intervention for improving health outcomes: The WiseApp for Spanish-speakers living with HIV study protocol. *BMC Public Health*, *24*(1). Advance online publication. DOI: 10.1186/s12889-023-17538-y PMID: 38233908

Oturu, K., O'Brien, O., & Ozo-Eson, P. I. (2024). Barriers and enabling structural forces affecting access to antiretroviral therapy in Nigeria. *BMC Public Health*, *24*(1). Advance online publication. DOI: 10.1186/s12889-023-17271-6 PMID: 38184516

Qayyum, S. F., Khan, H., & Rukh, G. (2024). Incidence of Opportunistic Infections in HIV Patients at Anti-Retroviral Therapy (ART) Adherence Unit, Islamabad Pakistan. *Journal of Health and Rehabilitation Research*, *4*(1). Advance online publication. DOI: 10.61919/jhrr.v4i1.542

Quaker, A. S., Shirima, L. J., & Msuya, S. E. (2024). Trend and factors associated with non-suppression of viral load among adolescents on ART in Tanzania: 2018–2021. *Frontiers in Reproductive Health*, *6*. Advance online publication. DOI: 10.3389/frph.2024.1309740 PMID: 38292142

Rietveld, C. A., & Patel, P. C. (2024). Antiretroviral Therapy Coverage, Entrepreneurship, and Development in Low- and Middle-Income Countries. *Business & Society*. Advance online publication. DOI: 10.1177/00076503241232070

Sadiq, E., Katzew, S., Nel, J., Tade, G., Woodiwiss, A., Norton, G., & Modi, G. (2024). Stroke, HIV and the Immune Reconstitution Inflammatory Syndrome in the absence of opportunistic infections. *Journal of the Neurological Sciences*, *457*. Advance online publication. DOI: 10.1016/j.jns.2024.122880 PMID: 38219384

Saleh, R. A. A., Ghaleb, M., & Shafik, W., & ERTUNÇ, H. M. (2024). Efficient white blood cell identification with hybrid inception-xception network. *The Journal of Supercomputing*, *80*(17), 25155–25187.

Saltini, P., Tassis, B., Ronchi, A., Tagliabue, C., Di Pietro, G., Dellepiane, R. M., Muscatello, A., Giacomelli, A., Pugni, L., Ferrazzi, E., Bandera, A., & Bozzi, G. (2024). Preventing HIV mother-to-child transmission in a vertically infected pregnant woman with multiclass drug resistance, role of bis-in-die dolutegravir and neonatal AZT prophylaxis: A case report. *Heliyon*, *10*(1). Advance online publication. DOI: 10.1016/j.heliyon.2023.e23072 PMID: 38163123

Shafik, W. (2024a). Artificial Intelligence-Enabled Internet of Medical Things for Enhanced Healthcare Systems. In *Smart Healthcare Systems* (pp. 119–134). CRC Press., DOI: 10.1201/9781032698519-9

Shafik, W. (2024b). Dissecting the Role of Women in Cybersecurity and Information Technology: A Medical Perspective. In *Next-Generation Cybersecurity: AI, ML, and Blockchain* (pp. 325–350). Springer. https://doi.org/DOI: 10.1007/978-981-97-1249-6_15

Shafik, W. (2024c). The Future of Healthcare: AIoMT—Redefining Healthcare with Advanced Artificial Intelligence and Machine Learning Techniques. In *Artificial Intelligence and Machine Learning in Drug Design and Development* (pp. 605–634). Wiley., DOI: 10.1002/9781394234196.ch19

Shafik, W. (2024d). The Future of Healthcare: Data-Driven Trends and Innovation. In *Advancing Healthcare through Data-driven Innovations* (pp. 166–185). CRC Press.

Shafik, W. (2025a). Revolutionizing Skin Cancer Diagnosis With Artificial Intelligence: Insights Into Machine Learning Techniques. In *Impact of Digital Solutions for Improved Healthcare Delivery* (pp. 167–194). IGI Global.

Shafik, W. (2025b). Smart biomedical devices for smart healthcare. In *Machine Learning Models and Architectures for Biomedical Signal Processing* (pp. 421–448). Elsevier.

Sheira, L. A., Ryan, K. P., Fahey, C. A., Katabaro, E. D., Sabasaba, A. N., Njau, P. F., & McCoy, S. I. (2024). The impact of cash incentives on mental health among adults initiating antiretroviral therapy in Tanzania. *AIDS Care*, *36*(2). Advance online publication. DOI: 10.1080/09540121.2023.2222576 PMID: 37321981

Shi, J., Ying, G., Zheng, R., & Zhang, Z. (2024). Clinical significance and management of low-level HIV viremia in the era of integrase strand transfer inhibitors. *HIV Medicine*, *25*(3). Advance online publication. DOI: 10.1111/hiv.13585 PMID: 37990782

Shimura, M., Higashi-Kuwata, N., Fujiwara, A., Taniguchi, M., Ichinose, T., Hamano, F., Uematsu, M., Inoue, T., Matsuyama, S., Suzuki, T., Ghosh, A. K., Shindou, H., Shimuzu, T., & Mitsuya, H. (2024). A lipid index for risk of hyperlipidemia caused by anti-retroviral drugs. *Antiviral Research*, *223*. Advance online publication. DOI: 10.1016/j.antiviral.2024.105819 PMID: 38272319

Slogrove, A. L., Bovu, A., De Beer, S., Phelanyane, F., Williams, P. L., Heekes, A., Kalk, E., Mehta, U., Theron, G., Abrams, E. J., Cotton, M. F., Myer, L., Davies, M. A., & Boulle, A. (2024). Maternal and birth outcomes in pregnant people with and without HIV in the Western Cape, South Africa. *AIDS*, *38*(1). Advance online publication. DOI: 10.1097/QAD.0000000000003728 PMID: 37720974

Tekle, A., Tsegaye, A., & Ketema, T. (2024). Adherence to Anti-Retroviral Therapy (ART) and Its Determinants Among People Living with HIV/ AIDS at Bonga, Kaffa, South-West Ethiopia. *Patient Preference and Adherence*, *18*. Advance online publication. DOI: 10.2147/PPA.S445164 PMID: 38476589

Trickey, A., Glaubius, R., Pantazis, N., Zangerle, R., Wittkop, L., Vehreschild, J., Grabar, S., Cavassini, M., Teira, R., D'Arminio Monforte, A., Casabona, J., Van Sighem, A., Jarrin, I., Ingle, S. M., Sterne, J. A. C., Imai-Eaton, J. W., & Johnson, L. F. (2024). Estimation of Improvements in Mortality in Spectrum among Adults with HIV Receiving Antiretroviral Therapy in High-Income Countries. *Journal of Acquired Immune Deficiency Syndromes*, *95*(1). Advance online publication. DOI: 10.1097/QAI.0000000000003326 PMID: 38180742

Tun, W., Conserve, D. F., Bunga, C., Jeremiah, K., Apicella, L., & Vu, L. (2024). Quality of Care is Perceived to be High with Community-based Antiretroviral Therapy (ART) Services for Female Sex Workers in Tanzania: Qualitative Findings from a Pilot Implementation Science Study. *AIDS and Behavior*, *28*(1). Advance online publication. DOI: 10.1007/s10461-023-04155-4 PMID: 37632605

Wagner, G. J., Bogart, L. M., Klein, D. J., Lawrence, S. J., Goggin, K., Gizaw, M., & Mutchler, M. G. (2024). Culturally Relevant Africultural Coping Moderates the Association Between Discrimination and Antiretroviral Adherence Among Sexual Minority Black Americans Living with HIV. *AIDS and Behavior*, *28*(2). Advance online publication. DOI: 10.1007/s10461-023-04233-7 PMID: 38060112

Wang, L., Muwonge, T. R., Simoni, J. M., Nambi, F., Nakabugo, L., Kibuuka, J., Thomas, D., Katz, I. T., Feutz, E., Thomas, K. K., Ware, N. C., Wyatt, M. A., Kadama, H., Mujugira, A., & Heffron, R. (2024). Behavioral Modeling and its Association with PrEP and ART Use in Ugandan HIV-Serodifferent Couples. *AIDS and Behavior*, *28*(5). Advance online publication. DOI: 10.1007/s10461-024-04286-2 PMID: 38361169

West, R. E., Oberly, P. J., Riddler, S. A., Nolin, T. D., & Devanathan, A. S. (2024). Development and validation of an ultra-high performance liquid chromatography-tandem mass spectrometry method to quantify antiretroviral drug concentrations in human plasma for therapeutic monitoring. *Journal of Pharmaceutical and Biomedical Analysis*, *240*. Advance online publication. DOI: 10.1016/j.jpba.2023.115932 PMID: 38198884

Wiche Salinas, T. R., Zhang, Y., Gosselin, A., Rosario, N. F., El-Far, M., Filali-Mouhim, A., Routy, J. P., Chartrand-Lefebvre, C., Landay, A. L., Durand, M., Tremblay, C. L., & Ancuta, P. (2024). Alterations in Th17 Cells and Non-Classical Monocytes as a Signature of Subclinical Coronary Artery Atherosclerosis during ART-Treated HIV-1 Infection. *Cells*, *13*(2). Advance online publication. DOI: 10.3390/cells13020157 PMID: 38247848

ENDNOTES

1 https://www.mayoclinic.org/diseases-conditions/hiv-aids/symptoms-causes/syc-20373524

2 https://my.clevelandclinic.org/health/diseases/4251-hiv-aids

3 https://en.wikipedia.org/wiki/Orthoretrovirinae

4 https://en.wikipedia.org/wiki/Flaviviridae

5 https://en.wikipedia.org/wiki/CCR5

6 https://en.wikipedia.org/wiki/Reverse-transcriptase_inhibitor

7 https://my.clevelandclinic.org/health/treatments/24937-protease-inhibitors

[8] https://www.unicef.org/indonesia/prevention-mother-child-transmission-hiv

Chapter 5
Artificial Intelligence (AI)-Powered Personalization in HIV Care:
From Diagnosis to Drug Response Optimization

Arpita Nayak
https://orcid.org/0000-0003-2911-0492
KIIT School of Liberal Studies, KIIT University, Bhubaneswar, India

Ipseeta Satpathy
https://orcid.org/0000-0002-0155-5548
KSOM, KIIT University, Bhubaneswar, India

Vishal Jain
https://orcid.org/0000-0003-1126-7424
School of Engineering and Technology, Vivekananda Institute of Professional Studies - Technical Campus, New Delhi, India

ABSTRACT

HIV is still a major health challenge worldwide, so introducing new solutions is required to improve diagnosis, treatment and control of the disease. Most people who need traditional ART are given the same doses, but this method can ignore how genes, risky behaviours and viruses differ from one patient to another. AI can help by analysing EHR data, genomic information, information collected by wearables and live patient input to design individual treatment plans. The chapter looks at applying machine learning and deep learning in early detection and assessing risk, mostly in places with limited resources. Moreover, the chapter points out the ethical

DOI: 10.4018/979-8-3373-2863-8.ch005

and technical problems faced when using AI in HIV care such as privacy of data, biased results from algorithms and how results can be explained. This chapter aims to add to the body of literature how AI impacts HIV care.

I. INTRODUCTION

With current estimates, HIV remains a major global issue because it affects 39 million people worldwide. Although there have been major developments in HIV treatment and health practises, this disease currently puts a heavier strain on groups in low- and middle-income countries in sub-Saharan Africa, Asia and Eastern Europe. Although certain infectious diseases are treatable, HIV is a lifelong disease that brings the need for lifelong medical care, adherence to treatment and careful management of additional health problems. Lingering HIV can become even more problematic because there is still a stigma, slowing down diagnosis, causing treatment to be interrupted and leading to distress for those affected. Therefore, healthcare providers aim to limit HIV growth and help PLHIV maintain high quality life and long-term health (Mereu et al.,2022).

Although standardised treatment works for many, it tends to not address the diverse ways that infection develops in PLHIV. Most often, ART treatment plans are based on information about groups of people instead of a thorough study of what individuals need, meaning important things like genetic factors, the immune system, certain types of viral infections and social influences are not taken into account. In addition such a broad approach fails to take into account the large variations seen in treatment responses, how patients stick to treatment and their daily surroundings. Frequently, it will result in drug resistance, people not taking medicines well, harm from medications and fatigue with the treatments. When there is a shortage of healthcare resources, the lack of monitoring equipment, adequate preparation of staff and efficient patient routes often gets worse. As a result of seeking more equity in care, there is an increased awareness that individualised treatment plans should be both effective and possible for many people (Keddem et al.,2023).

This difference between approved procedures and what individuals actually require has created a major need for technology, mainly through Artificial Intelligence (AI). AI which stands for the ability of machines to improve how people think, has quickly become important in healthcare. With AI, doctors and researchers can now handle a huge variety of data such as EHRs, lab findings, genomics and behavioural patterns, much faster compared to earlier clinical approaches. In HIV care, AI can make use of all this data to provide insights personally relevant for each patient that help through every step of their treatment. AI technology can improve accuracy, response time and the fitting of treatment plans early, during medication use, while checking adherence and when managing chronic diseases (Bekker et al.,2023).

Using machine learning, it is possible to analyse vast information about patients to help decide the most effective treatment courses for them. These algorithms can detect patients who may not stick with their treatment or respond well to it much earlier than symptoms can be seen by doctors. In particular, when used on imaging or genomic data, deep learning can discover concealed factors that influence resistance to treatments or reactions in patients. AI-enabled chatbots and mobile health apps are now regularly available to support patients with reminders, encouragement and advice to improve their on-going care. (Xiang et al.,2022).

In addition, AI offers more than just help for individual patients in HIV treatment. More generally, AI can make workflows in healthcare more efficient, ease the workload on overstretched systems and support better overall use of resources in the field. AI models help public health agencies spot places where infection is on the rise, forecast the progress of outbreaks and decide how best to manage resources used for both prevention and treatment. AI-based data can give policy-makers valuable insights to help choose funding options, build better programmes and see whether programmes are successful. As a result, AI helps make care personal for individual patients and also guides better, more thoughtful decisions at the level of larger organisations. Excitement for applying AI in HIV care is justified, but we need to be aware of its constraints, particularly when it comes to data ethics, understanding the models and giving all patients access to AI. What patients say about HIV, their treatment past and any risk factors should be dealt with the strictest confidentiality and be agreed upon by the patient beforehand. It is important that AI tools do not create algorithmic bias or health inequality may be reinforced when the data they use is not comprehensive. Mechanisms to explain, hold responsible and harmonise with human decision-making should accompany AI in clinical use, particularly when the results influence life-changing situations (Heerden et al.,2023; Olaboye et al.,2024).

Al's rise in the medical field has been revolutionising and reinventing how we identify, track, and care for patients. This state-of-the-art technology is propelling the industry's tremendous innovation, enabling quick breakthroughs in drug research and discovery while enabling medical professionals to deliver better, faster care.

Al's adoption in the healthcare sector has been further accelerated by the COVID-19 pandemic. The pandemic facilitated the broad acceptance and development of Al-based healthcare, allowing for its efficient application in clinical trials, diagnostics, detection, patient care, claims settlement, and virtual assistants. Statista estimates that the value of Al in healthcare was around $11 billion globally in 2021 and would rise at a compound annual growth rate (CAGR) of 37% from 2022 to 2030, reaching $188 billion as shown in figure 1. Improved patient care, chronic illness management, early risk assessment, process automation, and optimisation are just a few of the ways in which Al in healthcare may greatly help both patients and professionals. Data on the doctor, therapy, and medical facility may be easily retrieved as more and more healthcare invoices are converted to digital formats. Following data mining, hospitals can provide reports on the errors they consistently make when treating a certain ailment in order to assist patients get well and possibly prevent needless hospital stays when required. (Srivastava, 2018).

Figure 1. AI market size in healthcare 2021 to 2030

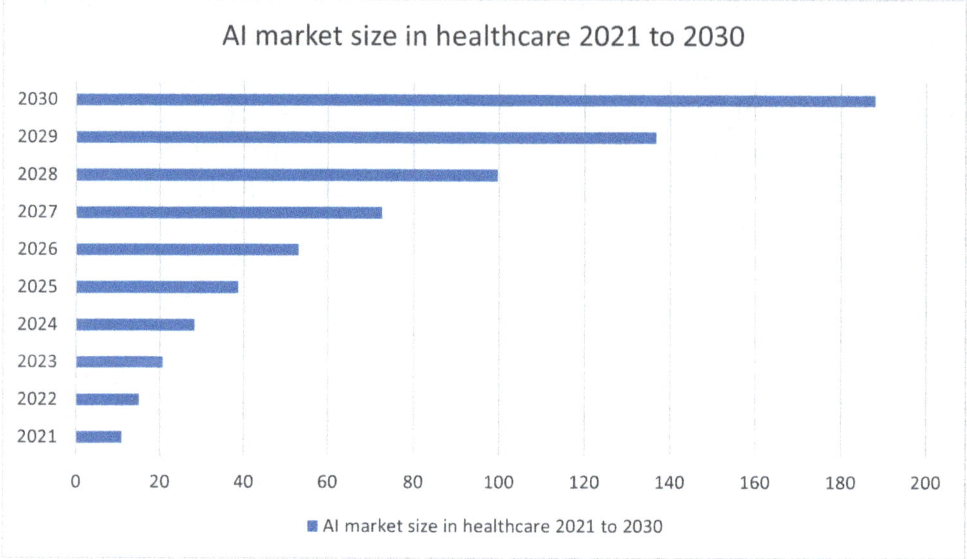

The chapter focuses on applying AI to HIV treatment such as in early spotting of the virus, creating optimum ART plans, monitoring adherence, prediction modelling and providing immediate aid to patients. In addition, the course considers how AI is used in monitoring public health and preventing epidemics. In this chapter, it explains possible issues such as those involving data privacy, along with the chance that some groups may miss out on the benefits.

II. RESEARCH QUESTIONS AND OBJECTIVES

Research Questions

- How can AI models be used to personalize antiretroviral therapy (ART) based on individual patient profiles in HIV treatment?

- What role do AI-powered tools play in predicting treatment adherence and clinical outcomes in people living with HIV?

Research Objectives

- To explore how AI technologies can enhance personalized HIV treatment by analyzing patient-specific data such as genomics, treatment history, and behavioral patterns.
- To evaluate the effectiveness of AI-driven tools in improving early diagnosis, drug adherence, and treatment outcome prediction in HIV care.

III. ARTIFICIAL INTELLIGENCE (AI) IN EARLY DIAGNOSIS OF HIV

Treating the disease and stopping its spread is much easier if HIV is spotted and caught early. If HIV is found quickly, ART begins at the right time which controls virus levels, helps the immune system and makes it less likely for the virus to pass to others. Yet, many difficulties are still preventing early diagnosis worldwide, mainly in areas where resources are scarce and the problem is widespread. They are made up of a lack of places to be tested, society's judgments against people sick with HIV, long delays in seeing symptoms and scarce experts to treat them. AI makes it possible to process a lot of detailed data and recognise patterns that people may miss, making it easier to find HIV cases earlier (Xiang et al.,2022).

AI methods, largely focused on machine learning (ML), are now being built to assess both health-related and demographic information to signal people who might be in danger of HIV. To create these models, people use big groups of patient records, lab test results and lifestyle risk factors. Pattern recognition allows the algorithm to guess the chances of HIV infection before the disease is confirmed. In practical terms, it is possible to develop supervised learning models that will associate certain groups of symptoms like unexplained weight loss, recurring infections or picking up infections along with demographic features like age, gender, sexual activity or geography, to help with predicting the risk of HIV infection (Roche et al.,2024).

Going beyond just tracking symptoms, AI tools are now used to analyse unstructured records such as electronic health records, doctors' notes and images. Because of NLP, machines can now understand human language in medical records and discover possible HIV risk cases that human reviewers could have missed. With the help of NLP technology, doctors are able to pick out patients whose EHR data show frequent viral infections, repeated fatigue or treatments for opportunistic infections and ensure they follow up properly. In many parts of the world where healthcare is limited, AI is being used to help people get screened for HIV. AI-powered mHealth apps are now being used to help people get screened for illnesses remotely. These apps let people report their own symptoms and actions via mobile, determine risk there and then using AI and recommend relevant guidance, like where to get a confirmation HIV test nearby. They are providing more people with access and also making it easier to have your health evaluated privately and discreetly (Williams et al.,2023).

Applications of machine learning in HIV testing seem to help reduce errors in classification. Although usual testing strategies are generally accurate, errors can happen at the start of exposure due to issues with early seroconversion. By teaching AI on several types of biological samples, the AI can help improve the accuracy of diagnosis by linking diverse data points that could be checked separately. When you combine various random forests and gradient boosting machines, you improve the accuracy of predicting HIV infection status. An area of great hope is AI-backed equipment that performs diagnostics by combining testing at the point of care with future possibilities. AI is being used to build rapid diagnostic devices that read samples of saliva or blood, apply ML algorithms and quickly assess the risk of HIV. They give results right away and can suggest advice that fits the patient's history, way of life and other conditions. In addition, CNNs and other deep learning models are being applied to analyse both medical images and microscopy slides to look for common HIV-related conditions such as Kaposi's sarcoma and some types of pneumonia (Obeagu et al.,2024).

Such models are important in public health planning because they help detect communities and people who are more likely to get HIV. Using such models allows analysing lots of data on society, disease rates, health system strength and travel behaviour to see where new infections are likely to develop. They can use the results to move resources where they are most needed, make testing more efficient and spotlight warning messages for high-risk populations. AI is now used for both heatmaps and geospatial analysis to arrange mobile testing units and outreach programmes in different countries, confirming that such approaches can work. Even though AI shows major promise for HIV diagnosis, there are some critical obstacles. Challenges with both data availability and quality are most noticeable in locations with poorly developed electronic health systems. In underserved locations, datasets needed for training AI models are generally difficult to access and poorly organised. Furthermore, collection of data with bias can cause wrong results that can harm some populations. If AI technology is mostly taught on urban examples, it likely won't recognize risks in places outside cities or among people who are underserved (Ma et al.,2025).

Artificial Intelligence brings up ethical matters when it is used to help with early HIV diagnosis.. The wrong use of prediction or leaks of private information may increase stigma and prevent individuals from getting help. As a result, adding AI to HIV diagnostics should be done alongside well-established governance, ongoing model evaluation and a commitment to being open about decisions. In short, AI has the capacity to increase accurate, fast and smart ways to identify HIV early on. Thanks to machine learning, NLP, mobile technology and predictive analytics helped by AI, it is possible to connect healthcare requirements with accessible and available solutions in challenging locations. Despite problems on both the technical and ethical sides, more progress, teamwork with various experts and safe application can let AI help find out about and address HIV as soon as possible.

IV. AI FOR PERSONALIZED ANTIRETROVIRAL THERAPY (ART)

Modern healthcare and especially treatments for diseases such as HIV, focuses strongly on personalised medicine. For over two decades, ART has been adapted and updated to become the top strategy for treating HIV infection. Yet, with a variety of drugs to use and mix, most standard treatment routines do not pay close attention to patients' specific genetics, viruses they carry or immune differences. Because treatment is not tailored, this can cause uneven results, unwanted reactions, an increase in drug resistance and undesirable long-term outcomes. As AI advances, there are growing chances to customise ART for each patient which can help improve HIV treatment and advance the idea of using precision medicine (Sah et al.,2025).

Having a good understanding of patient variability is essential to making ART personalised. A person's immune system, the kind of virus they have, their genes and existing medical conditions will influence their response to certain ART medicines. By way of illustration, if someone has a variant of HLA or cytochrome P450 genes, it could greatly affect the body's drug metabolism and make the chemicals more toxic for that person. Certain types of HIV may have mutations that make certain antiretrovirals less effective. Because of time and data difficulties, traditional clinical practise may miss or under-include these factors when planning treatment. AI addresses this need by examining multiple layers of data at the same time which exceeds people's ability to handle (Koh et al.,2024).

Information about ART treatments from the past and present, CD4 counts, viral loads, additional health issues, reported adverse effects and adherence is all stored in EHRs. By using both kinds of genomic information, AI models can use EHRs to discover patterns needed for precise treatment decisions. Machine learning works with data from EHRs to guide clinicians on selecting drug treatments that they believe will be effective for each patient. Algorithms such as decision trees, support vector machines or neural networks can extract knowledge from data sets in which labelled ART intervention results are provided. Life science models can guide clinicians toward recommending treatment courses to newly diagnosed patients with similar attributes (Jin, 2025).

Apart from analysing clinical records, AI is able to interpret unstructured data found in doctor notes, lab reports and what patients report. By using NLP, it becomes possible to learn about important details from the narrative, like past negative reactions, psychosocial matters or difficulty sticking to a treatment. These subtle details are very important for good treatment outcomes, though they are sometimes missing from old health data systems. When this information is added, AI can provide ART plans that fit a patient's health needs as well as their social habits and behaviour. In addition, AI is now helping by developing tools called clinical decision support systems (CDSS) that include AI-based advice in regular care routines. They give healthcare providers computerised advice on which ART regimen to use, boost or lower drug doses and look for possible drug interactions. If HIV and renal impairment are listed in a patient's profile, the system will list possible nephrotoxic medicines and provide safer alternatives. If both diseases are present, the CDSS includes this factor in choosing the right drugs. The goal of these tools is to support, not take over, the role of clinicians, giving them the ability to decide on better, more personalised care in a more efficient manner (Kumbale, 2021).

In addition to data stored in medical records, AI examines things such as doctor notes, lab results and what patients themselves report. NLP allows healthcare professionals to identify key points such as earlier troubles, social issues and problems with following treatment from the patient's storey. Even though they matter a lot for treatment effectiveness, these factors are often not stored in standard health data systems. AI can guide treatment choices by selecting ART that is right for the patient's body and is also suitable for the patient's everyday life. There has been an important development in creating clinical decision support systems that incorporate advice from AI into daily patient care by medical staff. Mechanisms in these systems offer healthcare providers guidance for selecting ART medications, changing treatment doses and predicting the chance of drug interactions. Should someone on HIV therapy also need dialysis, the system may note the risk with certain agents and provide safer suggestions. When patients have infections with both COVID-19 and hepatitis B or C, the CDSS allows for their needs in the selection of drugs. They aim to supplement, rather than substitute for, physician judgement, so that caregivers can make better and more confident choices quickly (Eissa, 2025).

Besides, AI models can be adjusted according to the patient's new health problems. HIV treatment has to keep changing, as changes in how a person follows the treatment, resistance to medications or infections can happen along the way. It is possible to adjust ART procedures better by using reinforcement learning which shapes actions automatically from data that is available fast. The use of adaptive models allows for early predictions of therapy changes which can prevent clinical worsening and support lifelong effective virus control. AI helps a lot by predicting the ability of microbes to resist drugs. It is especially important to use resistance testing when deciding which ART regimen to use for patients who did not respond well to earlier treatments. By analysing viral genetic sequences, AI algorithms can find out about known resistance mutations and guess how they might impact the action of antiretroviral drugs. Some researchers have seen that deep learning is more accurate than manual interpretation or rule-based systems in identifying complex patterns of drug resistance. Because of this, clinicians can select options that are potent despite any developing resistance. AI is also valuable in helping to bring about new options for ART medications and protocols. Investigating large-scale biomedical data about structures, results from research studies and drug interactions, AI is able to improve the process of finding and optimising drugs. Using generative models, we can create molecules with desirable characteristics and ML helps us estimate the results these compounds would have in patients. As a result, the process of making new effective, safe and easy-to-use ART medicines could be both faster and less expensive (Padhi et al.,2023).

Applying AI in personalised antiretroviral therapy greatly improves the way HIV is treated. The use of clinical, genetic and behavioural data by AI helps healthcare providers suggest the right ART treatment for each patient. HIV care is improved when decision support systems, predictive analytics and adaptive learning models are included. With the progress of these technologies and their ethical systems, health outcomes for those living with HIV globally should improve a lot.

V. DRUG ADHERENCE MONITORING AND INTERVENTION

People living with HIV (PLHIV) need to stay on their antiretroviral therapy (ART) to successfully control HIV infection. Advances in making ART easier to use and more effective do not fix the problem of patients not taking these drugs regularly. When people do not stick to taking their medicine as directed, the virus may come back and they may gain resistance to the drugs. This also supports the spread of the virus which runs counter to public health goals. Using self-reports, counting pills and seeing if there are refills is the standard, but it's not always truly accurate or complete. In this situation, technology is changing the approach to overseeing medication use and stepping in with timely assistance to support treatment (Whiteley et al.,2021).

Integrating AI into both wearable and mobile devices is making adherence monitoring much more reliable. Smartwatches, fitness bands and biosensor patches all collect information that can show whether or not a person is sticking to all their treatment regimens. A good example is that some devices can use sensors to cheque the user's activity, sleep behaviour, heart rate and other factors related to both taking medicine and general health. When this data is sent to AI tools, they cheque for deviations from normal practise and may flag the first signs of missing doses or tiring of treatment (Sekandi et al.,2023).

mHealth applications are important when it comes to supporting people to follow their treatments in real time. Using artificial intelligence, mobile apps can send notes about medications, cheque when users take their pills by picture or voice and track their daily compliance with usage. Apps that require people to use computer vision are able to see whether medication is taken by reviewing videos the user sends. Certain apps use GPS to double-cheque if a person has their medication at home or is late to get their refills. Because these applications are so well-developed, they help us notice subtle patterns in patient behaviour and require little continuous clinician supervision (Xiang et al.,2022).

Predictive analytics adds a valuable approach to fighting against non-adherence. Analysing data from the past with psychosocial and clinical information, AI models can spot people who might not follow their treatment plan. These models combine missed appointments, mood from mobile journals, social standing and medical conditions to develop full adherence risk profiles. All of these techniques are used to build models that can see relationships invisible to the usual analytical tools. If healthcare providers detect non-adherence early, they are able to stop problems from getting worse through counselling, reminder messages or modifying the patient's medication schedule (Stoner et al.,2022).

More organizations are now using chatbots and virtual health assistants using AI. They are created to have conversations with people, instruct them and motivate them. Chatbots, accessed on mobile devices or the internet, are able to remind patients about their medicine, answer questions about it and watch for side effects regularly. Unlike traditional alerts that stay the same, chatbots can personalise how often they remind patients and what they say which helps people stay interested. Thanks to NLP and sentiment analysis powered models, signs of emotional stress or treatment exhaustion may be identified, making it possible for help to be given to patients quicker if required. Aside from reminders, chatbots make it possible for patients to quickly talk to clinicians and share their important health details. Via the chatbot, if a user complains of feeling dizzy or sick, the information can be handled using AI and sent to the specified healthcare expert. It is most useful in places with many patients, short staffing or busy clinics, where continual monitoring by clinical staff might not work (Periáñez et al.,2024).

In addition, Amazon Alexa, Google Assistant and other types of voice assistants are being tried for supporting adherence with voice. Thanks to these tools, patients can have reminders speak to them, keep a log of their medications and get answers about any problems with their pills. For people who do not have good reading skills or would rather hear than read, interface tools make the process more approachable. Using them on smart home systems or mobile devices, people can enjoy support without the need for big technical know-how or new hardware. It also helps by offering treatments that change with the patient's needs over time. Reinforcement learning may be used to choose reminders that suit each patient according to their responses. If someone regularly avoids texts but tries to follow instructions in pictures, the system will adapt by adding video prompts. Just as with people and rules, machine learning lets reminders trigger at times that suit how a person works in their daily routine. By personalising medicine this way, users are more likely to follow the plan and are supported, instead of being closely tracked (Liu et al.,2021).

AI is helping to change the way drug adherence is tracked and treated in HIV patients. AI technologies, including sensors, mobile apps, analytics and chatbots, all help patients stick with ART. Healthcare technologies help clinics perform better and ensure patients receive timely, personalised and kind support. To keep these tools useful, they should always be used fairly, inclusively and with the principle of placing care under human control. Effective AI use can help solve one of the greatest ongoing challenges in managing HIV, moving us toward helping everyone with HIV stay virus-free and have a better quality of life.

VI. PREDICTIVE MODELLING FOR TREATMENT OUTCOMES

In recent changes to HIV care, predictive modeling is one of the most promising ways AI can be used. By using large, mixed sets of data, AI is able to predict treatment responses in each individual, expect possible problems and rank people according to their risk levels. Such insights allow healthcare providers to better customise treatments, boost health outcomes, lower the risk of failure and enhance how smoothly treatments are carried out. As a result, predictive modelling introduces a change from reactive care to proactive and individualised healthcare that depends on actual data patterns (Maskew et al.,2022).

Using ML-based AI, it is now possible to accurately forecast the reaction of HIV patients to ART. How effective ART is for someone can change a lot depending on their viral load, level of CD4 cells, history of treatment, certain genes, how well they adhere to therapy, health conditions and social circumstances. Simple statistical methods usually fail to show how many of these variables interact in detailed or nonlinear ways. In contrast, machines learning models are capable of dealing with these complexities and discover sensible patterns in multidimensional data (Seboka et al.,2023).

Previous patient data storage allows supervised learning algorithms to be trained on the difference between successful treatment and not. They are trained to recognise how important measures of CD4 count, medications chosen, adherence and patient characteristics are for different outcomes. With training completed, the model suggests likely outcomes for new patients and supports clinicians in determining which ART course to use and how often to increase patient monitoring. If virological response can be predicted early, doctors can make prompt and correct decisions, sparing patients the delay caused by guesswork (Fieggen et al.,2022).

AI helps find out whether patients are likely to suffer from adverse drug reactions before they develop, in addition to predicting the results of their overall treatment. ADRs often lead to people not taking their medicine as prescribed or leaving treatment, mainly for patients managing additional health problems or on multiple treatments. AI is able to notice links between the characteristics of patients and the side effects they experience after analysing data from pharmacovigilance, EHR and real-world evidence. Probability of ADRs can be estimated using logistic regression, Naive Bayes classifiers and other methods involving age, kidney or liver function, different drug combinations and genetic differences (Duthe et al., 2021).

In addition, as more pharmacogenomic information becomes accessible, AI can help explain how our genes determine how drugs are handled and what side effects they may cause. The appearance of HLA-B57:01 is linked with a heightened risk of hypersensitivity to abacavir, a drug often used to treat AIDS. Genomic and clinical data can train AI to spot patients with high risk such markers. This allows doctors to take preventive steps to avoid severe reactions. Because treatment decisions are personalised, they are both successful and safe for each patient. This modelling approach is also valuable for organising individuals into high- or low-risk groups. Grouping patients as low, moderate or high risk for treatment failure, side effects or hospitalisation helps the hospital distribute resources more effectively. High-risk patients may get top priority for things like more cheque-ups with their clinicians, help with following therapies or therapies for mental or social issues. Automated AI tools can handle stratification by staring new data and updating patients' risk categories smartly and in real time. The difference between this strategy and the past is that it tracks changing levels in patients, unlike static clinical guidelines that can ignore more refined changes (Lainjo, 2024).

Through predictive analytics, healthcare organisations can see what the ART outcomes will likely be across different age groups, locations or in different programmes. Officials in public health can use data from simulations to predict drug use, understand how resistance might develop and forecast the effects of changes in policy. Using AI-powered simulation models, we can know what to expect from new drugs or changes in compliance ahead of actual use. As a result, predictive modelling is useful in clinical care and also manages the broad health system. Using data sent real-time by digital adherence tools, wearables and mobile health apps improves the power of predictive models. Doctors are notified when their system identifies deviations in a patient's recovery, thanks to the analysis of up-to-date data. For example, a significant drop in daily steps, less restful sleep and failing to cheque in with healthcare can lead healthcare to recommend intervention for a potential increased chance of virus recurrence (Kamal et al.,2021).

Still, predictive modelling has many obstacles to overcome in HIV care. The accuracy of a model is based largely on how good, complete and representative the data is. Lacking data, inaccurate data and not fully including women, minorities or rural regions could result in bias and reduce the ability to apply the research to most people. In addition, most of these models are shaped in well-resourced nations and may not be effective in low- and middle-income countries because of other types of care, resources and public health trends. We must also deal with how easy it is to understand the outcomes of complex AI models. Algorithms for deep learning work extremely well, but because they are difficult to understand, it is challenging to explain their reasoning. A lack of transparency may lessen how much clinicians trust the industry and cause obstacles for approving products or therapies by regulators. XAI efforts are helping to tackle the problem by inventing models that show how a prediction is arrived at and the certainty behind it. The use of SHAP and LIME allows doctors to study and approve proposed decisions before putting them to use (Lai, 2023).

Ethics are very important when using predictive models. Making sure patients agree, guarding their personal information and ensuring unbiased decisions are most important. Predictive insights should be used to support people, rather than add to the discrimination and wrong ideas still found in HIV situations. Making sure that AI tools are responsible means involving patients, clinicians, ethicists and policymakers in the process. The conclusion is that predictive modelling has greatly strengthened our efforts to deliver and improve HIV treatment. An AI tool can forecast what works well for each patient, predict risks of side effects and sort patients by risk factors to support clinical decisions and result in better outcomes. HIV care should adopt these new technologies based on their accuracy, fairness, honesty and being patient-focused as they evolve. When done right, predictive modelling can support the development of a smarter, safer and more responsive system for addressing HIV.

VII. AI IN HIV EPIDEMIC SURVEILLANCE AND PUBLIC HEALTH STRATEGY

Controlling HIV around the globe has long depended on tracking the disease, catching it early and planning ahead with public health measures. Historically, these approaches have relied upon epidemiology method, occasional surveys and a review of old medical and behaviour data. Even though they give helpful results, delays in gathering information, problems with reporting and a lack of immediate risk detection are common issues. Artificial Intelligence (AI) is transforming the way we monitor HIV, so we can track outbreaks immediately, pinpoint growing risks among people and track both stigma and awareness of HIV using digital routes (Marcus et al.,2020).

AI is being used in public health to quickly spot outbreaks of HIV. Including many different kinds of data—for example, results from clinical tests, demographics, movement patterns and information on social habits—the models detect rapidly any anomalies pointing to an increase in HIV cases. If machine learning algorithms analyse the past records of TB and look at things like increased testing positivity, more people having several STIs at once and shifts in how a region uses health services, they can recognise the signs of an upcoming TB outbreak. Because of real-time surveillance, health authorities can jump in early with testing, brief communities and start treatments before things get worse (Zeng et al.,2021).

It is very important to detect outbreaks as early as possible. Not noticing clusters of cases in their early stages can cause officials to miss their chance to treat them easily and could lead to more cases and added pressure for healthcare providers. AI accelerates how timely this information is by handling the detection and forecasting with very little human support. Under conditions where public health expertise is not sufficient, AI models function alone and issue warnings about any problems right away. In addition to identifying new outbreaks, AI makes it possible to map areas that are at risk of more cases which helps organisations distribute resources wisely. Using the methods of years past, it's difficult to catch the ongoing changes in population behaviour or the reasons for differences in health. Alternatively, with the help of AI, modellers can include numerous real-time factors, like demographics, people's wealth, education, movement patterns and behavioural risks, to help predict where the next cases might be (Tshimula et al.,2024).

It's also possible for unsupervised learning to detect that certain groups of people who face similar risks may be dispersed around the world. In the same manner, supervised models are used to estimate risk for people or populations based on historical transmission information. These tools can help public health planners decide where to put most of their HIV prevention and testing efforts. Moreover, artificial intelligence enables improved map prediction that helps in humanitarian areas and in regions that lack regular surveillance. With AI, mobile data, imagery from satellites and remote sensing can be reviewed to estimate where there are people, what infrastructure is missing and which areas might be blocked from necessary healthcare. When combined with data on HIV health, these points guide decisions about mobile clinics, harm reduction services and places to distribute treatment (Eze et al.,2024).

Because of advances in natural language processing (NLP), following and understanding public conversations about HIV has become easier today. Misinformation and negative attitudes about HIV still make it hard for programmes to prevent and treat the disease in different parts of the world. Many people do not want to face discrimination and untrue tales shared online can further spread distrust about the virus. NLP, an AI area centred on language analysis, provides resources for following, understanding and reacting to social changes as they occur. Models that use NLP can extract HIV content from Twitter, Reddit, Facebook and health forums. They can be used to tag messages as stigma, support, misinformation or awareness and they detect public attitudes. Increased use of stigmatising language or negative thoughts in an area may indicate that fewer people are testing for HIV or sticking to their HIV medication, so that measures can be taken early. In addition, examining online discussions over time shows how awareness promotion, community work and policies are effective (Xiang et al.,2022).

AI-based monitoring of social media makes awareness tracking easier and also helps us to better understand groups in society that are often not seen in traditional health surveys. Systemic prejudice and anxiety about disclosing their status often stop LGBTQ+ communities, sex workers and people who inject drugs from having their health information included in official data. Still, there is a chance that these groups express themselves more openly on anonymous parts of the web which provides a way for AI to listen sensitively and spot problems, what they don't understand and what is important to them. AI systems that do this work should follow guidelines that protect privacy and do not use digital surveillance to create more stigma or distrust. Being able to predict the major impacts of policy and intervention changes is a key asset to public health strategy. With agent-based models and reinforcement learning algorithms, it is possible to simulate the actions of individuals in a scenario such as new PrEP or testing rules and estimate how they would change transmission of infections. With these tools, policymakers can examine potential interventions online which spares them the time and money required for hands-on testing. By using predictive modelling, policymakers can expect the results of each strategy and make decisions about where to invest resources most logically (Mody et al.,2024).

Even though AI looks very promising in HIV monitoring and public health, we must keep a few factors in mind. The most important issue is making sure that the data is correctly representative. AI models that have learned from datasets without including important populations or regions can produce biased and questionable results. Therefore, we have to intentionally work towards gathering data in inclusive and diverse ways. Being upfront and easy to understand about AI models guarantees we can trust them. Black-box algorithms in public health may not be accepted by stakeholders unless their use and results are made clearly visible and easy to understand. It is also important that data privacy and governance benefits the community and is developed effectively. AI-driven real-time systems should clearly show where their data comes from and how it is used, primarily when health information or groups at risk are concerned. It is just as important that local communities help determine how these technologies are used. Using community-based participatory research models allows AI tools to be effective, culturally sensitive and ethically developed. AI is playing a major role in changing how HIV epidemic surveillance and public health strategy are implemented. With real-time outbreak detection, mapping risks before they occur and analysing social opinions, AI provides various ways to address HIV. Rather than just giving isolated accounts of infections, these capabilities let the system watch for trends and shape actions to help people. If these innovations continue to improve, ensuring they are ethical, adapted to different places and used in communities will be important for making a bigger, positive impact on the world's HIV response.

VIII. CHALLENGES AND ETHICAL CONSIDERATION

When AI is included in both HIV treatment and public health, it brings new opportunities together with many difficult challenges and ethical problems. HIV-related problems are especially difficult because stigma, discrimination and a history of exclusion still affect many people seeking care. Since AI is starting to be used for diagnosis, organising treatments, checking on patient compliance and monitoring epidemics, it is necessary to examine its use in these areas from the perspectives of privacy, fairness, accountability and transparency. Ethical AI goes beyond technology and is also a duty towards those who might be at risk in healthcare (Garett et al.,2024).

HIV puts confidentiality at the forefront and due to the sensitivity of related information, data security has become a major issue. Health information linked to HIV status, ART adherence, sexual history, comorbid illnesses and social conditions is both private and in many settings is considered strongly stigmatised. Personal and social damages can be very high when unauthorised access, data breaches or inappropriate use of such information happen to anyone. Danger is greater for people living with HIV in places where the law does not protect them, causing them to face social rejection, unemployment or attack.AI systems need lots of patient data to operate properly, mostly when building and checking tools for predictions. Yet, the finer the detail in the data, the larger the risk of someone finding out who provided it, even after anonymization. Re-identification attacks which cross-cheque various datasets to find a person's identity, are now a major concern. Because of this, we need strong data governance frameworks. Such requirements should involve the best encryption, safe storage of data, tight access rules and legally put-together agreements for exchanging data. Patients must understand exactly how their data will be dealt with and used, be able to give clear consent and keep their choice to not use their data while still receiving the same care (Nichol et al.,2021).

Using data ethically goes beyond just improving security; it needs a sense of the surrounding social and political environment. Without proper regulation, artificial intelligence tools in heavily-controlled environments could cause human rights problems. Health data gathered for health purposes could be shared with criminal prosecutors and used to target members of the LGBTQ+, sex worker or drug user communities, if proper protections connecting health care and law enforcement are absent. A further significant problem is that AI models can unwittingly make unequal health problems worse. If information included in past data shows that certain parts of the population were treated differently, AI systems have the potential to replicate those differences. If, for instance, data from the past leaves out information about women, transgender people and racial minorities, AI tools could be less dependable for them. Models designed for rich countries are likely to struggle in low- and middle-income countries because care systems, resources and people are quite different (Senel & Beka,2025).

Bias in AI doesn't always appear on the surface. Sometimes, bias appears as different prediction results, unfair recommendations for care or lack of attention to social influences on health. A model that cheques for non-adherence by using prescription refill patterns from pharmacies isn't likely to identify barriers people from rural or less prosperous areas face and might not provide support when needed. We should intentionally create such applications, verify them with different data sets and strengthen our dedication to AI that promotes fairness on a continual basis. We also need to think about how fairly people can access AI tools and what benefits they receive. A lot of AI-based healthcare technologies are first built and tested in areas with advanced technology, but later introduced in countries with less access. If tools are not adapted to local situations, they may not help those who need them, leave some people even more cut off from the digital world or leave more people at risk. Making sure AI helps everyone is important and it comes from culturally sensitive design, local collaboration and improving skills. It is just as important that AI decisions in healthcare are easy to understand and transparent. AI models can be used in ART regimen choice, drug interaction prediction and risk grouping. However, they may fail to explain why certain actions are needed. Despite reaching high accuracy, these models often go unrecognised by clinicians because the underlying reasoning is unknown and this can also make their use difficult to justify to patients. If treatment choices depend on an algorithm's output, everyone important to the patient's care should review the reasons for those decisions and their basis in clinical studies (Heerden et al.,2023).

Being transparent is important for both regulation and keeping everyone legally accountable. Tools for HIV care should be regularly checked, errors detected and harm rectified when any imperfections are found. Standards and certification should be introduced and managed for AI in healthcare that uphold the same safety, assistance and good practises as the systems now used in pharmaceuticals and medical devices. Besides, institutions need to make it possible for patients and providers to bring up concerns, reconsider algorithmic results and get the help they require. Besides what individuals do, well-developed systems are needed to make sure AI is used properly in public health. For example, oversight should include multiple stakeholders, community boards and involve PLHIV in the building, using and evaluating of these AI systems. If those most influenced by AI are represented, frameworks have a greater chance of promoting human rights, linking to people's lives and ensuring the solutions respect people's dignity and right to self-determination.AI can greatly help in improving strategies for HIV treatment and public health, but its ethical and working challenges cannot be ignored. If issues of unguarded privacy, model inequities or obscured workings are left easily, they can challenge trust, make things more unbalanced for certain groups or lead to harm. To guarantee AI is used in HIV care ethically, experts from different fields, technical fields and cultures are needed. The main point is to ensure that, while AI learns, healthcare is also made fairer, open to all and more compassionate.

IX. PRACTICAL IMPLICATION

At last week's 13th International AIDS Society Conference on HIV Science (IAS 2025) in Kigali, Rwanda, artificial intelligence (AI) was a major topic. Experts were both excited and cautious about how developments in AI and digital technology might change HIV prevention and care services. It has already been proved quite successful, with Aimee, an AI chatbot created by women in South Africa, finding over 1500 active users monthly to communicate using over 30,000 messages. Aimee was created with the aim of providing understanding, private, and reachable assistance through WhatsApp and assists the user to share their sensitive issues like the HIV virus, relationship issues, and gender-based problems. Aimee, which is based on large language models such as ChatGPT and Gemini, focuses on developing trust via sentiment detection, progressive disclosure, and active listening. Her design allows her to react to emotional indicators- she listens more when users are upset and refers them to health practitioners where required. The statistics indicate that most of the users open over time, and the discussion is not on superficial questions but on personal issues, which result in significant behavioural outcomes, including, but not limited to, the adoption of associated health services in a quarter of users. By comparison, the Canadian chatbot MARVIN, which is an HIV self-management, has been improved to recognize and address emotional distress or academic language. The earlier versions have restricted responding to such messages, particularly self-harm or insults but the new MARVINs have demonstrated a high level of accuracy up to 95 percent in categorizing and responding to such messages according to their harm or insult character hence the safety and supportive attitude. Both Aimee and MARVIN show the increased importance of empathic AI in establishing trust, fostering mental health, and changing healthcare communication (Samuel n.d.,).

X. CONCLUSION

AI is adding unmatched efficiency, individualised care and prediction qualities to all aspects of treating HIV patients. AI is helping clinicians to detect problems faster and develop ART therapies that meet each person's individual needs. Regular monitoring with wireless devices, forecasts about disease outcomes and the use of AI in epidemic monitoring have together changed how HIV is handled and understood. At the same time, while we have many AI options, the real success in applying it to HIV care comes from ensuring ethical, inclusive and transparent health systems are put in place. Data privacy, removing bias from AI models and making AI decisions easy to understand are necessary to win the trust of patients and providers. It is important to ensure AI is available to all so that current differences in HIV results are not furthered. Effective future outcomes in AI-supported HIV care will rely on how strongly technologists, clinicians, public health experts, patients and policymakers can collaborate. For AI solutions to be useful, reliable and responsible, experts from different fields must work together. Since we are at the meeting point of new technologies and health equity, AI should be used to improve, open up and protect HIV care for all people.

REFERENCES

Bekker, L. G., Beyrer, C., Mgodi, N., Lewin, S. R., Delany-Moretlwe, S., Taiwo, B., & Lazarus, J. V. (2023). HIV infection. *Nature Reviews. Disease Primers*, *9*(1), 42. PMID: 37591865

Duthe, J. C., Bouzille, G., Sylvestre, E., Chazard, E., Arvieux, C., & Cuggia, M. (2021). How to identify potential candidates for HIV pre-exposure prophylaxis: An AI algorithm reusing real-world hospital data. In *Public Health and Informatics* (pp. 714–718). IOS Press.

Eissa, M. E. (2025). A BRIEF OVERVIEW OF HIV TREATMENT STRATEGIES: A FOCUSED LOOK AT CHALLENGES AND OPPORTUNITIES. *Universal Journal of Pharmaceutical Research.*

Eze, C. E., Igwama, G. T., Nwankwo, E. I., & Victor, E. (2024). AI-driven health data analytics for early detection of infectious diseases: A conceptual exploration of US public health strategies.

Fieggen, J., Smith, E., Arora, L., & Segal, B. (2022). The role of machine learning in HIV risk prediction. *Frontiers in Reproductive Health*, *4*, 1062387. PMID: 36619681

Garett, R., Kim, S., & Young, S. D. (2024). Ethical Considerations for Artificial Intelligence Applications for HIV. *AI*, *5*(2), 594–601.

Jin, R., & Zhang, L. (2025). AI applications in HIV research: Advances and future directions. *Frontiers in Microbiology*, *16*, 1541942. PMID: 40051479

Kamal, S., Urata, J., Cavassini, M., Liu, H., Kouyos, R., Bugnon, O., & Schneider, M. P. (2021). Random forest machine learning algorithm predicts virologic outcomes among HIV infected adults in Lausanne, Switzerland using electronically monitored combined antiretroviral treatment adherence. *AIDS Care*, *33*(4), 530–536. PMID: 32266825

Keddem, S., Agha, A., Morawej, S., Buck, A., Cronholm, P., Sonalkar, S., & Kearney, M. (2023). Characterizing Twitter Content about HIV Pre-exposure Prophylaxis (PrEP) for women: Qualitative content analysis. *Journal of Medical Internet Research*, *25*, e43596. PMID: 37166954

Koh, M. C. Y., Ngiam, J. N., Yong, J., Tambyah, P. A., & Archuleta, S. (2024). The role of an artificial intelligence model in antiretroviral therapy counselling and advice for people living with HIV. *HIV Medicine*, *25*(4), 504–508. PMID: 38169077

Kumbale, C. M., & Voit, E. O. (2021). Toward personalized medicine for HIV/AIDS. *Journal of AIDS and HIV treatment, 3*(2), 37.

Lai, J. (2023). Developing a predictive information system for determining the prognosis of HIV and tuberculosis co-infection in incarcerated individuals. *International Journal for Applied Information Management*, *3*(2), 101–110.

Lainjo, B. (2024). Original Research Article Artificial intelligence with machine learning and the enigmatic discovery of HIV cure. *Journal of Autonomous Intelligence*, *7*(2).

Liu, A. Y., Laborde, N. D., Coleman, K., Vittinghoff, E., Gonzalez, R., Wilde, G., & Buchbinder, S. (2021). DOT diary: Developing a novel mobile app using artificial intelligence and an electronic sexual diary to measure and support PrEP adherence among young men who have sex with men. *AIDS and Behavior*, *25*, 1001–1012. PMID: 33044687

Ma, Y., Achiche, S., Tu, G., Vicente, S., Lessard, D., Engler, K., & Lebouché, B. (2025). The first AI-based Chatbot to promote HIV self-management: A mixed methods usability study. *HIV Medicine*, *26*(2), 184–206. PMID: 39390632

Marcus, J. L., Sewell, W. C., Balzer, L. B., & Krakower, D. S. (2020). Artificial intelligence and machine learning for HIV prevention: Emerging approaches to ending the epidemic. *Current HIV/AIDS Reports*, *17*, 171–179. PMID: 32347446

Maskew, M., Sharpey-Schafer, K., De Voux, L., Crompton, T., Bor, J., Rennick, M., & Pisa, P. (2022). Applying machine learning and predictive modeling to retention and viral suppression in South African HIV treatment cohorts. *Scientific Reports*, *12*(1), 12715. PMID: 35882962

Mereu, A., Liori, A., Fadda, L., Puddu, M., Chessa, L., Contu, P., & Sardu, C. (2022). What do young people know about HIV? Results of a cross sectional study on 18-24-year-old students. *Journal of Preventive Medicine and Hygiene*, *63*(4), E541. PMID: 36891004

Mody, A., Sohn, A. H., Iwuji, C., Tan, R. K., Venter, F., & Geng, E. H. (2024). HIV epidemiology, prevention, treatment, and implementation strategies for public health. *Lancet*, *403*(10425), 471–492. PMID: 38043552

Nichol, A. A., Bendavid, E., Mutenherwa, F., Patel, C., & Cho, M. K. (2021). Diverse experts' perspectives on ethical issues of using machine learning to predict HIV/AIDS risk in sub-Saharan Africa: A modified Delphi study. *BMJ Open*, *11*(7), e052287. PMID: 34321310

Obeagu, E. I., Ubosi, N. I., Obeagu, G. U., & Akram, M. (2024). Early Infant Diagnosis: Key to Breaking the Chain of HIV Transmission. *Elite Journal of Public Health*, *2*(1), 52–61.

Olaboye, J. A., Maha, C. C., Kolawole, T. O., & Abdul, S. (2024). Artificial intelligence in monitoring HIV treatment adherence: A conceptual exploration. *International Medical Science Research Journal*, *4*(6), 681–692.

Padhi, A., Agarwal, A., Saxena, S. K., & Katoch, C. D. S. (2023). Transforming clinical virology with AI, machine learning and deep learning: A comprehensive review and outlook. *Virusdisease*, *34*(3), 345–355. PMID: 37780897

Periáñez, Á., Schmitz, K., Makhupula, L., Hassan, M., Moleko, M., del Río, A. F., . . . Tang, D. (2024). Optimizing HIV Patient Engagement with Reinforcement Learning in Resource-Limited Settings. *arXiv preprint arXiv:2408.07629.*

Roche, S. D., Ekwunife, O. I., Mendonca, R., Kwach, B., Omollo, V., Zhang, S., & Ortblad, K. F. (2024). Measuring the performance of computer vision artificial intelligence to interpret images of HIV self-testing results. *Frontiers in Public Health*, *12*, 1334881. PMID: 38384878

Sah, A. K., Elshaikh, R. H., Shalabi, M. G., Abbas, A. M., Prabhakar, P. K., Babker, A. M., & Agarwal, S. (2025). Role of Artificial Intelligence and Personalized Medicine in Enhancing HIV Management and Treatment Outcomes. *Life (Chicago, Ill.)*, *15*(5), 745. PMID: 40430173

Samuel, K. (n.d.). *Stepping into the AI-driven future of HIV prevention and care*. Aidsmap.com. Retrieved October 18, 2025, from https://www.aidsmap.com/news/jul-2025/stepping-ai-driven-future-hiv-prevention-and-care

Seboka, B. T., Yehualashet, D. E., & Tesfa, G. A. (2023). Artificial intelligence and machine learning based prediction of viral load and CD4 status of people living with HIV (PLWH) on anti-retroviral treatment in Gedeo Zone Public Hospitals. *International Journal of General Medicine*, , 435–451. PMID: 36760682

Sekandi, J. N., Shi, W., Zhu, R., Kaggwa, P., Mwebaze, E., & Li, S. (2023). Application of artificial intelligence to the monitoring of medication adherence for tuberculosis treatment in Africa: Algorithm development and validation. *JMIR AI*, *2*(1), e40167. PMID: 38464947

Sekandi, J. N., Shi, W., Zhu, R., Kaggwa, P., Mwebaze, E., & Li, S. (2023). Application of artificial intelligence to the monitoring of medication adherence for tuberculosis treatment in Africa: Algorithm development and validation. *JMIR AI*, *2*(1), e40167. PMID: 38464947

Senel, B., & Beka, H. (2025). Artificial Intelligence in HIV Diagnosis and Treatment: A Comprehensive Review. *Cumhuriyet Medical Journal*, *47*(1), 10–21.

Srivastava, S. (2018, February 15). How is AI in Healthcare Transforming the Industry? *Appinventiv*. https://appinventiv.com/blog/ai-in-healthcare/

Stoner, M. C., Maragh-Bass, A. C., Sukhija-Cohen, A. C., & Saberi, P. (2022). Digital directly observed therapy to monitor adherence to medications: A scoping review. *HIV Research & Clinical Practice*, *23*(1), 47–60. PMID: 35904111

Tshimula, J. M., Kalengayi, M., Makenga, D., Lilonge, D., Asumani, M., Madiya, D., . . . Kasoro, N. M. (2024). Artificial Intelligence for Public Health Surveillance in Africa: Applications and Opportunities. *arXiv preprint arXiv:2408.02575*.

Whiteley, L. B., Olsen, E. M., Haubrick, K. K., Odoom, E., Tarantino, N., & Brown, L. K. (2021). A review of interventions to enhance HIV medication adherence. *Current HIV/AIDS Reports*, *18*(5), 443–457. PMID: 34152554

Williams, E., Moso, M., Lim, C., Chibo, D., Nicholson, S., Jackson, K., & Williamson, D. A. (2023). Laboratory diagnosis of HIV: A contemporary overview in the Australian context. *Pathology*, *55*(5), 610–620. PMID: 37302942

Xiang, Y., Du, J., Fujimoto, K., Li, F., Schneider, J., & Tao, C. (2022). Application of artificial intelligence and machine learning for HIV prevention interventions. *The Lancet. HIV*, *9*(1), e54–e62. PMID: 34762838

Zeng, D., Cao, Z., & Neill, D. B. (2021). Artificial intelligence–enabled public health surveillance—from local detection to global epidemic monitoring and control. In *Artificial intelligence in medicine* (pp. 437–453). Academic Press.

Chapter 6
Impact of Digital Tools and Healthcare Technology in Enhancing HIV Treatment and Monitoring

S. Srinivasan
https://orcid.org/0009-0002-0179-9849
Department of Humanities and Social Sciences, Graphic Era University, Dehradun, India

R. Vallipriya
https://orcid.org/0009-0008-6692-603X
Department of Biochemistry and Biotechnology, Pavendar Bharathidasan College of Arts and Science, Bharathidasan University, Tiruchirappalli, India

Ajay Kumar Singh
https://orcid.org/0000-0003-0429-0925
Department of Humanities and Social Sciences, Graphic Era University, Dehradun, India

ABSTRACT

HIV remains a significant global public health concern, with nearly 39.9 million people affected worldwide by the end of 2023. Although there is no cure, early diagnosis, antiretroviral therapy (ART), and patient monitoring can improve life expectancy and reduce transmission. This study aims to assess the utilization of healthcare services, welfare benefits, and patient monitoring systems for HIV-infected individuals. Conducted in Trichy District, Tamil Nadu, the study used a

DOI: 10.4018/979-8-3373-2863-8.ch006

descriptive, cross-sectional design with a sample size of 90 HIV-infected individuals receiving treatment adherence in ICTCs. The study highlights gaps in healthcare technology, treatment management, and welfare assistance, particularly for marginalized communities. The findings aim to enhance treatment adherence, improve patient outcomes, and promote equitable access to services through technological interventions. The study recommends policy formulation, livelihood training, and awareness programs to improve the quality of life for HIV-affected individuals and reduce associated stigma.

INTRODUCTION

HIV remains a major global public health challenge, with an estimated 42.3 million people living with the infection worldwide (Achwoka, 2021) HIV can be prevented through diagnosis and by providing proper treatment and care, which can help manage opportunistic infections. HIV is a chronic health condition that can enable people living with HIV to have a long-term life expectancy (Masur et al., 2002). WHO, the Global Fund, and UNAIDS are working globally to reduce HIV. They are implementing multiple strategies to achieve HIV reduction as per the SDG target, which aims to end the HIV epidemic by 2030 (Assembly, 2021).

There will be people living with HIV in 2025, and 95% of them are expected to be diagnosed, with 95% receiving lifesaving ART therapy that can protect HIV-affected persons. People living with HIV, nearly 95% of whom are receiving treatment to achieve suppressed viral load, can benefit in terms of health and reduce HIV transmission (Laar, 2022). In 2023, the percentages respectively increased to 86%, 89%, and 93%. People living with HIV, nearly in 2023, had an HIV status known to 86% of them, 77% received ART, and 72% had suppressed viral loads. Human immunodeficiency virus (HIV) is a virus that attacks the human body, weakening the immune system (Haris & Abbas, 2024). In the advanced stage of infection, it becomes acquired immunodeficiency syndrome (AIDS). HIV targets the human body's white blood cells, which can decrease the immune system (German Advisory Committee Blood, 2016). This can increase diseases like TB and other kinds of infections, and sometimes it can also affect cancer. HIV can spread through body fluids and can affect an uninfected person (Bekker et al., 2023). It can include blood, breast milk, semen, and vaginal fluids. It does not spread through touching, kissing, hugging, living in the same places, or sharing food items. This can spread from a mother to her baby, but it can be prevented in the early stage. HIV can be prevented through ART, but if left untreated, it can lead to AIDS after many years (Posse et al., 2017). As per WHO's definition, advanced HIV disease (AHD) is identified when the CD4 cell count is less than 5 cells/mm^3 and classified as stage 3 or 4 in adults and adolescents (Mulumba et al., 2025). There are children under 5 years old living with HIV who can receive advanced HIV disease treatment (Nalwanga & Musiime, 2022).

AIDS is a major threat to public health. It is one of the most infectious diseases in the pandemic era of the late 20th and 21st centuries across the globe. This can improve the utilization of health services provided (Bloom & Cadarette, 2019). As per the WHO report and the Global HIV program, an initiative was launched for monitoring HIV-affected patients and ensuring the quality of care for their treatment. To provide service delivery for HIV services, it integrates HIV and TB, which can affect maternal women and children, ensuring safety for newborns in healthcare services. The HIV patient monitoring system can prevent severe illness in HIV patients and provide standardized treatment (McIntyre, 2005; Hawkins et al., 2005; Mutabazi et al., 2017).

Impact of Case Management on HIV Support Services

The case management of HIV-affected patients, when handled by healthcare workers, follows certain strategies to reduce unwanted outcomes and support their needs and services (Poindexter, 2010). The ambulatory services are provided at a lower cost for HIV-infected persons. This can showcase the HIV-affected persons with the support to receive the benefits of advocacy, psychological, and emotional services for HIV-infected persons. The previous study examined that providing proper counseling can benefit the infected person, improve treatment outcomes, and ensure they follow the record receipt of counseling sessions (Land, 2015). The infected person receives the receipt for Medicaid, and it can provide a record and case management system. The digital technology is used to store all the history of the patients' records, notified by the computer, and able to follow the periodical check-up. Whether they are regularly coming for the treatment, the previous visits are able to be tracked and monitored for the HIV-infected person (Singh et al., 2019; Mudrick et al., 2020; Herman, 2021).

Natural History of HIV infection

HIV-infected persons, their T cells help to find the macrophages, and the dendritic cells can identify the CD4 and chemokine for their organ. The early infection provides the targets for CCR5; it can provide the macrophages and the dendritic cells (Barmania & Pepper, 2013). This can provide the affected individual with CCR5, and for the polymorphism, there is 1% of the population that has protection. The HIV-affected persons have a high viral load; this can replicate to a detectable RNA viral level (Ji, 2007). The virus can provide antigens like p24. This can explain that viraemia indicates a response due to cytotoxic T cells, which has implications for non-lytic inhibition and the depletion of target cells; for the outcome, partial CD4+ recovery is required (Morvan et al., 2021). The study provides that replication continues in lymphoid tissue, leading to an increase in viraemia as the process progresses. The study provides a comprehensive understanding of the virus's plasma; it shows a half-life of two days, which indicates increased production and clearance (Dandri et al., 2008). Mutation can be driven by error-prone reverse transcription, leading to increased drug resistance and immune evasion; for example, mutated p24 can improve CXCR4 binding, enhancing CD4+ T cell infection (Madapuji Srinivasan, 2024). T cells provide the loss of syncytium formation, which can increase apoptosis in both thymic and peripheral regions, leading to increased T cell loss and causing impairment. The model provides a reflection of the in vivo outcome, showing falling CD4 counts and rising viral load, with up to 10^{10} HIV-infected persons producing 10^{8} CD4+ T cells lost in daily life (Février et al., 2011; Van der Berg, 2021; Westerdijk, 2024) .

Immune Monitoring

To monitor CD4 counts, the advanced stage of flow cytometry with monoclonal antibodies can provide the CD4+ T cell count and monitor the immune system. The CD4 count increases the CD4 percentage, and it can provide the CD4:CD8 ratio; it can be used in clinical studies to increase trial use. CD4:CD8 ratio can be improved by the physiological CD8+ expansions; it increases during HIV infection (Pattanapanyasat & Thakar, 2005; Li et al., 2023) . As per the increase in the cytometer, the increase in cell population is based on the size and is stained with fluorochrome-tagged antibodies. The early method used was the two-platform method; the CD4 level increased in percentage (Fedr et al., 2023). This means cytometry was used for lymphocytes in hematology, and with the increase in lymphocyte counts, it was called CD4 counts increase. These are methods that pose errors, such as calling non-lymphoid cells during manual gating (Vlad, 2019; McIntyre, 2024). These were caused by the following factors:

Double staining with CD3 and CD4/CD8 to exclude monocytes (CD3− CD4+) and NK cells (CD3− CD8+);

Two-colour cytometry using CD45+ and excluding CD14+ to purify lymphocyte populations (requires extra steps);

Three-colour cytometry using CD45 and side scatter for more accurate lymphocyte gating.[REMOVED HYPERLINK FIELD]

Virological Monitoring

The viral load is measured based on quantitative RT-PCR; it has been a strong predictor of HIV disease progression. The level more than 10^5 copies per ml ($\log_{10}$ 5.0) within six months of seroconversion increases the 10-fold risk over five years (Omondi et al., 2021). The patients are normal, the CD4 counts increase, and the signal viral load impacts the prediction of long-term treatment outcomes. The viral load provides a more effective measure for long-term prognosis, and it can indicate CD4 level increase better than risk (Korenromp et al., 2009). To reduce the viral load, the progress level should slowly decrease in alignment and there is a need to develop effective treatment. This study examines the patient's HAART level and viral load as the best way to predict survival; a level $< 10^5$/ml is connected with a delay in AIDS progression. This can impact the viral load test in central treatment adherence and monitoring support services (Drain et al., 2019; Balsamo, 2021; Pham et al., 2022) .

Viral load assays involve three factors to measure the viral RNA.

Quantitative RT–PCR converts viral RNA into DNA for quantification.

Monitoring Patients with HIV Disease

To monitor a person with HIV infection, it is important to prolong age, detect early diagnosis, provide on-time regular treatment, and avoid the spread of the infection, as it can cause opportunistic conditions. Immuno monitoring system to improve timely prophylaxis can reduce morbidity level (Nikolopoulos & Tsantes, 2022). The ART evolved for the challenges of the resistance level. This can increase the treatment regimen, the reason for the guidelines to provide the laboratory treatment, and it can establish the standard way (Zolopa, 2010). This existing literature provides the HIV history details, and it can provide a clear idea about the immunological and virological testing mechanisms and provide the monitoring recommendations. The recent literature review provides the effect of case management and provides the healthcare services to increase the HIV patients at the country level (WHO, 2021). The ART and prophylactic treatment reduce the mortality and morbidity rate. The case management impacts the unmet needs for healthcare services and supports the use and recommendation for HIV-infected persons over time (Meya et al., 2022).

Viral Load (VL) Monitoring Uptake

The study provides a comprehensive understanding of 12 relevant studies documented for the VL monitoring rate, nearly providing 11 intakes over 12 months of regular follow-up. There is a median level of 86%, with high levels reported in South

Africa and Kenya, where the majority—92% and 99% uptake respectively—was supported by dedicated research staff (Koss et al., 2020). The least value is 14.3%, which is retrospective for the rural area from Thailand where routine VL testing is not available (Kawichai et al., 2005). The study understands the centralized and decentralized care model for high levels of VL monitoring — it is centralized 99% vs 91%, and the lowest range is 29% vs 14%. This shows better uptake for the decentralized care support at 92% vs 90% and 61% vs 14% (Pham et al., 2017). In South Africa, the decentralized program is supported by NGOs, volunteer organizations, and positive networks to provide positive results. Finally, the study provides a clear understanding that the clinic offers higher Viral Load monitoring based on over 80% of the patients having VL after 6 to 24 months of treatment in South Africa (Tsondai, 2016).

Monitor and Evaluate Treatment Monitoring Challenges

Technology and Monitoring in Decentralized Care

The technology plays a vital role for affected persons with HIV in the treatment adherence monitoring process in decentralized settings. This can provide the centric care like point-of-care testing; this provides a lab to monitor for the ART patients (Plebani et al., 2025; Srinivasan, 2025). VL monitoring faces challenges without POC testing, and it can increase the requirement for effective sample collection, testing, and transport for the facility to get to know the result or diagnosis details (Lakshmanan & Liu, 2025). The CD4 can monitor the POC advanced technologies; it can be used for the decentralized private clinics, and this can provide reliable results. The improvement for the patient retention is compared with the testing based on lab testing (Heidt et al., 2020).

Human Resource Constraints

Challenges in Task-Shifting and Treatment Monitoring

There are challenges for the regular and routine monitoring by health professionals such as trained ART doctors to scale up the ART. This can lead to increasing tasks for physicians and nurses. The approach helps to expand access and represents support for HIV treatment and challenges in monitoring infected patients (Hermann et al., 2009). The primary care services provide the nurses and counselors to interact with patients and provide motivational talk to support the affected individuals. This can provide better patient care, and this can increase treatment adherence in the continuous process (Zuckoff, 2012; Searight, 2018). The regular monitoring is a challenging task; there are some staff nurses unable to provide the services and unable to refer patients, and this can cause treatment failure (Iedema et al., 2012). This may cause two VL test results, and it also indicates failure. The lack of training and lack of confidence to interpret the VL, and the inability to manage the data for the second-line therapy for the affected individual, are challenges for the healthcare workers (Kalemeera et al., 2022). Second-line therapy ART provides the effort for treatment adherence, and it can signal the uncertainty of the clinical conditions. To switching the treatment adherence for the risk ineffective for second-line outcomes. The critical issues address the limited treatment and low cost for the second and third line regiments (Hoffmann et al., 2023).

BACKGROUND

HIV treatment has evolved significantly with advances in digital healthcare technologies (Singh et al., 2025). Despite this, the global HIV burden remains a major public health challenge, particularly in developing countries (Banda, 2024; Srinivasan, 2025). Digital healthcare provides better health interventions to increase better solutions for treatment adherence and monitoring for patient engagement (Nyamboga & Obeagu, 2024). The digital tools provide support for HIV treatment in various aspects to help—mobile health (mHealth), telemedicine support, electronic health record services (EHRs), AI-driven support and diagnosis for HIV treatment—and AI can support laser operations and treatment plans (Beecroft et al., 2024). It can provide real-time support to monitor affected HIV patients. The technology enhances communication between patients and health professionals, and also healthcare workers.

This can increase better understanding. To improve the rapport and continue hospital visits, support the decision-making process, and increase treatment on time and on a regular basis. To provide virtual counseling and address Adverse Drug Reaction (ADR) issues, and for patients to get clarifications (Vallée, & Arutkin, 2024). The virtual communication provides the patient regular treatment and reduces the viral load complications for people living with HIV (PLHIV). The government and non-governmental organizations support and provide digital health innovation in the broader spectrum of public health. The digital health advancement provides digital literacy, data accuracy, strengthens the infrastructure, and supports equitable access for rural and underserved communities. The impact of digital healthcare technology is to enhance HIV treatment and monitor outcomes. To transform HIV care and service delivery to provide a better understanding for the healthcare settings (Cuadros et al., 2024).

HIV remains a major global health challenge, with 38 million people affected worldwide and 2.4 million in India. Despite ART progress, barriers like limited access, stigma, and poor adherence remain. Digital tools—mobile apps, telemedicine, EHRs, and SMS reminders—support awareness, testing, adherence, and monitoring, improving HIV care outcomes.

OBJECTIVES

- To assess the utilization of services and the medical care support received by HIV-infected persons.
- To find out the various welfare benefits and support received by HIV patients from the government and non-governmental organizations.
- To identify effective HIV treatment and patient monitoring systems.
- To know the benefits of healthcare technology for HIV-affected patients in multiple aspects.

RESEARCH QUESTIONS

1. How are they utilizing health services while living with HIV-infected persons?
2. What are the types of medical services and medical care support received by HIV-infected persons?
3. What are the HIV treatment methods that are more effective and improve patient outcomes?
4. How does it provide an effective patient monitoring system for HIV management?
5. What are the types of welfare assistance benefits and support that living with HIV patients receive from government services?
6. How do HIV patients benefit from various assistance and support provided by non-governmental organizations?
7. How does it enhance healthcare technology to improve outcomes for HIV-affected patients?
8. What are the healthcare technologies to increase the quality of life for HIV-affected patients?

RELEVANT LITERATURE

Health Care Utilization in HIV-Infected Households

HIV (Human Immunodeficiency Virus) affected for those who have low level immune system this is can target for the CD4 cells it is left and untreated. AIDS (Acquired Immunodeficiency Syndrome) is the stage when damage to the immune system increases. People living with HIV need support from family members for caregiving. This can influence the health services to be properly utilized within the household. When an HIV-affected person needs a long-term life, they can take lifetime antiretroviral therapy (ART) to control the virus and maintain the immunity level in the body (Land, 2015). This can include regular and routine checks for the viral load as well as the CD4 counts. Mental health needs to be enhanced to cope with situational stress and stigma for HIV-affected individuals. This can increase the opportunity for diseases like TB and pneumonia (Obeagu & Obeagu, 2024). Due to an HIV-affected person, the family members are often impacted. This needs to be addressed by providing awareness to close contacts and family members about the consequences of HIV risk. This can lead to providing regular counseling support and reducing the need for PrEP and PEP. The infected person faces lots of fear and stigma. This can increase the need for care and support for the vulnerable and neglected communities (Sousa et al., 2021). They can face the problem of financial burden for the treatment and drug adverse reactions (ADR). This complication they can face additionally when they want to buy drugs and medicines, and they need to increase their immune system. They eat some healthy food for that and need financial support (Keter, 2023). The public health perspective is to integrate the support for the patient and their family, to support and increase the community outreach activities to reduce the stigma level. To provide the policy and promote household-centered HIV care, it is crucial for the affected individual. HIV-affected persons can manage the household. This can address the gaps in medical, psychological, and economic needs for the HIV-infected person and improve stigma-free healthcare services (Nkambule, 2022).

Health Care Services and Support for HIV-Infected People

HIV-infected persons receive medical care and services. This can aim to manage the virus level and maintain overall healthcare services. The core service is Antiretroviral Therapy (ART); this helps to suppress the virus and strengthen the immune system. To regularly monitor the required healthcare services and detect the viral load and CD4 count, it is related to health issues (Obeagu, 2024). There is a high probability for opportunistic infections such as TB, fungal infections, and other related diseases like pneumonia (Srinivasan, & Praba Lama, 2025).

Effective Treatment Improving Outcomes

Effective HIV treatment depends on Antiretroviral Therapy (ART). This can involve a combination of medical support, and it can suppress the virus to prevent the disease and increase the immune system. The modern ART provides integrase strand transfer inhibitors (INSTIs); it can be combined with nucleoside reverse transcriptase inhibitors (NRTIs) (Zhao et al., 2022).

Maintain an Effective HIV Patient Monitoring System

The early screening and creation of awareness help reduce opportunistic infections, drug resistance, and co-morbid diseases, and can provide early intervention services. Electronic health records (EHRs) and mobile health clinics (mHealth) help in tracking patient records and providing a continuous monitoring system (Armstead et al., 2021). This can provide healthcare workers with a systematic way, such as on-time reminders and communication between healthcare workers and affected individuals. The counseling provides psychological well-being improvement and offers comprehensive system improvement. This can emphasize patient-centered care service support for PLHIV individuals (Chinyandura et al., 2022).

Welfare Assistance Programs for HIV Patients

PLHIV persons receive various welfare assistance from the government, which can increase their health and well-being. The services provide vocational training support and livelihood support (Hosaka et al., 2021). This can provide subsidized antiretroviral therapy (ART) through public healthcare service support facilities for regular health check-ups and ongoing treatment. The government also provides nutritional support, transport allowances, and financial support. This can support vulnerable PLHIV individuals. The affected individuals who have disabilities receive pension support (Amadhila & Shawapala, 2022). This service is more useful during times of illness. To provide psycho-social support, counseling services, and legal support against stigma and discrimination. The affected individual may benefit from housing assistance support, skill development events, and employment opportunities. This can improve the quality of life (Greifinger & Dick, 2011). The central government provides affected PLHIV with train fare reduction and concession support. The financial support of Rs. 1000 per month can be availed, which is more useful for the PLHIV. These are the benefits to increase continuity of care and support, reduce economic hardship, and increase social inclusion for PLHIV individuals; finally, it can improve their quality of life (Odame-Takyi, 2016).

Aid and Support are Provided by Non-Governmental Organizations for HIV Patients

There are some volunteer organizations that provide support and services for PLHIV individuals. This can be done with the help of government funding to offer a wide range of services. This can include various awareness programs and screening tests in peripheral areas and provide free-of-cost testing and counseling services (Cornman et al., 2005). This can attribute the antiretroviral medication to the concerned health departments. NGOs provide support services for affected individuals such as psycho-social support, peer counseling, and strengthening and creating support group networks. This can help individuals who are affected to cope with the situation and address stigma and mental health challenges (Mlambo, 2021). There are many Non-Governmental Organizations that provide affected individuals with nutritional support, home-based services, and transport to healthcare facilities through mobile clinics and counseling services in a home-based system. NGOs advocate for the rights of PLHIV and provide legal assistance (Olaleye et al., 2023). This can address their problems and barriers with the support services. The community engagement activities aim to promote awareness among the general public and reduce the stigma faced by HIV-affected individuals. This can improve the quality of life of PLHIV and the overall well-being of affected individuals (Hlaing, 2024).

Cost-effectiveness and Sustainability

Economic feasibility of digital HIV interventions was assessed via cost-effectiveness and budget-impact analyses from healthcare payer and societal perspectives over 10 years (3% discount rate). Outcomes included QALYs and HIV cascade indicators such as retention and viral suppression. Costs encompassed start-up, operational, and health system expenses. Sensitivity analyses tested uncertainties, while a 5-year budget-impact assessment estimated scale-up requirements. Implementation and sustainability were guided by NASSS, RE-AIM/PRISM, and WHO Digital Health Strategy, focusing on governance, financing, workforce capacity, and interoperability (Gashu, 2024).

ETHICAL CONSIDERATIONS

Data privacy and digital tracking for vulnerable HIV populations were carefully managed. Tools used secure, encrypted storage, unique identifiers, and role-based access. Informed consent explained data usage, tracking, and withdrawal rights. Systems adhered to national laws and WHO ethics guidance, ensuring confidentiality, autonomy, and equitable access, with continuous monitoring for breaches (Tiffin et al., 2019).

Influence of Digital Tools on HIV Care

Digital technologies support all HIV treatment stages. In diagnosis, mobile apps and reporting systems enhance awareness, self-testing, and linkage to care. For adherence, SMS reminders, apps, and telehealth improve medication intake, engagement, and identification of non-compliance. Monitoring and follow-up via EHRs and remote tracking enable timely interventions, better viral load monitoring, and reduced loss to follow-up, improving continuity of care and outcomes, especially in rural settings (Jones-Esan et al., 2024; Rosen et al., 2024; Peeriga & Manubolu, 2025).

Figure 1. Influence of digital tools on HIV treatment stages

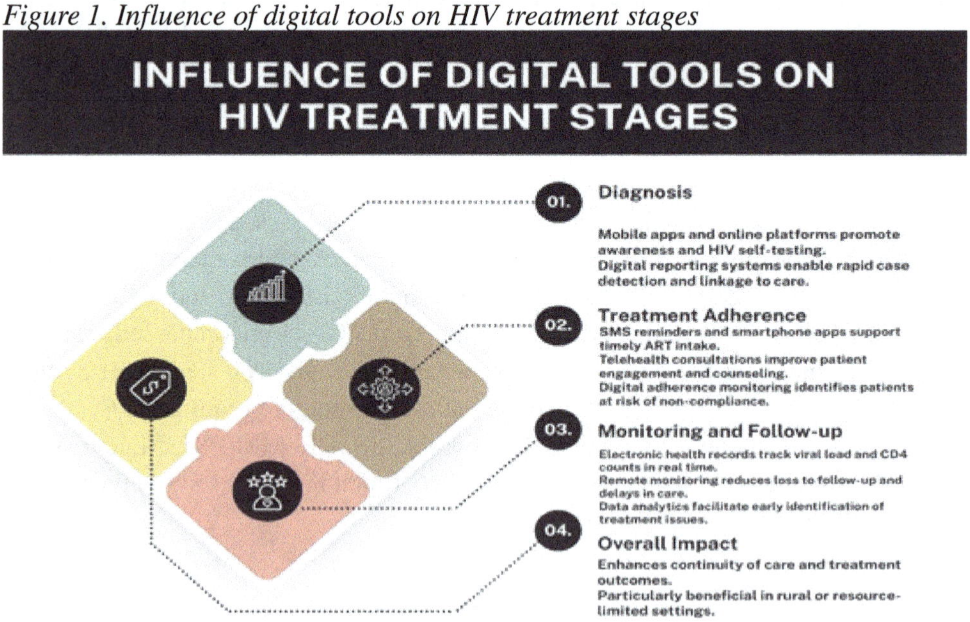

Telehealth Scalability in HIV Care

Telehealth enhances HIV care continuity and adherence but faces scalability challenges due to poor digital infrastructure, limited broadband, and weak policy support. Expanding connectivity, affordable devices, and interoperable platforms via public–private partnerships can strengthen community-based HIV programs (Ezenwaji et al., 2025).

Integration Challenges within Legacy Healthcare Systems

Outdated systems lack interoperability and secure data-sharing, hindering coordinated HIV care. Modernizing EHRs, adopting cloud-based solutions, and aligning data protection policies are vital. National initiatives should promote seamless telehealth integration with traditional HIV surveillance (Bhardwaj et al., 2024).

Training Gaps among Rural Healthcare Workers

Limited digital literacy restricts telehealth adoption. Regular training, certification, and mentorship, along with integration into medical curricula, enhance workforce preparedness and long-term scalability (Hilty et al., 2020).

Interoperability and Digital Literacy

Interoperable systems enable seamless patient data exchange, while digital literacy among providers and patients ensures proper use of telehealth tools, improving efficiency, access, and sustainability, especially in resource-limited settings (Cuadros et al., 2024).

Promoting Equitable HIV Telehealth Access

Elderly, uneducated, and remote populations face digital exclusion due to low literacy, poor connectivity, and unaffordable devices. Community-based training, simplified platforms, and targeted outreach improve inclusivity and care adherence (Miriti et al., 2025; Mekonnen, 2024).

Comparing Centralized and Decentralized HIV Care Models

Centralized models offer streamlined data management but may limit remote access. Decentralized models improve local engagement but face interoperability challenges. Hybrid approaches integrating both can optimize reach, ART retention, viral suppression, and equitable access (Liang et al., 2024; Fox et al., 2019).

METHODS

The study used a descriptive, cross-sectional design to examine healthcare utilization, medical support, and welfare benefits for HIV-affected individuals, focusing on treatment adherence, patient monitoring, and healthcare technology. Data were collected from 90 purposively sampled HIV-infected individuals across five blocks in Trichy District, Tamil Nadu, using a structured questionnaire. Analysis was conducted with SPSS v21, including descriptive statistics, frequencies, factor analysis, and chi-square tests. Consent and confidentiality were ensured, with permissions obtained from participants and the ICTC team.

Figure 2. Trichy district block wise map is covered

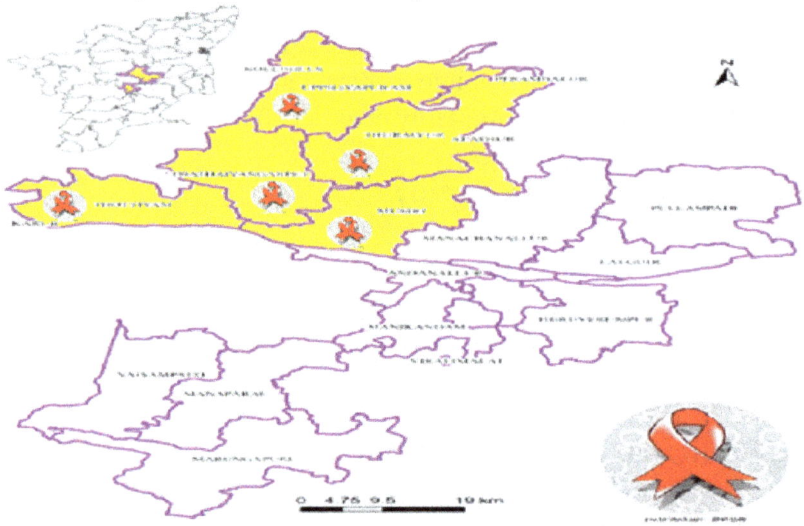

RESULT

Figure 3. Age

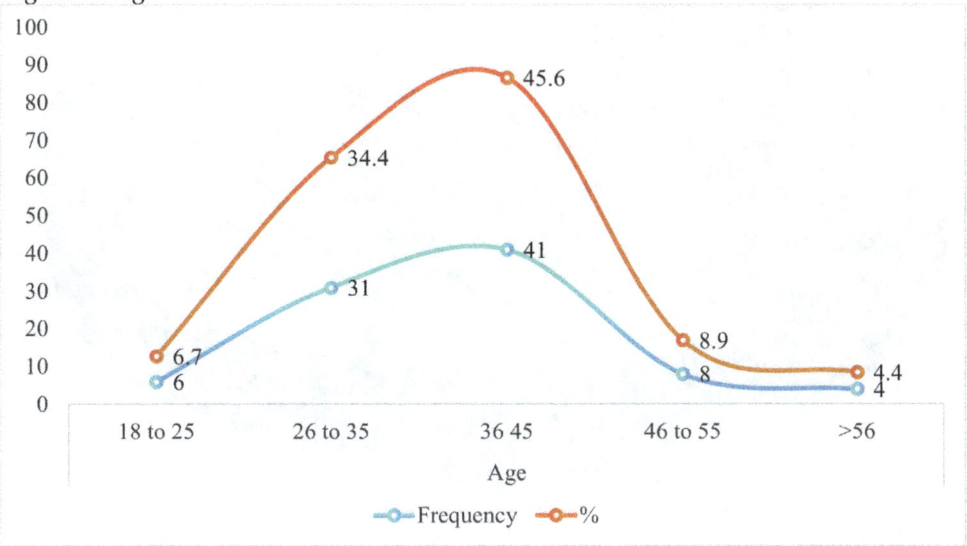

Most respondents were aged 36–45 years (45.6%), followed by 26–35 years (34.4%). Smaller proportions were 46–55 years (8.9%), 18–25 years (6.7%), and above 56 years (4.4%), indicating that most participants were in their prime working and productive years.

Figure 4. Gender

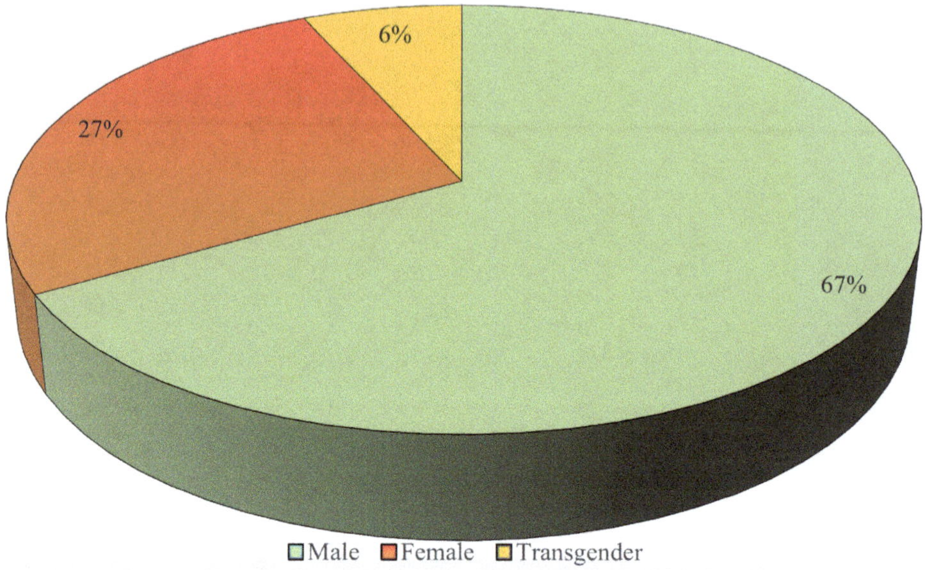

The majority of respondents were male (66.7%), followed by females (26.7%) and transgender individuals (6.7%), indicating predominance of men and lower participation from women and transgender participants.

Figure 5. Monthly income

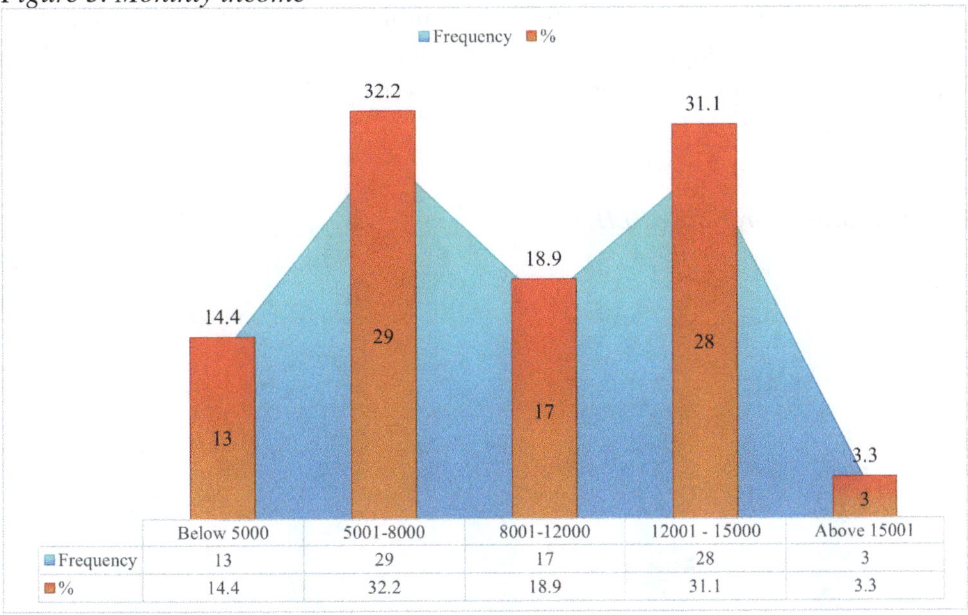

Most respondents earned 5,001– 8,000 (32.2%) or 12,001– 15,000 (31.1%), with smaller proportions earning 8,001– 12,000 (18.9%), below 5,000 (14.4%), or above 15,000 (3.3%), indicating predominantly low-income participants.

Tale 1. Demographic and socio-economic characteristics of respondents

Descriptions	Options	Frequency	%	Mean	SEM	SD	Range
Marrital Status	Single	8	8.9	2.155	0.668	0.634	3.00
	Married	64	71.1				
	Widow	14	15.6				
	Divorce	4	4.4				
	Total	90	100				
Employment Status	Employed	21	23.3	1.900	0.633	0.600	'2.00
	Unemployed	57	63.3				
	Self	12	13.3				
	Total	90	100				
Area of Residence	Rural	56	62.2	1.455	0.673	0.638	2.00
	Urban	27	30				
	Semi-Urban	7	7.8				
	Total	90	100				

Most respondents were married (71.1%), widowed (15.6%), single (8.9%), or divorced (4.4%) (mean 2.155 ± 0.668). Regarding employment, 63.3% were unemployed, 23.3% employed, and 13.3% self-employed (mean 1.900 ± 0.633). Most participants resided in rural areas (62.2%), followed by urban (30%) and semi-urban (7.8%) locations (mean 1.455 ± 0.673).

Figure 6. Block of residing PLHIV

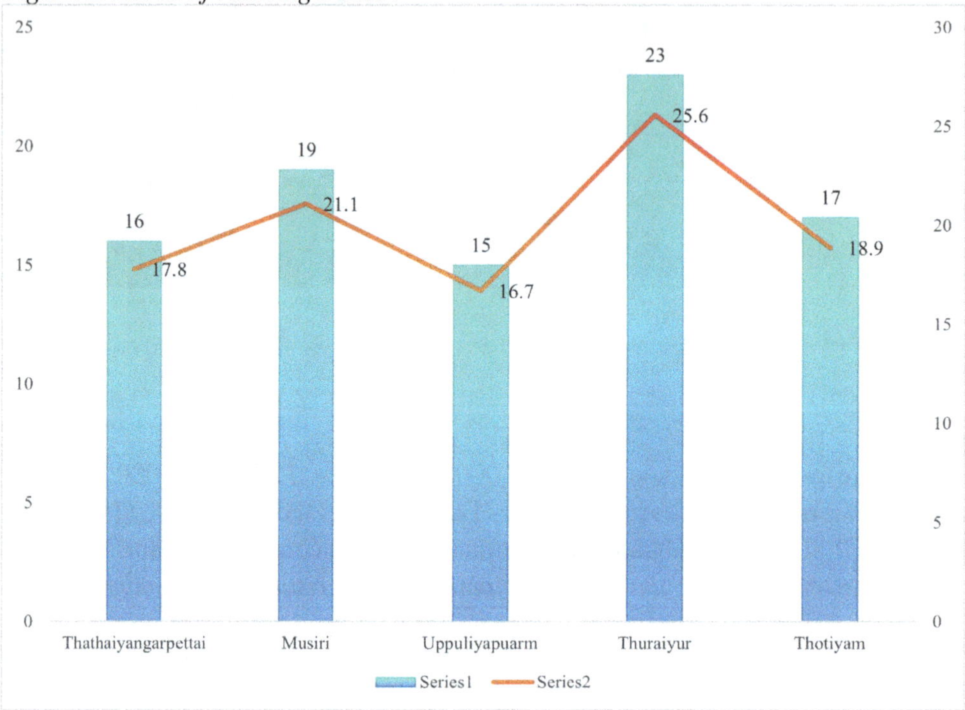

Most respondents were from Thuraiyur (25.6%), followed by Musiri (21.1%), Thotiyam (18.9%), Thathaiyangarpettai (17.8%), and Uppuliyapuram (16.7%), indicating fairly balanced geographic coverage and effective ART outreach.

Table 2. Access to Antiretroviral Therapy (ART) and related healthcare services among HIV patients

Descriptions	Options	Frequency	%
	Yes	77	85.6
	No	13	14.4
Currently Receiving (ART)	Total	90	100
	Below 2 years	17	18.9
	3 to 5 years	32	35.6
Years of ART	6 to 8 years	31	34.4
	Above 8 years	10	11.1
	Total	90	100
	Government Hospital	63	70
Where Receive ART Services	Private Clinic	13	14.4
	NGO based facility	14	15.6
	Total	90	100
	Monthly	58	64.4
	Every 3 moths	15	16.7
Frequency of HIV-Related Healthcare Check-Ups	Every 6 months	13	14.4
	Only when sick	4	4.4
	Total	90	100
	Distance to Health Facility	24	26.7
	Cost of Transportation	41	45.6
Challenges in Accessing Medical Care	Stigma and Discrimination	17	18.9
	Lack of Information	8	8.9
	Total	90	100

A majority (85.6%) of respondents are on antiretroviral therapy (ART), mostly for 3–8 years (70%), primarily through government hospitals (70%), with NGOs (15.6%) and private clinics (14.4%) also contributing. Regular follow-up is common (64.4% monthly), though some face delays. Main barriers include transport costs (45.6%), distance (26.7%), stigma (18.9%), and lack of information (8.9%).

Table 3. Access to health, welfare, and technological support services among people living with HIV

Descriptions	Yes	%	No	%	Total	%
Receive counseling or mental health support	65	72.2	25	27.8	90	100
Treated for opportunistic infections	27	30	63	70	90	100
Regularly monitored for CD4 count and viral load	66	73.3	24	26.7	90	100
Access to nutritional support or supplement	28	31.1	62	68.9	90	100
Aware of government/NGO programs supporting HIV patients	70	77.8	20	22.2	90	100
Received financial or welfare support related to your condition	64	71.1	26	28.9	90	100
Receiving any government support related to HIV care	49	54.4	41	45.6	90	100
Financial assistance/disability pension	20	22.2	70	77.8	90	100
Nutritional supplements	65	72.2	25	27.8	90	100
Transport Allowance	43	47.8	47	52.2	90	100
Housing Support	21	23.3	69	76.7	90	100
Receiving support from NGOs/community-based organizations	67	74.4	23	25.6	100	100
					Partially	%
Welfare support sufficient for your needs	47	52.2	26	28.9	90	18.9
Receive reminders for appointments/medications	61	67.8	29	32.2	90	100
Experienced barriers in continuing treatment	18	20	72	80	90	100
Used healthcare technology tools (apps, SMS, teleconsultation)	42	46.7	48	53.3	90	100
Mobile app for medication reminders	14	15.6	76	84.4	90	100
SMS alerts for appointments	46	51.1	44	48.9	90	100
Telemedicine services	12	13.3	78	86.7	90	100
Electronic Health Record system	36	40	54	60	90	100
Wearable devices for health monitoring	9	10	81	90	90	100
Technologies helped in managing condition	58	64.4	32	35.6	90	100
Improved medication adherence	48	53.3	42	46.7	90	100
Reduced need to travel	76	84.4	14	15.6	90	100
Better access to doctors/specialists	35	38.9	55	61.1	90	100
Increased confidence in self-care	71	78.9	19	21.1	90	100
No impact	15	16.7	75	83.3	90	100

About 72% of participants received counseling, while over one-fourth did not. Treatment for opportunistic infections was low (30%), and 73% had regular CD4/viral load monitoring. Nutritional support was limited (31%), but 78% were aware of welfare programs, with 71% receiving financial aid. Access to government support was moderate (54%), while disability pensions (22%) and housing assistance (23%)

were low. NGO and community support reached 74%, and 68% received treatment reminders. Only 20% reported barriers to care.

Use of healthcare technology was reported by 47%, mainly SMS alerts (51%) and EHRs (40%), while mobile apps (16%), telemedicine (13%), and wearables (10%) were less common. Technology helped reduce travel for 84%, improved adherence for 53%, and increased self-care confidence for 79%, though 17% saw no benefit.

DISCUSSION

Most participants were aged 36–45 (46%) and 26–35 (34%), mostly male (67%), from diverse locations, indicating wide outreach. ART coverage was high (86%), primarily through government hospitals (70%), with 70% on treatment for 3–8 years. Monthly follow-ups were common (64%), though barriers included transport (46%), distance (27%), stigma (19%), and limited information (9%). Socio-demographically, 71.1% were married, 63.3% unemployed, earning mostly 5,001–8,000 (32.2%) or 12,001–15,000 (31.1%), with 62.2% in rural areas. Counseling (72.2%) and regular CD4/viral load monitoring (73.3%) indicate good care, but support for opportunistic infections (30%) and nutrition (31.1%) was limited. Welfare awareness was high (77.8%), with 71.1% receiving financial aid, though government benefits, disability pensions, and housing support were underutilized. Community support is strong (74.4%). Digital tools aid treatment adherence (46.7% usage), SMS (51.1%) and EHRs (40%) are most used, reducing travel (84.4%), improving adherence (53.3%), and increasing confidence (78.9%). Expansion of digital interventions and literacy support is needed to enhance inclusive HIV care.

FEATURE IMPLICATIONS

Healthcare services enable policymakers to empower healthcare providers to increase effective support for patient services. This can lead to better allocation of medical care support for HIV-affected individuals. Effective treatment provides support to HIV-affected individuals and includes monitoring services to refine the treatment. To provide effective treatment and monitor patients' treatment adherence, track maintenance can reduce loss to follow-up, increase long-term care services, and lead to better outcomes (Ukoaka et al., 2024). HIV-affected individuals can benefit through various welfare assistance and support from non-governmental organizations to receive services and social support benefits. Healthcare benefits, with the support of technologies, provide easy access to telemedicine services, mobile health services (mHealth), and the maintenance of e-health records (EHRs) to enhance treatment services and monitor HIV patients' treatment adherence (Rufu et al., 2022). Digital tools can facilitate communication between healthcare providers and HIV-affected individuals to increase treatment adherence, support diagnosis services, and enhance healthcare services and support.

Digital tools enhance communication, early diagnosis, and treatment efficiency. The study recommends policies addressing socio-economic conditions of PLHIV, livelihood support, and skill development for healthcare workers. Patient-centered technology, awareness campaigns, advocacy, and sensitization reduce stigma, encourage early testing, and enhance quality of life (Srinivasan et al., 2025; Ehrenkranz et al., 2021).

CONCLUSION

Digital tools and healthcare technology transform HIV care by enabling timely, patient-centered treatment and improving adherence. Mobile apps, telemedicine, and electronic health records support monitoring, personalized care, and real-time tracking, enhancing quality of life for PLHIV and advancing SDG 3 on good health and well-being.

REFERENCES

Achwoka, D. E. (2021). *Non-communicable Diseases (NCDS) Burden Among People Living With HIV/AIDS (PLHIV) in Kenya* (Doctoral dissertation, University of Nairobi). https://erepository.uonbi.ac.ke/handle/11295/157294

Amadhila, E. M., & Shawapala, T. (2022). Are social protection grants alleviating poverty among vulnerable groups in Namibia?–The case of older persons and persons with disabilities. *African Review of Economics and Finance*, *14*(2), 119–141. https://journals.co.za/doi/abs/10.10520/ejc-aref_v14_n2_a8

Armstead, A. B., Wilkerson, J. M., Gemeinhardt, G., Nyitray, A., & Collins, D. M. (2021). Antiretroviral therapy adherence, functional independence, and falls among people with HIV. *Occupational Therapy in Health Care*, *35*(3), 318–335. DOI: 10.1080/07380577.2021.1938337 PMID: 34137654

Assembly, U. G. (2021). Political declaration on HIV and AIDS: ending inequalities and getting on track to end AIDS by 2030. In *74th Plenary Meeting* (Vol. 8). https://www.unaids.org/sites/default/files/media_asset/2021_political-declaration-on-hiv-and-aids_en.pdf

Balsamo, A. (2021). Study of deferiprone-induced agranulocytosis in β-thalassemic patients through a metabolomics approach. https://iris.unica.it/handle/11584/316317

Banda, J. H. (2024). *Achieving the 2030 Goal of Ending HIV: An Advanced Analysis of Strategic Intervetnitions*. Socio Economic Challenges, and Biomedical Progress., DOI: 10.61784/wjbs3013

Barmania, F., & Pepper, M. S. (2013). CC chemokine receptor type five (CCR5): An emerging target for the control of HIV infection. *Applied & Translational Genomics*, *2*, 3–16. DOI: 10.1016/j.atg.2013.05.004 PMID: 27942440

Beecroft, A., Vaikla, O., & Pant Pai, N. (2024). Digital HIV self-testing as an exemplar: A perspective on benefits, challenges, and opportunities. *Expert Review of Molecular Diagnostics*, *24*(10), 913–925. DOI: 10.1080/14737159.2024.2406974 PMID: 39323182

Bekker, L. G., Beyrer, C., Mgodi, N., Lewin, S. R., Delany-Moretlwe, S., Taiwo, B., Master, M. C., & Lazarus, J. V. (2023). HIV infection. *Nature Reviews. Disease Primers*, *9*(1), 42. DOI: 10.1038/s41572-023-00452-3 PMID: 37591865

Bhardwaj, K., Soryan, I., Saxena, D., Gandhi, D., & Viswas, S. (2024). Breaking Down Barriers: How Cloud Computing Drives Interoperability in Health Care. In *International Conference on Information and Communication Technology for Intelligent Systems* (pp. 101-111). Singapore: Springer Nature Singapore. doi:DOI: 10.1007/978-981-97-6678-9_9

Bloom, D. E., & Cadarette, D. (2019). Infectious disease threats in the twenty-first century: Strengthening the global response. *Frontiers in Immunology*, *10*, 549. DOI: 10.3389/fimmu.2019.00549 PMID: 30984169

Chinyandura, C., Jiyane, A., Tsalong, X., Struthers, H. E., McIntyre, J. A., & Rees, K. (2022). Supporting retention in HIV care through a holistic, patient-centred approach: A qualitative evaluation. *BMC Psychology*, *10*(1), 17. DOI: 10.1186/s40359-022-00722-x PMID: 35093165

Cornman, H., Grimm, C. D., & Rana, S. (2005). Engaging Local Non-Governmental Organizations (NGOs) in the Response to HIV/AIDS. https://scholars.unh.edu/anth_facpub/2/

Cuadros, D. F., Huang, Q., Mathenjwa, T., Gareta, D., Devi, C., & Musuka, G. (2024). Unlocking the potential of telehealth in Africa for HIV: Opportunities, challenges, and pathways to equitable healthcare delivery. *Frontiers in Digital Health*, *6*, 1278223. DOI: 10.3389/fdgth.2024.1278223 PMID: 38500968

Dandri, M., Murray, J. M., Lutgehetmann, M., Volz, T., Lohse, A. W., & Petersen, J. (2008). Virion half-life in chronic hepatitis B infection is strongly correlated with levels of viremia. *Hepatology (Baltimore, Md.)*, *48*(4), 1079–1086. https://aasldpubs.onlinelibrary.wiley.com/doi/pdf/10.1002/hep.22469 PMID: 18697217

Drain, P. K., Dorward, J., Bender, A., Lillis, L., Marinucci, F., Sacks, J., Bershteyn, A., Boyle, D. S., Posner, J. D., & Garrett, N. (2019). Point-of-care HIV viral load testing: An essential tool for a sustainable global HIV/AIDS response. *Clinical Microbiology Reviews*, *32*(3), 10–1128. DOI: 10.1128/cmr.00097-18 PMID: 31092508

Ehrenkranz, P., Grimsrud, A., Holmes, C. B., Preko, P., & Rabkin, M. (2021). Expanding the vision for differentiated service delivery: a call for more inclusive and truly patient-centered care for people living with HIV. *JAIDS Journal of Acquired Immune Deficiency Syndromes, 86*(2), 147 152. doi: DOI: 10.1097/QAI.0000000000002549

Ezenwaji, C. O., Alum, E. U., & Ugwu, O. P. C. (2025). Bridging the gap: Telemedicine as a solution for HIV care inequities in rural and vulnerable communities. *International Journal for Equity in Health*, *24*(1), 205. DOI: 10.1186/s12939-025-02584-2 PMID: 40660269

Fedr, R., Kahounová, Z., Remšík, J., Reiterová, M., Kalina, T., & Souček, K. (2023). Variability of fluorescence intensity distribution measured by flow cytometry is influenced by cell size and cell cycle progression. *Scientific Reports*, *13*(1), 4889. DOI: 10.1038/s41598-023-31990-1 PMID: 36966193

Février, M., Dorgham, K., & Rebollo, A. (2011). CD4+ T cell depletion in human immunodeficiency virus (HIV) infection: Role of apoptosis. *Viruses*, *3*(5), 586. DOI: 10.3390/v3050586 PMID: 21994747

Fox, M. P., Pascoe, S., Huber, A. N., Murphy, J., Phokojoe, M., Gorgens, M., Rosen, S., Wilson, D., Pillay, Y., & Fraser-Hurt, N. (2019). Adherence clubs and decentralized medication delivery to support patient retention and sustained viral suppression in care: Results from a cluster-randomized evaluation of differentiated ART delivery models in South Africa. *PLoS Medicine*, *16*(7), e1002874. DOI: 10.1371/journal.pmed.1002874 PMID: 31335865

Gashu, K. D. (2024). The Digital Ecosystem and Major Public Health Informatics Initiatives in Resource-Limited Settings. In *Public Health Informatics: Implementation and Governance in Resource-Limited Settings* (pp. 97-140). Cham: Springer Nature Switzerland. doi:DOI: 10.1007/978-3-031-71118-3_4

German Advisory Committee Blood (Arbeitskreis Blut), Subgroup 'Assessment of Pathogens Transmissible by Blood. (2016). Human immunodeficiency virus (HIV). *Transfusion Medicine and Hemotherapy; Offizielles Organ der Deutschen Gesellschaft für Transfusionsmedizin und Immunhämatologie*, *43*(3), 203–222. DOI: 10.1159/000445852 PMID: 27403093

Greifinger, R., & Dick, B. (2011). Provision of psychosocial support for young people living with HIV: Voices from the field. *SAHARA J : Journal of Social Aspects of HIV/AIDS Research Alliance*, *8*(1), 33–41. DOI: 10.1080/17290376.2011.9724982 PMID: 23237644

Haris, M., & Abbas, R. (2024). Four decades of HIV: Global trends, testing assays, treatment, and challenges. *Zoonoses*, *4*(1), 997. DOI: 10.15212/ZOONOSES-2023-0039

Hawkins, D., Blott, M., Clayden, P., De Ruiter, A., Foster, G., Gilling-Smith, C., Layall, G. H., Mercey, D., Newell, M. L., O'Shea, S., Smith, R., Sunderland, J., Wood, C., & Taylor, G. (2005). Guidelines for the management of HIV infection in pregnant women and the prevention of mother-to-child transmission of HIV. *Virology Papers*, 151.

Heidt, B., Siqueira, W. F., Eersels, K., Diliën, H., van Grinsven, B., Fujiwara, R. T., & Cleij, T. J. (2020). Point of care diagnostics in resource-limited settings: A review of the present and future of PoC in its most needed environment. *Biosensors (Basel)*, *10*(10), 133. DOI: 10.3390/bios10100133 PMID: 32987809

Herman, T. (2021). *Impact of Integrating Directly Observed Therapy with Care Coordination in Improving Anti-Retroviral Therapy Adherence for Patients Who Are HIV Positive and Non-Suppressed* (Doctoral dissertation, D'Youville College).

Hermann, K., Van Damme, W., Pariyo, G. W., Schouten, E., Assefa, Y., Cirera, A., & Massavon, W. (2009). Community health workers for ART in sub-Saharan Africa: Learning from experience–capitalizing on new opportunities. *Human Resources for Health*, *7*, 1–11. DOI: 10.1186/1478-4491-7-31 PMID: 19358701

Hilty, D. M., Gentry, M. T., McKean, A. J., Cowan, K. E., Lim, R. F., & Lu, F. G. (2020). Telehealth for rural diverse populations: Telebehavioral and cultural competencies, clinical outcomes and administrative approaches. *mHealth*, *6*, 20. DOI: 10.21037/mhealth.2019.10.04 PMID: 32270012

Hlaing, M. M. (2024). *The Effect of Social Support on HIV-related Stigma among People Living with HIV/AIDS (Case Study of Myeik Township)(Mi Mi Hlaing, 2024)* (Doctoral dissertation, MERAL Portal).

Hoffmann, C. J., Gonzalez, C. J., & Stein, D. K. (2023). Second-line ART after treatment failure or for regimen simplification. *Medical Care*, *2*, 2–25.

Hosaka, K. R., Kang, E., Huff, J., Shaw, S., & Duomai, S. (2021). Livelihood intervention and mental well-being among women living with HIV in Delhi. *AIDS Care*, *33*(8), 1037–1043. DOI: 10.1080/09540121.2020.1837336 PMID: 33103920

Iedema, R., Allen, S., Britton, K., & Gallagher, T. H. (2012). What do patients and relatives know about problems and failures in care? *BMJ Quality & Safety*, *21*(3), 198–205. DOI: 10.1136/bmjqs-2011-000100 PMID: 22178930

Ji, H. (2007). Association of interferon regulatory factor-1 polymorphisms with resistance to infection by HIV-1 in Kenyan female sex workers.

Jones-Esan, L., Somasiri, N., & Lorne, K. (2024). Enhancing healthcare delivery through digital health interventions: a systematic review on telemedicine and mobile health applications in Low and Middle-Income Countries (LMICs). *Research Square*. doi: DOI: 10.21203/rs.3.rs-5189203/v1

Kalemeera, F., Ndevahoma, S., Mubita, M., & Godman, B. (2022). Evaluation of Namibia's antiretroviral therapy guidelines' recommendations for switching from first-line to second-line, using predictors of first-line treatment failure: An exploratory study. *Expert Review of Anti-Infective Therapy*, *20*(6), 915–921. DOI: 10.1080/14787210.2022.2015325 PMID: 34878350

Kawichai, S., Nelson, K. E., Natpratan, C., Celentano, D. D., Khamboonruang, C., Natpratan, P., & Beyrer, C. (2005). Personal history of voluntary HIV counseling and testing (VCT) among adults aged 19–35 years living in peri-urban communities, Chiang Mai, northern Thailand. *AIDS and Behavior*, *9*, 233–242. DOI: 10.1007/s10461-005-3904-0 PMID: 15933842

Keter, G. (2023). *The Impact of Demographic Factors on Adverse Drug Reactions and Survival Rates Among Hiv Patients in Nairobi County From 2015 to 2021* (Doctoral dissertation, University of Nairobi). https://erepository.uonbi.ac.ke/handle/11295/164239

Korenromp, E. L., Williams, B. G., Schmid, G. P., & Dye, C. (2009). Clinical prognostic value of RNA viral load and CD4 cell counts during untreated HIV-1 infection—A quantitative review. *PLoS One*, *4*(6), e5950. DOI: 10.1371/journal.pone.0005950 PMID: 19536329

Koss, C. A., Charlebois, E. D., Ayieko, J., Kwarisiima, D., Kabami, J., Balzer, L. B., Atukunda, M., Mwangwa, F., Peng, J., Mwinike, Y., Owaraganise, A., Chamie, G., Jain, V., Sang, N., Olilo, W., Brown, L. B., Marquez, C., Zhang, K., Ruel, T. D., & Havlir, D. V. (2020). Uptake, engagement, and adherence to pre-exposure prophylaxis offered after population HIV testing in rural Kenya and Uganda: 72-week interim analysis of observational data from the SEARCH study. *The Lancet. HIV*, *7*(4), e249–e261. https://www.thelancet.com/journals/lanhiv/article/PIIS2352-3018(19)30433-3/fulltext PMID: 32087152

Laar, A. (2022). Access to Life-Saving Public Health Goods by Persons Infected with or Affected by HIV. In *Balancing the Socio-political and Medico-ethical Dimensions of HIV: A Social Public Health Approach* (pp. 51–63). Springer International Publishing., DOI: 10.1007/978-3-031-09191-9_4

Lakshmanan, K., & Liu, B. M. (2025). Impact of point-of-care testing on diagnosis, treatment, and surveillance of vaccine-preventable viral infections. *Diagnostics (Basel)*, *15*(2), 123. DOI: 10.3390/diagnostics15020123 PMID: 39857007

Land, H. (2015). Diverse people affected by HIV/AIDS. *Transformative Social Work Practice, 25.*

Li, R., Duffee, D., & Gbadamosi-Akindele, M. F. (2023). CD4 count. In *StatPearls* [Internet]. StatPearls Publishing., https://www.ncbi.nlm.nih.gov/sites/books/NBK470231/

Liang, X., Alam, N., Sultana, T., Bandara, E., & Shetty, S. (2024). Designing A Blockchain-Empowered Telehealth Artifact for Decentralized Identity Management and Trustworthy Communication: Interdisciplinary Approach. *Journal of Medical Internet Research, 26*, e46556. DOI: 10.2196/46556 PMID: 39320943

Madapuji Srinivasan, M. (2024). *Molecular Mechanisms and Host Factors Involved in HIV-1 Latency* (Doctoral dissertation, Université d'Ottawa/University of Ottawa). https://ruor.uottawa.ca/server/api/core/bitstreams/1aa1292f-c82e-4cbe-88ed-ebc6e9a450ce/content

Masur, P. B. H., Kaplan, J. E., & Holmes, K. K. (2002). Guidelines for preventing opportunistic infections among HIV-infected persons—2002: Recommendations of the US Public Health Service and the Infectious Diseases Society of America. *Annals of Internal Medicine, 137*(5_Part_2), 435–478. DOI: 10.7326/0003-4819-137-5_Part_2-200209031-00002 PMID: 12617574

McIntyre, A. (2024). *The role of CD4+ help in promoting CD8+ T cell function following allogeneic haematopoietic stem cell transplantation* (Doctoral dissertation, UCL (University College London)). https://discovery.ucl.ac.uk/id/eprint/10188958/

McIntyre, J. (2005). Maternal health and HIV. *Reproductive Health Matters, 13*(25), 129–135. DOI: 10.1016/S0968-8080(05)25184-4 PMID: 16035606

Mekonnen, Z. A. (2024). Public Health Informatics: An Overview. *Public Health Informatics: Implementation and Governance in Resource-Limited Settings*, 27-61. doi:DOI: 10.1007/978-3-031-71118-3_2

Meya, D. B., Kiragga, A. N., Nalintya, E., Banturaki, G., Akullo, J., Kalyesubula, P., Sessazi, P., Bitakalamire, H., Kabanda, J., Kalamya, J. N., Namale, A., Bateganya, M., Kagaayi, J., Gutreuter, S., Adler, M. R., & Mitruka, K. (2022). Impact of an intensive facility-community case management intervention on 6-month HIV outcomes among select key and priority populations in Uganda. *AIDS Research and Therapy, 19*(1), 62. DOI: 10.1186/s12981-022-00486-9 PMID: 36471321

Miriti, D., Marwa, I., & Muriuki, J. (2025). Clinical factors Associated with Viral Load Suppression Among HIV and AIDS-Positive Children (0–14 Years) Attending Meru County Referral Hospital, Meru County, Kenya.

Mlambo, N. (2021). *A Non-Governmental Organistion's Psycho-Social and Educational Support for Orphans and Vulnerable Children in Soweto*. University of Johannesburg., https://www.proquest.com/openview/16788e444b4dbe9be04a69d4144ab366/1?cbl=2026366&diss=y&pq-origsite=gscholar

Morvan, M. G., Teque, F. C., Locher, C. P., & Levy, J. A. (2021). The CD8+ T Cell noncytotoxic antiviral responses. *Microbiology and Molecular Biology Reviews : MMBR*, *85*(2), 10–1128. DOI: 10.1128/mmbr.00155-20 PMID: 33980586

Mudrick, N. R., Breslin, M. L., Nielsen, K. A., & Swager, L. C. (2020). Can disability accommodation needs stored in electronic health records help providers prepare for patient visits? A qualitative study. *BMC Health Services Research*, *20*, 1–18. DOI: 10.1186/s12913-020-05808-z PMID: 33066788

Mulumba, E. M., Kayembe, M. F., Chewe, W. C., Chanda, C., Dube, N., Chituta, C., Hamooya, B. M., Kasweka, F. T., Matabishi, M., & Assani, M. B. (2025). Performance of the VISITECT® CD4 Test for Rapid Identification of Advanced HIV Disease at AHF-Supported Sites in Zambia: A Diagnostic Accuracy Analysis in a Zambian Population. medRxiv, 2025-01. doi:DOI: 10.1101/2025.01.06.25320078

Mutabazi, J. C., Zarowsky, C., & Trottier, H. (2017). The impact of programs for prevention of mother-to-child transmission of HIV on health care services and systems in sub-Saharan Africa-A review. *Public Health Reviews*, *38*, 1–27. DOI: 10.1186/s40985-017-0072-5 PMID: 29450099

Nalwanga, D., & Musiime, V. (2022). Children living with HIV: A narrative review of recent advances in pediatric HIV research and their implications for clinical practice. *Therapeutic Advances in Infectious Disease*, *9*, 20499361221077544. DOI: 10.1177/20499361221077544 PMID: 35186289

Nikolopoulos, G. K., & Tsantes, A. G. (2022). Recent HIV infection: Diagnosis and public health implications. *Diagnostics (Basel)*, *12*(11), 2657. DOI: 10.3390/diagnostics12112657 PMID: 36359500

Nkambule, B. S. (2022). *Factors Associated With Access to HIV Care in East and Southern Africa* (Doctoral dissertation, National Yang Ming Chiao Tung University).

Nyamboga, T. O., & Obeagu, E. I. (2024). Sustainable Solutions: Strategic Management for Long-Term HIV Care in At-Risk Populations. *Elite Journal of Public Health*, *2*(7), 63-74. https://kiu.ac.ug/assets/publications/3245_sustainable-solutions-strategic-management-for-long-term-hiv-care-in-at-risk-populations.pdf

Obeagu, E. I. (2024). Reducing Viral Load Impact: Blood Transfusions as a Complementary Approach in HIV Treatment. *International Journal of Medical Sciences and Pharma Research, 10*(3), 56–62. DOI: 10.22270/ijmspr.v10i3.115

Obeagu, E. I., & Obeagu, G. U. (2024). Mental Health and Psychosocial Effects of natural disaster on HIV Patients. *The Sciences, 4*(1), 38–44. https://kiu.ac.ug/assets/publications/1401_mental-health-and-psychosocial-effects-of-natural-disaster-on-hiv-p-atients.pdf

Odame-Takyi, K. T. (2016). *Implementation of HIV/AIDS policy in the Gauteng Department of Roads and Transport*. University of the Witwatersrand., https://www.proquest.com/openview/3204e91daeae914b9d16279f7ca8e739/1?cbl=2026366&diss=y&pq-origsite=gscholar

Olaleye, S. A., Sanusi, I. T., Salo, J., & Olaleye, E. O. (2023). Home care and mobile health services provision for rural dwellers: a conceptual framework of poverty alleviation and rural development. https://aisel.aisnet.org/iceb2023/34/

Omondi, F. H., Sudderuddin, H., Shahid, A., Kinloch, N. N., Jones, B. R., Miller, R. L., & Brumme, Z. L. (2021). HIV proviral burden, genetic diversity, and dynamics in viremic controllers who subsequently initiated suppressive antiretroviral therapy. *mBio, 12*(6), e02490–e21. PMID: 34781741

Pattanapanyasat, K., & Thakar, M. R. (2005). CD4+ T cell count as a tool to monitor HIV progression & anti-retroviral therapy. *The Indian Journal of Medical Research, 121*(4), 539–549. PMID: 15817962

Peeriga, R., & Manubolu, K. (2025). Pioneering Technologies to Revolutionize Antiviral Treatment. In *Global Perspectives on Antiviral Drug Development* (pp. 175–216). IGI Global Scientific Publishing., DOI: 10.4018/979-8-3693-9276-8.ch005

Pham, M. D., Nguyen, H. V., Anderson, D., Crowe, S., & Luchters, S. (2022). Viral load monitoring for people living with HIV in the era of test and treat: Progress made and challenges ahead–a systematic review. *BMC Public Health, 22*(1), 1203. DOI: 10.1186/s12889-022-13504-2 PMID: 35710413

Pham, M. D., Romero, L., Parnell, B., Anderson, D. A., Crowe, S. M., & Luchters, S. (2017). Feasibility of antiretroviral treatment monitoring in the era of decentralized HIV care: A systematic review. *AIDS Research and Therapy, 14*, 1–18. DOI: 10.1186/s12981-017-0131-5 PMID: 28103895

Plebani, M., Nichols, J. H., Luppa, P. B., Greene, D., Sciacovelli, L., Shaw, J., Khan, A. I., Carrar, P., Freckmann, G., Dimech, W., Zaninotto, M., Spannagl, M., Huggett, J., Kost, G. J., Trenti, T., Padoan, A., Thomas, A., Banfi, G., & Lippi, G. (2025). Point-of-care testing: State-of-the art and perspectives. [CCLM]. *Clinical Chemistry and Laboratory Medicine, 63*(1), 35–51. PMID: 38880779

Poindexter, C. C. (2010). *Handbook of HIV and social work: Principles, practice, and populations*. John Wiley & Sons., https://books.google.co.in/books?hl=en&lr=&id=w4M2vh_0Cs4C&oi=fnd&pg=PT24&dq=The+case+management+of+HIV-affected+patients,+when+handled+by+healthcare+workers,+follows+certain+strategies+to+reduce+unwanted+outcome&ots=-FpQcofbLl&sig=pec_J_Rgvoa5B-jZQiZWzkKbcRg&redir_esc=y#v=onepage&q&f=false

Posse, J. L., Dios, P. D., & Scully, C. (2017). Viral diseases transmissible by kissing. *Saliva Protection and Transmissible Diseases, 53*. Advance online publication. DOI: 10.1016/B978-0-12-813681-2.00004-4

Rosen, J. G., Ddaaki, W. G., Nakyanjo, N., Chang, L. W., Vo, A. V., Zhao, T., & Galiwango, R. M. (2024). The potential promise and pitfalls of point-of-care viral load monitoring to expedite HIV treatment decision-making in rural Uganda: A qualitative study. *BMC Health Services Research, 24*(1), 1265. DOI: 10.1186/s12913-024-11747-w PMID: 39434090

Rufu, A., Chitindingu, K., Chinofunga, S., Dupwa, B., & Mugurungi, O. (2022). Designing, Developing, pilot implementation and evaluation of a mobile android based tool to improve health outcomes in adolescents and young adults living with HIV: An Agile model Human-Centered Design Science three-phase Methodology. doi:DOI: 10.21203/rs.3.rs-1914197/v1

Searight, H. R. (2018). Counseling patients in primary care: Evidence-based strategies. *American Family Physician, 98*(12), 719–728. PMID: 30525356

Singh, A. K., Srinivasan, S., & Jyoti, B. (2025). Implications of Digitalization on Public Health Sector Across Countries. In *Digitalization and the Transformation of the Healthcare Sector* (pp. 359–394). IGI Global Scientific Publishing., DOI: 10.4018/979-8-3693-9641-4.ch013

Singh, Y., Jackson, D., Bhardwaj, S., Titus, N., & Goga, A. (2019). National surveillance using mobile systems for health monitoring: Complexity, functionality and feasibility. *BMC Infectious Diseases, 19*, 1–10. DOI: 10.1186/s12879-019-4338-z PMID: 31526387

Sousa, L. R. M., Elias, H. C., Fernandes, N. M., Gir, E., & Reis, R. K. (2021). Knowledge of PEP and PrEP among people living with HIV/aids in Brazil. *BMC Public Health*, *21*, 1–9. DOI: 10.1186/s12889-020-10135-3 PMID: 33413241

Srinivasan, S. (2025). A Comparative Performance of Digitalization and Health Sector in Selected Non-OECD Countries: Digitalization and Health Sector. In *Digitalization and the Transformation of the Healthcare Sector* (pp. 65–114). IGI Global Scientific Publishing., DOI: 10.4018/979-8-3693-9641-4.ch003

Srinivasan, S. (2025). Patient-Centric Care in Tuberculosis Management: Addressing Challenges and Improving Health Outcomes. In *Convergence of Population Health Management, Pharmacogenomics, and Patient-Centered Care* (pp. 265-282). IGI Global. doi: DOI: 10.4018/979-8-3693-3260-3.ch012

Srinivasan, S., & Praba Lama (2025). Patient-Centered Care for TB Patients: An Effective Approach to Corporate Social Responsibility. In Corporate Social Responsibility in Health and Social Care (pp. 183-218).IGI Global. doi:DOI: 10.4018/979-8-3693-5991-4.ch008

Srinivasan, S., Vallipriya, R., & Singh, A. K. (2025). Integrated Public-Private Partnerships to Combat Tuberculosis for Improving Economic Development. In *Public Private Partnership Dynamics for Economic Development* (pp. 323–356). IGI Global Scientific Publishing., DOI: 10.4018/979-8-3693-9153-2.ch015

Tiffin, N., George, A., & LeFevre, A. E. (2019). How to use relevant data for maximal benefit with minimal risk: Digital health data governance to protect vulnerable populations in low-income and middle-income countries. *BMJ Global Health*, *4*(2), e001395. PMID: 31139457

Tsondai, P. R. (2016). *HIV viral load monitoring in HIV-infected pregnant women established on antiretroviral therapy in Cape Town.*

Ukoaka, B. M., Ugwuanyi, E. A., Ukueku, K. O., Ajah, K. U., Udam, N. G., Daniel, F. M., Wali, T. W., & Gbuchie, M. A. (2024). Digital tools for improving antiretroviral adherence among people living with HIV in Africa. *Journal of Medicine, Surgery, and Public Health*, ●●●, 100077.

Vallée, A., & Arutkin, M. (2024). The Transformative Power of Virtual Hospitals for Revolutionising Healthcare Delivery. *Public Health Reviews*, *45*, 1606371. DOI: 10.3389/phrs.2024.1606371 PMID: 38962359

Van der Berg, A. (2021). *Investigating the effects of treatment in HIV disease models* (Doctoral dissertation, Stellenbosch: Stellenbosch University). https://scholar.sun.ac.za/items/7e137126-b5d0-4652-8000-d391fbe7b097

Vlad, G. (2019). Sources of errors in flow cytometry. In *Accurate Results in the Clinical Laboratory* (pp. 401–422). Elsevier., DOI: 10.1016/B978-0-12-813776-5.00027-3

Westerdijk, T. (2024). *Decoding HIV Dynamics: The Role of Modeling in Understanding Viral Load Decay under Retroviral Therapy* (Master's thesis). https://studenttheses.uu.nl/handle/20.500.12932/47716

World Health Organization. (2021). *Consolidated guidelines on HIV prevention, testing, treatment, service delivery and monitoring: recommendations for a public health approach.* World Health Organization.

Zhao, A. V., Crutchley, R. D., Guduru, R. C., Ton, K., Lam, T., & Min, A. C. (2022). A clinical review of HIV integrase strand transfer inhibitors (INSTIs) for the prevention and treatment of HIV-1 infection. *Retrovirology, 19*(1), 22. DOI: 10.1186/s12977-022-00608-1 PMID: 36273165

Zolopa, A. R. (2010). The evolution of HIV treatment guidelines: Current state-of-the-art of ART. *Antiviral Research, 85*(1), 241–244. DOI: 10.1016/j.antiviral.2009.10.018 PMID: 19883695

Zuckoff, A. (2012). "Why won't my patients do what's good for them?" Motivational interviewing and treatment adherence. *Surgery for Obesity and Related Diseases, 8*(5), 514–521. DOI: 10.1016/j.soard.2012.05.002 PMID: 22704048

APPENDIX

Abbreviations

Acquired Immunodeficiency Syndrome (AIDS)
Advanced HIV disease (AHD)
Adverse Drug Reaction (ADR)
Antiretroviral therapy (ART)
C-C Chemokine reporter type 5 (CCR5)
Cluster of Differentiation 4 (CD4)
C-X-C chemokine receptor (CXCR)
Deoxyribonucleic acid (DNA)
Electronic health records (EHRs)
Highly Active Antiretroviral Therapy (HAART)
Human Immunodeficiency Virus (HIV)
Integrated Counselling and Testing Centre (ICTCs)
Integrase strand transfer inhibitors (INSTIs)
Joint United Nations Programme on HIV/AIDS (UNAIDS)
Mobile health clinics (mHealth)
Non Governmental Organizations (NGOs)
Nonadoption, Abandonment, and challenges to the Scale-up, Spread, and Sustainability (NASSS)
Nucleoside reverse transcriptase inhibitors (NRTIs)
Practical, Robust Implementation and Sustainability Model (PRISM)
Pre-Exposure Prophylaxis (PrEP)
Point-of-care (POC)
People living with HIV (PLIV)
Post-Exposure Prophylaxis (PEP)
Quality-Adjusted Life Years (QALYs)
Reach, Effectiveness, Adoption, Implementation, and Maintenance (RE-AIM)
Reverse transcription polymerase chain reaction **(RT-PCR)**
Ribonucleic acid (RNA)
Short Message Service (SMS)
Sustainable Development Goals (SDGs)
Tuberclosis (TB)
World Health Organization (WHO)

Chapter 7
Enhancing Mental Health and Treatment Adherence in HIV/AIDS Patients Through Strengthened Social Networks

S. Srinivasan
https://orcid.org/0009-0002-0179-9849
Department of Humanities and Social Sciences, Graphic Era University, Dehradun, India

R. Vallipriya
https://orcid.org/0009-0008-6692-603X
Department of Biochemistry and Biotechnology, Pavendar Bharathidasan College of Arts and Science, Bharathidasan University, Tiruchirappalli, India

Jipson Joseph
https://orcid.org/0009-0005-1795-5051
School of Law, Christ University, Bangalore, India

ABSTRACT

The study explores how social networks and support enhance the health and treatment adherence of HIV patients. HIV/AIDS affects not only physical health but also leads to social stigma, discrimination, and emotional challenges. A strong social network improves the quality of life, reduces psychological issues like anxiety and depression, and promotes overall well-being. Strengthening network sustainability for vulner-

DOI: 10.4018/979-8-3373-2863-8.ch007

able HIV/AIDS patients can enhance emotional support, self-care, and treatment adherence. Conducted in Pudukottai District, Tamil Nadu, the study involved 120 samples, with data collected through the Positive Network and NGO support. The findings offer policy implications, assist healthcare providers in managing affected individuals effectively, and highlight the role of NGO services in improving mental health outcomes and creating a supportive environment for PLHIV.

INTRODUCTION

HIV-affected individuals face health challenges, including physical problems, as well as social issues like stigma and discrimination (Jaspal et al., 2021). Social and psychological support can further improve physical health and motivate treatment adherence. Self-care behaviors play a key role in preventing and reducing HIV transmission (Areri et al., 2020). Most PLHIV are connected to social support networks (SSNs), which enhance their social and emotional well-being. This can support various aspects such as financial aid, guidance support, career counseling, job opportunities, and advocacy support to provide a variety of services (Cox & Brennan, 2017). The network provides a stronger association with PLHIV people, which can increase relationships with peer groups, family, friends, and relatives to provide social support. The aim of the study is to present social networks and social support to enhance mental health among HIV/AIDS persons (Ajuna et al., 2021; De Andrade et al., 2022).

The study mainly emphasizes the social network associated with people affected with HIV/AIDS. Social support involves their mental health well-being among PLHIV people. The study provides significant improvement for the social network to enhance the quality of social support among HIV/AIDS patients. Social network and social support improve their psychological well-being, mental health wellness, and reduce the anxiety and depression levels of PLHIV people (Birore et al., 2022; Muwonge et al., 2022; Zhang et al., 2023).

The internationally "90-90-90" target calls for 90% of people living with HIV (PLHIV) to be diagnosed, 90% of those diagnosed to receive combination antiretroviral therapy (ART), and 90% of those on ART to achieve virological suppression (Ndashimye & Arts, 2019). The target aimed to be achieved by the year 2020 to 2023, but it decreased, and it can reduce the global burden of HIV/AIDS, which was 90% in 2010. HIV care is a continuous model and can treat HIV cases Payagala & Pozniak, 2024). This can provide various processes and phases involved in HIV treatment and can support the transition from diagnosis to achieving viral suppression. The above proportion refers to PLHIV who are in the initial stage. There is a parallel optimism that nearly 90-90-90 targets can be focused under the GFATM

(Frescura et al., 2025). The research study emphasizes PLHIV-affected individuals and reinforces the risk of drug use behaviour, which can increase sexual risk behaviour. Consequently, it leads to poor treatment outcomes among PLHIV individuals (Pontes-Pereira et al., 2023). To provide awareness on self-reported condom use, it can improve positive thoughts regarding condom use within social networks, and this can increase social support and engagement in the community (Craddock et al., 2022). The existing study gives a clear picture of the relationship between high-risk sexual behaviour and HIV infection through modes of HIV transmission and increased drug usage. The networks involved, such as bridge populations, are identified to equally contribute to both sexual and high injection drug user-related HIV transmission, as well as centrality and core-periphery relationships (Laymouna, 2023). Social networks play a vital role in reaching key populations and providing proper sensitization among affected individuals, who can also reach other key populations. This can prevent HIV transmission and support social network services. The social network plays a dual role in HIV transmission: it serves as both a route for virus transmission and as a means to disseminate communication related to HIV prevention and treatment support services (Pagkas-Bather et al., 2020; Yang et al., 2020; Stojanovski et al., 2021).

Social Support Network people are involved in various activities to provide counseling services, emotional support services, financial support, guidance services, and advocacy support for the affected individual (Li et al., 2006). The Social Network stabilizes and empowers the affected individuals, particularly PLHIV people, and provides resource support and transition for normative life changes, which can support the affected individuals (Hlaing, 2024). The social network can involve the PLHIV's family, friends, and their relatives, who can access various sources of social support and receive different forms of support and services (Knight & Schatz, 2022). The previous study on social support provides little information about the social network and its impact on the lives of PLHIV (Mwabenga, 2019).

India is a country with a population of 1.02 billion individuals living across thirty-five states and union territories, of which 82% reside in rural areas. HIV infection has been reported in all the states, with the highest rates reported in the southern part, especially in Tamil Nadu and Karnataka, and the western part, particularly Maharashtra Heterosexual transmission is dominant in all regions of India (Thirumalai, 2017). The prevalence of sexually transmitted diseases (STD) in the community is increasing, and there is a high prevalence rate of HIV among STD patients (Castro & Alcaide, 2016). National HIV prevention reports indicate that affected individuals engage in safer sexual behaviours, and nearly 2% of infections nationwide are attributed to injecting drug usage (IDU) (Kumar et al., 2018).

Injecting drug users (IDUs) in the northern part of India show a higher prevalence compared to the southern part of India. The prevalence rate among IDUs is nearly

19%. HIV transmission continues, and there is a need to provide interventions for HIV-affected individuals (Gupta & Barman, 2021). Men who have sex with men (MSM) are also at increasing risk of HIV in the country. As per the MSM survey, nearly 8.7% of them are HIV positive, and they need attention and advocacy for their particular community to ensure safety and security, which can highlight the importance of prevention in the community (Hess et al., 2017; Miller et al., 2021). A recent study was conducted on HIV transmission among heterosexuals under the NIMH HIV/STD prevention trial. On a trial basis, a community-based prevention intervention was implemented in Chennai to provide awareness among alcohol addicts and to sensitize bar and wine shops (Sivaram et al., 2009).

Network Dynamics

Network is based on membership and their relationships over the course of life. HIV prevention is a broader concept; the network starts largely with those who are at risk for health behaviours during adolescence and adulthood (Kaufman et al., 2014). Network changes may reflect their intention and intensity in terms of function, regularity, and frequency of interaction, both of which contribute to the spread or prevention of HIV. Network is not unstable for IDUs; it is the network ties that have been shown to promote HIV transmission. Social networks require structural changes to address network shifts over time (Shelton et al., 2019; Ward & Fauk, 2025).

Structural Factors and Social Networks

Social network is involved in both physical and social spaces based on its structure. Network members meet one another, share their experiences, face problems, and overcome issues, which helps motivate affected PLHIV (Zhang et al., 2013). Risk behaviour can change among affected individuals. Many studies show that injecting drug users (IDUs) face high risk due to injection-related involvement (Degenhardt et al., 2023). On the other hand, neighbourhood factors involve racial and socioeconomic issues, which can impact the availability of network members. The network also involves gender influences related to incarceration practices; they may have drug use and sex work-related social ties, contributing to HIV transmission under vulnerable conditions (Krüsi & Shannon, 2022). Stigma among affected individuals is another concern, and the network plays a vital role in advocating for them. They are able to talk and share issues like stigma and discrimination, and the network provides appropriate hand holding support for affected individuals. Social network dynamics contribute to reducing HIV transmission and providing care and support services for PLHIV (Treves-Kagan et al., 2015; Salmen et al., 2015; Obeagu et al., 2024).

Networks Strength

Social networks' strong-based approach is focused on health-affected individuals and provides both positive and negative aspects. The strong social network is associated with providing better health outcomes and enhancing social access to information. The negative and individual-based approach increases stress and leads to poor health performance and worse health outcomes. The negative and individual-based approach increases stress and leads to poor health performance and worse health outcomes. The social network process functions through individuals connected within an organization, represented as "nodes," associated with one or more types of interdependent people such as friends, co-workers, individuals with common interests, similar knowledge, equal status, and other related types. Social networks involve individuals and small groups of people. The network may function in various aspects through their families and within the same population group of a place. This can involve solving individual issues and providing advocacy support for the affected individuals.

Expertise Involved in Social Network

i. Social Network involves their physical connection.
ii. Digital connection is established globally through Facebook, LinkedIn, Twitter, and other types of media networks.
iii. Health apps connect through social networks such as healthcare networks and forums.
iv. Medical network involves non-professionals through the internet.
v. Scientific Social Network

Support Quality

Social Network provides quality support for individuals who need psychological assistance. The support must be provided by spouses, partners, and family members, and should include information beyond family circumstances. To provide sensitization to friends and community social support for people living with HIV. The social support must involve the workplace, family relationships, and health workers to provide quality support for the affected individuals. The social support might provide emotional support for the affected individuals and address the impact of

HIV diagnosis, treatment adherence, and regular treatment continuity. The effect of social stigma affects individuals in their daily lives, contributing to how they cope with stress and address issues related to their quality of life in day-to-day activities.

Problems Encountered by the Research

A significant challenge was obtaining permission to conduct research in certain centers. Similarly, no establishments permit an outsider to investigate internal problems, especially when the findings might be published. Non-cooperation among the respondents was another challenge. Although adequate sampling was available, respondents were not cooperative in completing the interview schedule.

The use of Western scales posed additional difficulties. Since the scales used by the researcher were developed for Western cultures, they were not easily applicable to the local context. Therefore, the study had to be conducted with extra care to achieve the desired objectives. Additionally, a comparative study was initially planned to assess Members of the HIV/AIDS community in the community and in institutions. However, due to the unavailability of permission, this comparison could not be conducted. Restrictions by NGOs also posed challenges. Although NGOs granted permission to carry out the research, some questions were required to be removed from the interview schedule as they pertained to the NGOs and their involvement. These were among the challenges encountered by the researcher during the course of this study. The research primarily focused on specific aspects, including the social network and social support of individuals living with HIV/AIDS. However, the scope of this field is extensive, leaving numerous other areas available for future exploration.

Scope of the Study

This research will be of great use to the Government Health Departments, Non-Governmental Organizations, Community Organizations, and Researchers who will be doing research in the same area. This will help them to identify the various tools and techniques and various types of training programme to these vulnerable sections of the society. This study deals with the social network and social support that which is available and their needs and wants of the people infected HIV from the network (Chen & Shi, 2015).

Background of the Study

HIV/AIDS is a global public health challenge affecting both physical and mental health. People living with HIV/AIDS (PLHIV) often face depression, anxiety, stress, and social isolation, which can disrupt treatment adherence. Social support from family, peers, and community groups is vital for mental well-being and consistent use of Antiretroviral Therapy (ART). These networks reduce stigma, provide emotional support, empower PLHIV to manage their condition, and improve quality of life. In vulnerable communities, they also counter harmful behaviors and support livelihoods. Strengthening social networks enhances resilience, mental health, and HIV treatment outcomes.

RESEARCH GAP, OBJECTIVE AND RESEARCH QUESTIONS

Research Gap

The study significantly provides the strengths and proper structure for social networks to increase the mental health outcomes for HIV/AIDS patients. The study emphasizes social support to increase physical health, mental confidence, intersection of social networks, quality of support, and improvement in mental health and well-being for affected individuals. This study can identify an in-depth investigation and provide quality of life, reduce stigma, and enhance advocacy support when promoting social networks and social support systems. This can improve mental health and reduce anxiety and depression among HIV-affected people.

Objectives

1. To evaluate the social network of individuals living with HIV/AIDS.
2. To explore the types of social support available to respondents
3. To examine the relationship between social networks and the quality of social support provided to PLHIV.
4. To investigate how social networks and social support enhance the mental health of PLHIV patients, specifically in reducing anxiety and depression.

Research Questions

1. In what ways do social networks impact the lives of infected individuals?
2. What is the structure and effectiveness of social networks for HIV/AIDS affected persons?
3. What kinds of social support are accessible to individuals HIV persons?
4. How effective is the social support in meeting the emotional and practical needs of affected vulnerable persons?

5. What is the nature of social networks available to HIV/AIDS individuals, and how do these networks affect their well-being?
6. How does the quality of social support within these networks influence the mental and emotional health of people have HIV/AIDS?
7. In what ways do social networks and social support help reduce anxiety and depression among People experiencing HIV/AIDS?
8. What is the correlation between the strength of social networks, the quality of social support, and the mental health outcomes of HIV/AIDS patients?

RELEVANT REVIEW

There are hundreds of thousands of people living with HIV/AIDS (PLHIV) who are involved in social networks. These social support groups share emotional feelings. The study mainly emphasizes healthcare interventions across various cultural differences and religions, which can play a vital role in improving the HIV care process (Airhihenbuwa et al., 2014). Global trends have identified the role of social networks among PLHIV and healthcare workers. Positive network effects help to intervene in health communication, empower patient well-being, and engage the community (Devy, 2020; Obeagu & Obeagu, 2024).

Figure 1. The impact of social support network structure and function on health and well-being

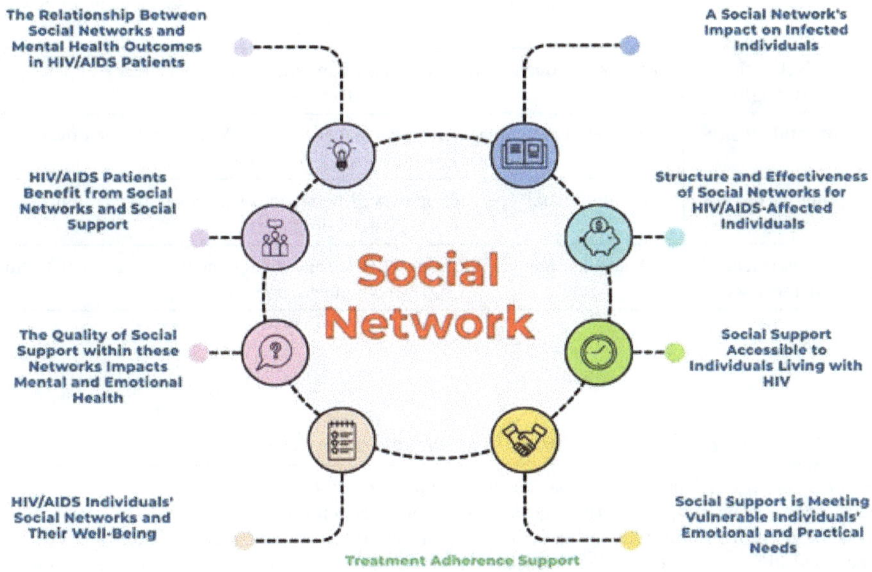

A Social Network's Impact on Infected Individuals

1. Structure and Effectiveness of Social Networks for HIV/AIDS-Affected Individuals
2. Social Support Accessible to Individuals Living with HIV
3. Social Support Meets Vulnerable Individuals' Emotional and Practical Needs
4. HIV/AIDS Individuals' Social Networks and Their Well-Being
5. The Quality of Social Support within These Networks Impacts Mental and Emotional Health
6. HIV/AIDS Patients Benefit from Social Networks and Social Support
7. The Relationship between Social Networks and Mental Health Outcomes in HIV/AIDS Patients.

Table 1. Operational definitions of constructs

Sl. No	Variables	Operational Definitions
1	**Social Support**	Perceived availability and adequacy of emotional, informational, and instrumental support measured through the Lubben Social Network Scale (LSNS).
2	**Network Strength**	The size, frequency, and closeness of an individual's social ties with family and friends.
3	**Mental Health**	The level of emotional well-being and absence of depressive symptoms assessed using standardized psychological scales.
4	**Quality of Life**	The individual's perception of well-being across physical, psychological, and social domains.
5	**Treatment Adherence**	The consistency with which PLHIV follow ART medication and counseling recommendations.

Table 2. Conceptual model of hypothesized relationships

1. Social network strength positively influences social support quality.
2. Social support quality improves mental health and treatment adherence.
3. Mental health mediates the relationship between social support quality and quality of life.
4. Gender and stigma moderate these relationships, affecting the level and effectiveness of received support.

Figure 2. Benefits of social networks

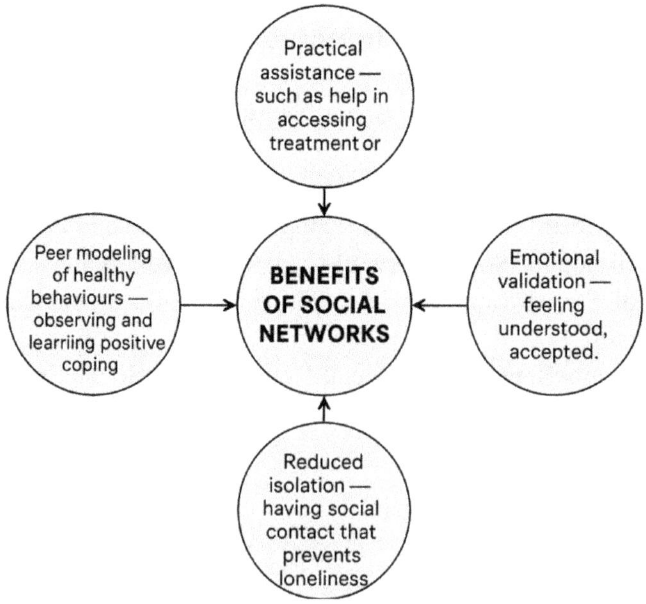

Practical assistance — help in accessing treatment and managing daily needs.

- Emotional validation — feeling understood, accepted, and supported.
- Reduced isolation — social contact that prevents loneliness.
- Peer modeling — learning positive coping and treatment behaviors from others.

Identifying these pathways is crucial for developing targeted and effective interventions to enhance the mental health of people living with HIV.

Digital Platform and Social Networks

The social network provides a wealth of opportunities for affected communities to deliver HIV/Sexually Transmitted Infection (STI) interventions at a minimal level of expenditure, which can reach unlimited geographical areas (Chesson et al., 2017). Social media platforms like Facebook, Twitter, Instagram, and WhatsApp have the potential to utilize social networks for HIV prevention. The social network is convenient for PLHIV individuals for face-to-face interaction in online mode. There is a study on African American and Hispanic men who have sex with men, where participants were identified through social media, although it may lead to bias in the sample (Threats & Bond, 2021; Ibrahim et al., 2024; Kiirya et al., 2025).

The digital platform is used for research-based questions and to identify the nature of social networks. There is a study where a person with 400 friends on Facebook was used to identify how friends influence behaviour (Wolf, 2022). This can provide a comparison of social networks through digital communication versus face-to-face interviews. The social network is more effective when it is target-oriented. The information and behaviour changes occur within the social network itself. Social network interventions can combine both face-to-face and online approaches from different and similar perspectives (Tso et al., 2016; Brandner, 2021).

Education Shapes Network Access and Support Quality

Education provides individuals with broader network opportunities to improve the knowledge of the affected person and their family. To increase peer support contact in professional aspects and promote better communication and understanding for emotional support and healthcare services. Education provides better communication, skills, knowledge, and confidence, helping individuals cope with stigma and engage in social groups. Education restricts network services of lower quality. Education strengthens the network to increase treatment adherence for mental health services.

Network Dynamics and Health Interdependence after Diagnosis

After diagnosis, networks may weaken due to stigma and emotional distress but can strengthen through peer and community support. Health and network participation are bidirectional—better health enables engagement, while supportive networks reduce stress, improve adherence, and enhance well-being.

Volunteer Counseling and Testing Social Networks

Volunteers who are living with HIV can support in identifying people and referring them for testing at the ICTC. This kind of volunteer work provides awareness in the community and in crowded places, and once individuals are identified, they can be referred to the ICTC center (Chellaiyann et al., 2018; George et al., 2024). An effective approach for newly HIV-infected individuals is to raise awareness about HIV infection status, provide counseling, and motivate them to take regular treatment. Providing counseling and referring them to testing centers and social networks is an effective way to support newly HIV-infected persons (WHO, 2021). The network-based services can alleviate barriers for those who face challenges in accessing HIV testing. Peer support groups can encourage and motivate individuals to get tested for HIV. Through social networks, HIV testing can be increased, and although there are no randomized controlled trials (RCTs), the emphasis on social network approaches remains strong (Hu, 2024; Monroe-Wise et al., 2025).

Social Support Networks, HIV Medical Care, and Medication Adherence

Social networks provide resources such as transportation services, access to medical facilities, appointments with health professionals, and emotional support for PLHIV individuals who are impoverished. Social support is a strong factor in the utilization of health care services and in supporting treatment adherence (Oliveeira et al., 2020; Waterfield et al., 2021). For those affected by HIV, the network initiates contact with close individuals, such as sex partners, to encourage testing and provide early diagnosis support services. There is a higher number of individuals affected among IDUs, and it is associated with HIV infections, as results have proven (Chiou et al., 2022). Networks can identify the impact of partner gender-related issues among impoverished populations who are affected. Main partners affected by HIV infections are also associated with treatment adherence among persons. Peer support groups play a role in supporting HIV-infected persons with treatment adherence services (Hill, 2019; Berg et al., 2021).

Social Network Interventions

Social networks provide intervention-based support and reduce long-term costs for affected individuals. This is achieved by promoting social norms and including considerations for sex and drug users (Broadhead et al., 2002). This can be particularly focused on marginalized and stigmatized vulnerable groups. Social networks play a key role in preventing HIV and reducing its transmission by promoting behavior change through support groups (Veinot, 2009; Conyers et al., 2017; West, 2019).

Treatment Adherence

The study emphasizes the role of social networks in improving treatment adherence and health outcomes for people living with HIV/AIDS. Volunteer-based networks strengthen health literacy, self-efficacy, and coping, while also reducing stigma and enhancing ART effectiveness.Families play a vital role in providing care, raising awareness, and supporting treatment. Engaging family members and neighbors ensures timely treatment monitoring, better health outcomes, and an overall improved quality of life for PLHIV.

Integrating Men and Alcohol Users in HIV Prevention: A Social Network Approach

Social network approach scientifically to involving men in HIV prevention. The nation should prevent the social network access to those involved in alcohol use among men, to target and provide various intervention strategies. This can focus on various indicators such as selecting vulnerable geographical locations, planning, implementation, evaluation, and involving private and public collaboration.

Figure 3. Preventing HIV/AIDS among alcohol users through social networks

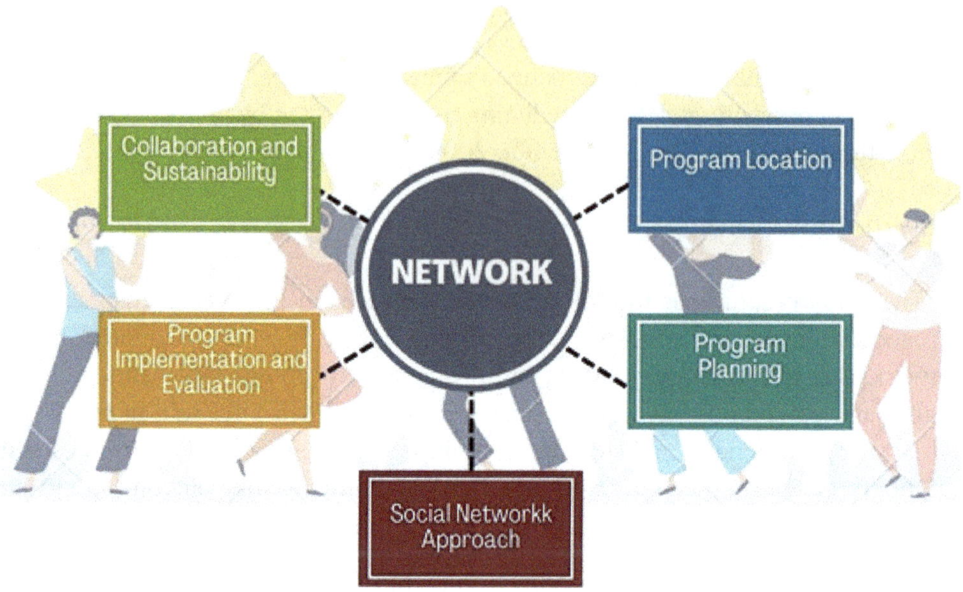

Program Location

To provide the community-based prevention activities to sensitize the community-driven. Provide mass media campaigns so they can reach and make an impact on the community (Aidoo-Frimpong et al., 2025). The targeted intervention should focus on the area, especially men, to engage through networks such as vulnerable areas, wine shops, youth clubs, sports groups, fun clubs, and other related groups. Venues like slum areas and public crowded places should be used to conduct health camps, such as testing for ICTC, involving people from public health centers (Ntiboneka, 2015).

Table 3. Healthcare delivery services

Sl. No	ART Healthcare Delivery	NGO Healthcare Services
1	ART centers are run by the government	It is run by a Non-Governmental Organization
2	Providing drugs and clinical services such as diagnosis, ART, and medical care.	Providing counseling services, psychosocial support, and community-based services.
3	Maintaining standard protocol services, especially for medical and clinical support.	This might provide social connection, emotional support services, and education for their needs.
4	Free and subsidized.	Funded through specific funds, donations, and voluntary services.
5	The target group is people living with HIV (PLHIV) who register under the government.	The target groups are vulnerable populations, including women, children, and high-risk individuals.
6	To control co-infections such as TB and other types of diseases.	To create awareness, prevent HIV, and provide treatment adherence support.

Gender-Specific Network Patterns

Gender roles play a vital role in social networks, especially among people living with HIV (PLHIV). Women affected by HIV are a smaller proportion, mainly due to family-centered networks. They often face societal norms and carry multiple responsibilities. Gender involves the type of services received and how it impacts mental health, treatment support, and enhances the quality of life.

Transgender PLHIV Experiences

The transgender regularly face challenges in their family and society, and they prefer peer support groups such as transgender community services. Gender-sensitive services provide counseling and community-based involvement, which can increase treatment adherence and mental health support for transgender individuals.

Social Support Dimensions

Social support involves various functions such as emotional and informational support to enhance health and well-being. Social support demonstrates various dimensions that help build resilience, enhance mental health support, and improve treatment adherence among PLHIV individuals.

Gender Considerations

Gender can influence the network, as women are highly affected by stigma, while men face fewer stigma-related issues. Transgender individuals face dual problems—discrimination in society and healthcare facilities—and advocate for peer network support. Gender sensitivity helps enhance mental health wellness and treatment continuation.

Social Support Theory

Social Support Theory highlights social relationships and emotional behavioral support to reduce stress levels and provide better health support for affected individuals. Affected individuals need support at the family level and from peer networks to ensure regular treatment adherence and improve their quality of life.

Stress and Coping Theory

Affected individuals need to learn how to manage stressful situations and cope with social support services. Stress affects mental health, and social support helps protect HIV-affected individuals by identifying their levels of stigma and depression.

Social Network Theory

Social Network Theory emphasizes the structure of relationships to build strong network access for better resources and information. Affected individuals involved in better-quality social networks experience improved emotional well-being and greater healthcare engagement.

Collaboration and Sustainability

Public and private collaboration should involve private business people, such as those running wine shops, as they can contribute to program sustainability. Clarify their doubts, and engage wine shop workers and staff members who frequently interact with high-risk individuals (Sivaram et al., 2007; Douglas-Jones, 2014). Support them in identifying at-risk populations.

Psychometric Properties

The Lubben's Social Network Scale (LSNS) explains the value of reliability and validity for various target populations. The LSNS explains the Cronbach's alpha value, which ranges from 0.80 to 0.92, and it is associated with different age groups. Social network can correlate with loneliness and depression among affected individual groups. This might validate the ability to understand depressive symptoms and their impact on quality of life. The variable analysis includes two factors: one is family and friendship networks, and the other is emotional and instrumental support.

Cultural Appropriateness for Tamil Nadu

The LSNS was developed in the West, but it is used universally to assess social support and its availability. The cultural adaptations for HIV-affected persons in Tamil Nadu are as follows:

Figure 4. Cultural adaptation and relevance of LSNS-6 in the Tamil Nadu context

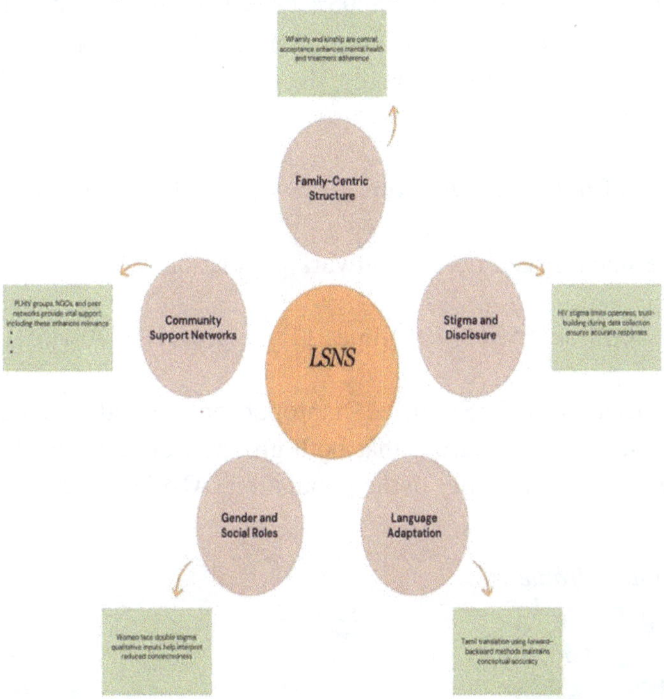

Family and kinship are central in Tamil culture, supporting mental health and treatment adherence. HIV-related stigma limits disclosure, making trust vital for accurate responses. The Tamil LSNS, translated via the forward–backward method, ensures linguistic and conceptual clarity. Gender norms influence social connectedness, with women experiencing double stigma from HIV and societal expectations. Community groups, PLHIV networks, and NGOs provide essential emotional and social support. The LSNS is a reliable, culturally adaptable tool for assessing social isolation and support quality, offering valuable insights into the psychosocial wellbeing of PLHIV in Tamil Nadu.

RESEARCH METHODLOGY

The total population (N) consists of 770 individuals, combining two groups: the NGO population and the Positive Network population. The NGO population includes 115 individuals, with 65 females and 50 males. The Positive Network population includes 655 individuals, comprising 333 males, 333 females, and 322 individuals classified as unclassified. To reduce the sample size while maintaining reasonable accuracy, the margin of error (E) was increased from 5% to 7% (0.07), and the confidence level (Z) was lowered from 95% (Z = 1.96) to 90% (Z = 1.645). These adjustments led to a reduction in the minimum sample size to 118.

To allocate the sample proportionally, the sample size for the NGO population was calculated as:

115770×118≈18\frac{115}{770} \times 118 \approx 18770115×118≈18

The sample size for the Positive Network population was calculated as:

655770×118≈100\frac{655}{770} \times 118 \approx 100770655×118≈100

The researcher adopted the Stratified Disproportionate Random Sampling method to identify the sampling, ensuring that both groups were adequately represented while considering the variability in the population (Al-Worafi, 2024).

Figure 5. Sampling framework

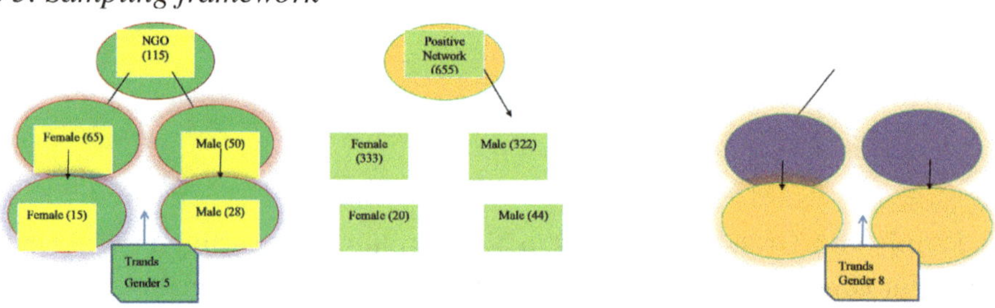

Tools of Data Collection

The researcher prepared a self-prepared interview schedule to relevant data on the following factors contributing to the spread of HIV/AIDS and standardized rating scales. They are - Characteristics of the respondents such as Age, Gender, Marital status, Knowledge about HIV/AIDS, Family Details, Economic Status, Clinical Details, General Health Conditions and Impact of HIV status on Social Life.

Inclusion Criteria

Adults above the age of 18 are included for the study.

Both male and female respondents are included for the study.

Respondents with or without spouse are included for the study.

Respondents with or without children are included for the study.

Respondents with or without job are included for the study.

Respondents under ART and Non ART treatment are included for the study.

Exclusion Criteria

Adults above the age of 60 are excluded from the study.

Respondents who are not identified as HIV positive by the Government are excluded from the study.

Relatives living with HIV/AIDS are excluded from the study.

Respondents who take medicines outside Pudukottai District are excluded from the Study.

Respondents who are outside Pudukottai District are not included in the study.

Respondents who are not enrolled in the 2 NGO's are excluded from the study.

RESULT

Table 4. Demographic and socio-economic profile of respondents (N = 120)

Descriptions	Options	Frequency	Valid Percent
Age	16 - 35	*22*	*18.3*
	36-40	*39*	*32.5*
	41-50	*55*	*45.8*
	51-60	*4*	*3.3*
	Total	***120***	***100***
Gender	Male	*72*	*60*
	Female	*35*	*29.2*
	Transgender	*13*	*10.8*
	Total	***120***	***100***
Marital Status	Single	*18*	*15*
	Married	*51*	*42.5*
	Separated	*28*	*23.3*
	Widowed	*14*	*11.7*
	Divorced	*9*	*7.5*
	Total	***120***	***100***
Education Qualification	No formal education	*45*	*37.5*
	Primary	*37*	*30.8*
	Secondary	*27*	*22.5*
	Graduate	*7*	*5.8*
	Postgraduate	*4*	*3.3*
	Total	***120***	***100***
Occupation	Laobur	*32*	*26.7*
	Agriculture	*30*	*25*
	Self-Employee	*37*	*30.8*
	Government	*8*	*6.7*
	Private	*13*	*10.8*
	Total	***120***	***100***

continued on following page

Table 4. Continued

Descriptions	Options	Frequency	Valid Percent
Monthly Income	below 5000	*40*	*33.3*
	5000 - 10000	*34*	*28.3*
	10001 - 15000	*28*	*23.3*
	15001 - 20000	*13*	*10.8*
	Above 20,001	*5*	*4.2*
	Total	***120***	***100***
Duration since HIV Diagnosis	Below 2 years	*42*	*35*
	3 - 5 yrs	*30*	*25*
	6 to 8 yrs	*21*	*17.5*
	9 to 10yrs	*17*	*14.2*
	Above 11 years	*10*	*8.3*
	Total	***120***	***100***
Location	Urban	*56*	*46.7*
	Rural	*64*	*53.3*
	Total	*120*	*100*
Name of the Block	Annavasal	*13*	*10.8*
	Aranthangi	*15*	*12.5*
	Avudaiyarkoil	*23*	*19.2*
	Karambakkudi	*26*	*21.7*
	Viralimalai	*27*	*22.5*
	Manamelkudi	*16*	*13.3*
	Total	***120***	***100***

Age Distribution

The majority of respondents are in the 41–50 years age group (45.8%), followed by 36–40 years (32.5%). Younger individuals (16–35 years) make up 18.3%, while those aged 51–60 are the least represented (3.3%). Gender Male respondents constitute the majority at 60%, with females at 29.2% and transgender individuals at 10.8%. Marital Status Most participants are married (42.5%), followed by separated (23.3%). Single (15%), widowed (11.7%), and divorced (7.5%) statuses are also noted. Educational Qualification A significant portion of respondents have no formal education (37.5%) or only primary education (30.8%).Secondary education accounts for 22.5%, while only a small proportion have graduate (5.8%) or postgraduate (3.3%) qualifications. Occupation The dominant occupations are self-employed (30.8%), labourers (26.7%), and those involved in agriculture (25%).Fewer respondents work in the private sector (10.8%) or government jobs (6.7%). Monthly Income A large majority earn below 10,000 per month (61.6%), with 33.3% earning below 5,000. Only 15% earn above 15,000, with just 4.2% earning above 20,000. Duration Since HIV Diagnosis 60% of participants have been diagnosed within the past 5 years, while 40% have been living with HIV for over 6 years. 35% were diagnosed less than 2 years ago, indicating a relatively recent increase in diagnoses. Slightly more participants are from rural areas (53.3%) compared to urban (46.7%). Geographical Distribution The largest groups are from Viralimalai (22.5%), Karambakkudi (21.7%), and Avudaiyarkoil (19.2%) Other blocks like Manamelkudi (13.3%), Aranthangi (12.5%), and Annavasal (10.8%) also contribute.

Table 5. Communication patterns on health condition among respondents (N = 120)

Descriptions	**Options**	**Frequency**	**Valid Percent**
Number of People Regularly Talked to About Health Condition	1 to 2 member	*50*	*41.7*
	3 members	*29*	*24.2*
	4 members	*19*	*15.8*
	More than 4 members	*22*	*18.3*
	Total	***120***	***100***
Type of People Regularly Talked	Family	*38*	*31.7*
	Friends	*22*	*18.3*
	Partner/Spouse	*28*	*23.3*
	Healthcare provider	*14*	*11.7*
	Support group members	*18*	*15*
	Total	***120***	***100***
Frequency of Communication	Daily	*23*	*19.2*
	Weekly	*24*	*20*
	Monthly	*33*	*27.5*
	Occasionally	*27*	*22.5*
	Never	*13*	*10.8*
	Total	***120***	***100***

continued on following page

Table 5. Continued

Descriptions	Options	Frequency	Valid Percent
Frequency of Interaction	In person	*40*	*33.3*
	Phone calls	*27*	*22.5*
	Text messages	*19*	*15.8*
	Social media	*19*	*15.8*
	Support group meetings	*15*	*12.5*
	Total	***120***	***100***
Number Who Know About HIV Status	1 to 2 member	*41*	*34.2*
	3 members	*34*	*28.3*
	4 members	*23*	*19.2*
	Nonof them not knowing	*22*	*18.3*
	Total	***120***	***100***

Number of People Regularly Spoken To

Majority (41.7%) talk to 1–2 people, while 24.2% talk to 3 members. 15.8% speak with 4 people, and 18.3% with more than 4. Type of People Consulte Most respondents talk to family (31.7%), followed by partners/spouses (23.3%) and friends (18.3%). Support group members (15%) and healthcare providers (11.7%) were also consulted. Frequency of Communication: Communication is monthly (27.5%) or occasionally (22.5%) for nearly half. 19.2% interact daily, while 20% do so weekly; 10.8% never discuss their condition. Mode of Interaction Interaction is mostly in person (33.3%), followed by phone calls (22.5%). Text messages and social media are used equally (15.8% each), with support group meetings at 12.5%. Number Aware of HIV Status 1–2 people are aware in 34.2% of cases; 3 people in 28.3%, and 4 people in 19.2%. 18.3% said no one knows about their status.

Table 6. Social network and support for people living with HIV/AIDS (N = 120)

Descriptions	Yes	%	No	%	Sometimes	%	Total	%
Network Involvement	*46*	*38.3*	*56*	*46.7*	*18*	*15*	*120*	*100*
Emotional Support	*68*	*56.7*	*29*	*24.2*	*23*	*19.2*	*120*	*100*
Descriptions	**Govt**		**NGO**		**Other Services**		**Total**	%

continued on following page

Table 6. Continued

Descriptions	Yes	%	No	%	Sometimes	%	Total	%
Practical Support Providers	*28*	*23.3*	*77*	*64.2*	*15*	*12.5*	*120*	*100*
Descriptions	**Weekly**		**Monthly**		**Occasionally**		**Total**	%
Participation Frequency	*39*	*32.5*	*58*	*48.3*	*23*	*19.2*	*120*	*100*
Descriptions	**Yes**		**No**		**Not sure**		**Total**	%
Help in Managing HIV/AIDS	*52*	*43.3*	*41*	*34.2*	*27*	*22.5*	*120*	*100*
Descriptions	**Yes**		**No**		**Maybe**		**Total**	%
Network Expansion	*49*	*40.8*	*50*	*41.7*	*21*	*17.5*	*120*	*100*
Descriptions	**Yes**		**No**		**Totla**	%		
Receiving Practical Support	*88*	*73.3*	*32*	*26.7*	*120*	*100*		
Judgment/Discrimination	*29*	*24.2*	*91*	*75.8*	*120*	*100*		
Support Group Participation	*85*	*70.8*	*35*	*29.2*	*120*	*100*		
Member of Organization	*83*	*69.2*	*37*	*30.8*	*120*	*100*		
Digital Connectivity	*88*	*73.3*	*32*	*26.7*	*120*	*100*		

Network Involvement & Emotional Support

46 (38.3%) are actively involved in a network; 56 (46.7%) are not. 68 (56.7%) feel emotionally supported by their network; 29 (24.2%) do not, and 23 (19.2%) feel supported sometimes. Practical Support Received Mainly received from NGOs (64.2%), followed by government (23.3%), and other services (12.5%). 88 (73.3%) receive practical support; 32 (26.7%) do not.

Participation Frequency Participation

Participation is monthly (48.3%), weekly (32.5%), and occasionally (19.2%). Network's Role in HIV Management 52 (43.3%) report their network has helped manage HIV/AIDS. 41 (34.2%) say no; 27 (22.5%) are unsure.

Support Network Expansion

49 (40.8%) expanded their network; 50 (41.7%) did not; 21 (17.5%) maybe. Perceived Discriminatio 29 (24.2%) feel judged or discriminated against; 91 (75.8%) do not. Support Group Membership 85 (70.8%) are part of an HIV/AIDS support group/ community; 83 (69.2%) are members of a formal organization. Digital Connectivity 88 (73.3%) use social media or mobile apps to stay in touch; 32 (26.7%) do not.

Table 7. Understanding the role of social networks and healthcare in supporting PLHIV

Descriptions	Strongly Disagree	%	Disagree	%	Neutral		Agree	%	Strongly Agree	%	Total	%
Someone to talk to when sad/ overwhelmed	*18*	*15*	*12*	*10*	*18*	*15*	*44*	*36.7*	*28*	*23.3*	*120*	*100*
Family supports my HIV status emotionally	*9*	*7.5*	*15*	*12.5*	*24*	*20*	*38*	*31.7*	*34*	*28.3*	*120*	*100*
Feel cared for by someone close	*8*	*6.7*	*14*	*11.7*	*15*	*12.5*	*35*	*29.2*	*48*	*40*	*120*	*100*
Can share fears with someone trusted	*12*	*10*	*25*	*20.8*	*24*	*20*	*28*	*23.3*	*31*	*25.8*	*120*	*100*
Receive encouragement in tough times	*27*	*22.5*	*22*	*18.3*	*21*	*17.5*	*28*	*23.3*	*22*	*18.3*	*120*	*100*
Get accurate HIV/AIDS treatment info	*8*	*6.7*	*28*	*23.3*	*27*	*22.5*	*32*	*26.7*	*25*	*20.8*	*120*	*100*
Healthcare providers explain clearly	*16*	*13.3*	*16*	*13.3*	*30*	*25*	*38*	*31.7*	*20*	*16.7*	*120*	*100*
Aware of support services/programs	*14*	*11.7*	*18*	*15*	*26*	*21.7*	*37*	*30.8*	*25*	*20.8*	*120*	*100*
Receive helpful health advice	*14*	*11.7*	*22*	*18.3*	*30*	*25*	*33*	*27.5*	*21*	*17.5*	*120*	*100*
Support groups offer useful guidance	*14*	*11.7*	*18*	*15*	*22*	*18.3*	*39*	*32.5*	*27*	*22.5*	*120*	*100*
Help with clinic/ hospital transport	*21*	*17.5*	*28*	*23.3*	*39*	*32.5*	*23*	*19.2*	*9*	*7.5*	*120*	*100*
Receive financial aid when needed	*24*	*20*	*28*	*23.3*	*22*	*18.3*	*28*	*23.3*	*18*	*15*	*120*	*100*
Help with daily tasks when unwell	*30*	*25*	*46*	*38.3*	*26*	*21.7*	*14*	*11.7*	*4*	*3.3*	*120*	*100*
Access to nutritious food via support	*12*	*10*	*21*	*17.5*	*33*	*27.5*	*42*	*35*	*12*	*10*	*120*	*100*
NGOs/community give practical help	*9*	*7.5*	*19*	*15.8*	*23*	*19.2*	*42*	*35*	*27*	*22.5*	*120*	*100*
Get feedback to know my strengths	*12*	*10*	*21*	*17.5*	*33*	*27.5*	*42*	*35*	*12*	*10*	*120*	*100*
Encouraged to stay positive	*12*	*10*	*28*	*23.3*	*46*	*38.3*	*21*	*17.5*	*13*	*10.8*	*120*	*100*
Respected in support group/ community	*24*	*20*	*25*	*20.8*	*25*	*20.8*	*28*	*23.3*	*18*	*15*	*120*	*100*
Get advice to improve my situation	*15*	*12.5*	*14*	*11.7*	*19*	*15.8*	*36*	*30*	*36*	*30*	*120*	*100*
Reminded of my value and worth	*23*	*19.2*	*27*	*22.5*	*22*	*18.3*	*32*	*26.7*	*16*	*13.3*	*120*	*100*

continued on following page

Table 7. Continued

Descriptions	Strongly Disagree	%	Disagree	%	Neutral		Agree	%	Strongly Agree	%	Total	%
Feel emotionally supported socially	*16*	*13.3*	*14*	*11.7*	*23*	*19.2*	*26*	*21.7*	*41*	*34.2*	*120*	*100*
Have someone to discuss feelings	*15*	*12.5*	*25*	*20.8*	*34*	*28.3*	*19*	*15.8*	*27*	*22.5*	*120*	*100*
Feel accepted, not judged	*23*	*19.2*	*28*	*23.3*	*18*	*15*	*24*	*20*	*27*	*22.5*	*120*	*100*
Get accurate HIV management info	*23*	*19.2*	*7*	*5.8*	*16*	*13.3*	*29*	*24.2*	*45*	*37.5*	*120*	*100*
Social circle helps with treatment info	*11*	*9.2*	*15*	*12.5*	*15*	*12.5*	*38*	*31.7*	*41*	*34.2*	*120*	*100*
Learn from others' HIV experience	*9*	*7.5*	*8*	*6.7*	*18*	*15*	*43*	*35.8*	*42*	*35*	*120*	*100*
Receive financial help when needed	*15*	*12.5*	*9*	*7.5*	*15*	*12.5*	*45*	*37.5*	*36*	*30*	*120*	*100*
Help with medical visit transport	*35*	*29.2*	*19*	*15.8*	*19*	*15.8*	*26*	*21.7*	*21*	*17.5*	*120*	*100*
Others help me see my strengths	*15*	*12.5*	*14*	*11.7*	*27*	*22.5*	*25*	*20.8*	*39*	*32.5*	*120*	*100*
Strong network improves support quality	*21*	*17.5*	*13*	*10.8*	*14*	*11.7*	*33*	*27.5*	*39*	*32.5*	*120*	*100*
Social ties boost confidence in managing HIV	*25*	*20.8*	*19*	*15.8*	*19*	*15.8*	*28*	*23.3*	*29*	*24.2*	*120*	*100*
Mental health benefits from social support	*13*	*10.8*	*9*	*7.5*	*20*	*16.7*	*42*	*35*	*36*	*30*	*120*	*100*
Support helps with treatment adherence	*10*	*8.3*	*9*	*7.5*	*20*	*16.7*	*45*	*37.5*	*36*	*30*	*120*	*100*

Emotional Support & Social Connection

56.6% agree or strongly agree they have someone to talk to when sad or overwhelmed. 60% feel emotionally supported by their family regarding their HIV status. 69.2% feel cared for by someone close. Only 49.1% say they can confidently share fears and anxieties with someone trusted. 41.6% feel encouraged during tough times — while 40.8% disagree or are neutral.

Access to Information & Services

47.5% report getting accurate HIV/AIDS treatment info. 48.4% agree that healthcare providers explain their condition clearly. 51.6% are aware of available support services/programs. 45% receive helpful health advice. 55% find support groups useful in guidance.

Practical Support

26.7% get transport help for clinic visits; 40.8% do not. 38.3% receive financial aid; 43.3% do not. Only 15% get help with daily tasks when unwell.45% have access to nutritious food via support services. 57.5% agree NGOs and community workers give practical help.

Recognition, Acceptance & Empowerment

45.8% get feedback that helps them know their strengths. 28.3% feel encouraged to stay positive; 61.6% are neutral or disagree. 38.3% feel respected in their support group or community. 60% receive advice to improve their situation. 40% feel reminded of their value and worth.

Judgment, Acceptance & Belonging

55.9% feel emotionally supported in their social circle. 38.3% feel they can discuss their feelings openly. 42.5% feel accepted and not judged — but 42.5% disagree or are neutral.

Knowledge Sharing & Learning

1.7% say they receive accurate HIV management information. 66% say social contacts help them stay informed. 70.8% learn from others' experiences in managing HIV.

Impact of Network & Social Ties

67.5% say they receive financial help when needed. 39.2% get transport support for medical visits. 53.3% say others help them recognize their strengths. 60% feel a strong network improves the quality of support. 47.5% feel more confident managing HIV because of social ties.65% say social support benefits their mental health.67.5% agree that social support helps maintain treatment adherence.

Table 8. The influence of social support on anxiety, depression, and isolation

Descriptions	Not at all	%	Several days	%	More than half the days	%	Nearly every day	%	Total	%
Mental Health and Social Support	*24*	*20*	*32*	*26.7*	*34*	*28.3*	*30*	*25*	*120*	*100*
Emotional Well-being and Social Ties	*32*	*26.7*	*48*	*40*	*24*	*20*	*16*	*13.3*	*120*	*100*
Psychological Distress and Support Systems	*19*	*15.8*	*56*	*46.7*	*14*	*11.7*	*31*	*25.8*	*120*	*100*
Anxiety, Depression, and Social Support	*24*	*20*	*37*	*30.8*	*19*	*15.8*	*40*	*33.3*	*120*	*100*
Impact of Social Connections on Mental Health	*32*	*26.7*	*48*	*40*	*24*	*20*	*16*	*13.3*	*120*	*100*
Support Networks and Emotional Health	*24*	*20*	*44*	*36.7*	*19*	*15.8*	*33*	*27.5*	*120*	*100*
Mental Health Relief Through Social Support	*13*	*10.8*	*53*	*44.2*	*15*	*12.5*	*39*	*32.5*	*120*	*100*
Role of Social Ties in Mental Well-being	*10*	*8.3*	*56*	*46.7*	*14*	*11.7*	*40*	*33.3*	*120*	*100*
Social Ties Ease Isolation	*24*	*20*	*28*	*23.3*	*30*	*25*	*38*	*31.7*	*120*	*100*

Many respondents experience persistent mental health challenges, with 28.3% facing issues more than half the days and 25% nearly every day, highlighting the importance of social support. Most individuals (66.7%) feel emotionally supported, though 13.3% report frequent struggles, suggesting that social relationships help but do not fully prevent distress. Psychological distress is common, affecting 46.7% for several days and 25.8% nearly daily, while 33.3% report near-daily anxiety or depression, emphasizing the need for strong support systems. A majority of respondents (66.7–80%) benefit from social ties, which help reduce isolation (56.7%) and provide relief from distress (44.2% several days, 32.5% nearly daily). The quality and depth of these connections significantly influence mental well-being, demonstrating that social support plays a key role in alleviating psychological distress, anxiety, and isolation.

DISCUSSION

The majority of respondents are aged 41–50 (45.8%), followed by 36–40 (32.5%), with youth (16–35) representing 18.3% and those above 50 only 3.3% (Bennin, 2024; Nsanzimana et al., 2022). Males constitute 60%, females 29.2%, and transgender individuals 10.8%. Most are married (42.5%), while others are separated (23.3%), single (15%), widowed (11.7%), or divorced (7.5%) (Didi, 2014). Educational levels are low, with 68.3% having no or primary education and 9.1% holding graduate/postgraduate degrees (Nwosu, 2024). Employment is mainly self-employment (30.8%), labor (26.7%), or farming (25%), with fewer in private (10.8%) or government (6.7%) jobs. Most earn below 10,000/month (61.6%), including 33.3% under 5,000, while only 4.2% earn above 20,000 (Hiremath, 2021).

Regarding HIV, 60% were diagnosed within five years and 35% within two, indicating recent increases. Slightly more participants are from rural areas (53.3%), particularly Viralimalai (22.5%), Karambakkudi (21.7%), and Avudaiyarkoil (19.2%) (Dagnaw, 2024). Social interaction is limited: 41.7% regularly talk to 1–2 people, mostly family (31.7%) or partners (23.3%), while 34.2% disclose their HIV status to 1–2 individuals and 18.3% to none (Mugerwa, 2023). Communication is mainly in-person (33.3%) or by phone (22.5%). Participation in social networks is moderate (38.3%), with 46.7% not involved. Emotional support is reported by 56.7%, and practical NGO support by 64.2% (financial aid 38.3%, transportation 26.7%, food 45%) (Derkinderen, 2017). Networks aid HIV management: 43.3% report benefits, 41.7% note expanded social connections, 70.8% join support groups, 69.2% participate in formal organizations, and 73.3% use digital platforms (Dulli et al., 2020). Mental health challenges persist, with 25% experiencing daily distress, but 66.7% receive emotional support, 65% report improved mental health, and 67.5% say support aids treatment adherence (Aunon, 2020; Ridgeway, 2024). About 42.5% feel accepted, 45.8% receive encouraging feedback, and 80% acknowledge social ties enhance overall well-being (Cederbaum et al., 2017; Teixeira da Silva et al., 2020).

CONCLUSION

Social Network Approach

The social network approach delivers cost-effective services and reaches hidden populations. It identifies risks among vulnerable communities, enabling targeted support for those affected or at risk of HIV (Board on Population Health, 2011; Amirkhanian, 2014). Key elements include leveraging networks to influence behavior, supporting network dynamics, empowering PLHIV, and addressing transmission patterns (Veenstra et al., 2013; Masila, 2024). Social networks optimize HIV care, reduce transmission, and protect future generations (Wambaire, 2019).

REFERENCES

Aidoo-Frimpong, G. A., Adekunle, T., Abu'Baare, G. R., & Adu, C. (2025). Community-Driven Recommendations for Developing Culturally Aligned Messaging to Improve Pre-Exposure Prophylaxis Acceptability and Uptake Among US-Based African Immigrants. *AIDS Patient Care and STDs*. Advance online publication. DOI: 10.1089/apc.2025.0020 PMID: 40106264

Airhihenbuwa, C. O., Ford, C. L., & Iwelunmor, J. I. (2014). Why culture matters in health interventions: Lessons from HIV/AIDS stigma and NCDs. *Health Education & Behavior*, *41*(1), 78–84. DOI: 10.1177/1090198113487199 PMID: 23685666

Ajuna, N., Tumusiime, B., Amanya, J., Awori, S., Rukundo, G. Z., & Asiimwe, J. B. (2021). Social networks and barriers to ART adherence among young adults (18–24 years) living with HIV at selected primary health facilities of South-Western Uganda: A Qualitative Study. *HIV/AIDS (Auckland, N.Z.)*, •••, 939–958. PMID: 34675686

Al-Worafi, Y. M. (2024). Medical and Health Sciences in Developing Countries: Sample Size Calculations and Sampling Techniques. In *Handbook of Medical and Health Sciences in Developing Countries: Education, Practice, and Research* (pp. 1–10). Springer International Publishing.

Amirkhanian, Y. A. (2014). Social networks, sexual networks and HIV risk in men who have sex with men. *Current HIV/AIDS Reports*, *11*, 81–92. DOI: 10.1007/s11904-013-0194-4 PMID: 24384832

Areri, H. A., Marshall, A., & Harvey, G. (2020). Interventions to improve self-management of adults living with HIV on antiretroviral therapy: A systematic review. *PLoS One*, *15*(5), e0232709. DOI: 10.1371/journal.pone.0232709 PMID: 32392245

Aunon, F. M. (2020). *Development and evaluation of a theory-informed mHealth intervention to promote viral suppression among women living with HIV who engage in sex work in Mombasa, Kenya: the role of text messaging, social support and stigma*. University of Washington.

Bennin, L. (2024). *Mental Health And Psychological Well-Being Assessment Of People Living With Hiv/Aids In Cape Coast Teaching Hospital* (Doctoral dissertation, University of Cape Coast). https://ir.ucc.edu.gh/xmlui/handle/123456789/11632

Berg, R. C., Page, S., & Øgård-Repål, A. (2021). The effectiveness of peer-support for people living with HIV: A systematic review and meta-analysis. *PLoS One*, *16*(6), e0252623. DOI: 10.1371/journal.pone.0252623 PMID: 34138897

Birore, C. M., Wu, L., Abrefa-Gyan, T., & Lewis, M. W. (2022). Social support and quality of life among people living with HIV/AIDS (PLWHA) in Ghana. *Journal of Family Issues, 43*(8), 2159–2180. DOI: 10.1177/0192513X21103004

Board on Population Health, Public Health Practice, Committee on HIV Screening, & Access to Care. (2011). *HIV Screening and Access to Care: Exploring the Impact of Policies on Access to and Provision of HIV Care.*

Brandner, L. O. U. (2021). The social capital of creative freelancers. Networking practices in digital and urban spheres. https://iris.uniroma1.it/handle/11573/1568978

Broadhead, R. S., Heckathorn, D. D., Altice, F. L., Van Hulst, Y., Carbone, M., Friedland, G. H., O'Connor, P. G., & Selwyn, P. A. (2002). Increasing drug users' adherence to HIV treatment: Results of a peer-driven intervention feasibility study. *Social Science & Medicine, 55*(2), 235–246. DOI: 10.1016/S0277-9536(01)00167-8 PMID: 12144138

Castro, J. G., & Alcaide, M. L. (2016). High rates of sexually transmitted infections in HIV-infected patients attending an STI clinic. *Southern Medical Journal, 109*(1), 1. DOI: 10.14423/SMJ.0000000000000389 PMID: 26741862

Cederbaum, J. A., Rice, E., Craddock, J., Pimentel, V., & Beaver, P. (2017). Social networks of HIV-positive women and their association with social support and depression symptoms. *Women & Health, 57*(2), 268–282. DOI: 10.1080/03630242.2016.1157126 PMID: 26910637

Chellaiyan, V. G., Raut, D. K., & Khokhar, A. (2018). Integrated counseling and HIV testing centers of Delhi: An evaluation. *Journal of Family Medicine and Primary Care, 7*(4), 791–795. DOI: 10.4103/jfmpc.jfmpc_128_17 PMID: 30234055

Chen, L., & Shi, J. (2015). Social support exchanges in a social media community for people living with HIV/AIDS in China. *AIDS Care, 27*(6), 693–696. DOI: 10.1080/09540121.2014.991678 PMID: 25532704

Chesson, H. W., Mayaud, P., & Aral, S. O. (2017). *Sexually transmitted infections: impact and cost-effectiveness of prevention*. The International Bank for Reconstruction and Development.

Chiou, P. Y., Hung, C. C., & Chen, C. Y. (2022). Sexual partner referral for HIV testing through social networking platforms: Cross-sectional study. *JMIR Public Health and Surveillance, 8*(4), e32156. DOI: 10.2196/32156 PMID: 35380540

Conyers, L. M., Richardson, L. A., Datti, P. A., Koch, L. C., & Misrok, M. (2017). A critical review of health, social, and prevention outcomes associated with employment for people living with HIV. *AIDS Education and Prevention*, *29*(5), 475–490. DOI: 10.1521/aeap.2017.29.5.475 PMID: 29068719

Cox, L. E., & Brennan-Ing, M. (2017). Medical, social and supportive services for older adults with HIV. *Interdisciplinary Topics in Gerontology and Geriatrics*, *42*, 204–221. DOI: 10.1159/000448563 PMID: 27875834

Craddock, J. B., Franke, N. D., & Kingori, C. (2022). Associations of social network- and individual-level factors with HIV testing, condom use, and interest in PrEP among young black women. *Archives of Sexual Behavior*, *51*(5), 2473–2483. DOI: 10.1007/s10508-022-02306-7 PMID: 35676567

Dagnaw, L. (2024). *Prevalence and Associated Risk Factors of Tuberculosis (Tb) Among Adult Human Immunodeficiency Virus (Hiv)/Acquired Immunodeficiency Syndrome (Aids) Patients Attending Health Facilities of South Achefer District Northwestern Ethiopia* (Doctoral dissertation). http://ir.bdu.edu.et/bitstream/handle/123456789/16079/Dagnaw.pdf?sequence=1

De Andrade, S. L. E., Moreira Freire, M. E., Collet, N., Brandão, G. C. G., Souza, M. H. D. N., & Nogueira, J. D. A. (2022). Structure of social networks of people living with HIV and AIDS. *Revista da Escola de Enfermagem da USP*, *56*, e20210525. DOI: 10.1590/1980-220X-REEUSP-2021-0525 PMID: 35201256

Degenhardt, L., Webb, P., Colledge-Frisby, S., Ireland, J., Wheeler, A., Ottaviano, S., Willing, A., Kairouz, A., Cunningham, E. B., Hajarizadeh, B., Leung, J., Tran, L. T., Price, O., Peacock, A., Vickerman, P., Farrell, M., Dore, G. J., Hickman, M., & Grebely, J. (2023). Epidemiology of injecting drug use, prevalence of injecting-related harm, and exposure to behavioural and environmental risks among people who inject drugs: A systematic review. *The Lancet. Global Health*, *11*(5), e659–e672. https://www.thelancet.com/journals/langlo/article/PIIS2214-109X(23)00057-8/fulltext PMID: 36996857

Derkinderen, N. (2017). *Knowledge Attitude and Practice towards HIV/AIDS Prevention among Myanmar Female Sex Workers in Maesot District, Tak.* Province., DOI: 10.58837/CHULA.THE.2017.484

Devy, S. R. (2020). Community Health Worker-Based Empowerment Against Stigmatization of People Living with HIV/AIDS: A Meta-Synthesis. *Systematic Reviews in Pharmacy*, *11*(5).

Didi, N. P. (2014). *Predictors of HIV Self Disclosure to Sexual Partners by Sero-Positive Adults in Informal Settlements: A Case of Central Division, Nairobi County, Kenya* (Doctoral dissertation, Kenyatta University).

Douglas-Jones, I. M. (2014). *The willingness of tavern and shebeen owners in Gqebera, Port Elizabeth to implement or strengthen existing HIV prevention efforts and measures in their establishments* (Doctoral dissertation, Stellenbosch: Stellenbosch University). https://scholar.sun.ac.za/items/28fa9e67-9ac5-472c-afd5-1dcf07246b85

Dulli, L., Ridgeway, K., Packer, C., Murray, K. R., Mumuni, T., Plourde, K. F., Chen, M., Olumide, A., Ojengbede, O., & McCarraher, D. R. (2020). A social media–based support group for youth living with HIV in Nigeria (SMART Connections): Randomized controlled trial. *Journal of Medical Internet Research*, *22*(6), e18343. DOI: 10.2196/18343 PMID: 32484444

Frescura, L., Godfrey-Faussett, P., Feizzadeh, A., El-Sadr, W., Syarif, O., & Ghys, P. D. (2025). Testing Treatment Target Working Group. (2022). Achieving the 95 95 95 targets for all: A pathway to ending AIDS. *PLoS One*, *17*(8), e0272405. DOI: 10.1371/journal.pone.0272405 PMID: 35925943

George, G., Chaturvedi, S., Corbishley, C., & Atun, R. (2024). Relational coordination and stigma at work: How frontline employees compensate for failures in public health systems. *Journal of Management Studies*, *61*(3), 752–784. DOI: 10.1111/joms.12813

Gupta, I., & Barman, K. (2021). Health, development, and HIV in India. In *Oxford Research Encyclopedia of Asian History*. DOI:DOI: 10.1093/acrefore/9780190277727.013.424

Hess, K. L., Crepaz, N., Rose, C., Purcell, D., & Paz-Bailey, G. (2017). Trends in sexual behavior among men who have sex with men (MSM) in high-income countries, 1990–2013: A systematic review. *AIDS and Behavior*, *21*, 2811–2834. DOI: 10.1007/s10461-017-1799-1 PMID: 28555317

Hill, M. (2019). *Characterizing the Social Networks & Art Adherence Behaviors of Trans Women Living with HIV* (Doctoral dissertation, University of Georgia).

Hiremath, R. N. (2021). *A Prospective Study To Assess The Factors Affecting Nutritional Status Of People Living With Hiv/Aids (Plha) Receiving Anti-Retroviral Therapy (Art)* (Doctoral dissertation, BLDE (Deemed to be University)). https://digitallibrary.bldedu.ac.in/handle/123456789/4166

Hlaing, M. M. (2024). *The Effect of Social Support on HIV-related Stigma among People Living with HIV/AIDS (Case Study of Myeik Township)(Mi Mi Hlaing, 2024)* (Doctoral dissertation, MERAL Portal).

Hu, S., Jing, F., Fan, C., Dai, Y., Xie, Y., Zhou, Y., Lv, H., He, X., Wu, D., Tucker, J. D., & Tang, W. (2024). Social network strategies to distribute HIV self-testing kits: A global systematic review and network meta-analysis. *Journal of the International AIDS Society*, *27*(7), e26342. DOI: 10.1002/jia2.26342 PMID: 39048927

Ibrahim, K., Kahle, E. M., Christiani, Y., & Suryani, S. (2024). Utilization of social media for the prevention and control of HIV/AIDS: A scoping review. *Journal of Multidisciplinary Healthcare*, •••, 2443–2458. https://www.tandfonline.com/doi/full/10.2147/JMDH.S465905#references-Section PMID: 38799010

Jaspal, R., Eriksson, P., & Nynäs, P. (2021). Identity, threat and coping among gay men living with HIV in Finland. *Cogent Psychology*, *8*(1), 1878980. DOI: 10.1080/23311908.2021.1878980

Kaufman, M. R., Cornish, F., Zimmerman, R. S., & Johnson, B. T. (2014). Health behavior change models for HIV prevention and AIDS care: Practical recommendations for a multi-level approach. *JAIDS Journal of Acquired Immune Deficiency Syndromes*, *66*, S250–S258. DOI: 10.1097/QAI.0000000000000236 PMID: 25007194

Kiirya, Y., Kitaka, S., Kalyango, J., Rujumba, J., Obeng-Amoako, G. A. O., & Amollo, M., Nan gendo, J., Karamagi, C., Musooke, P., & Katahoire, A. (2025). Acceptability of an online peer support group as a strategy to improve antiretroviral therapy adherence among young people in Kampala district, Uganda: Qualitative findings. *BMC Infectious Diseases*, *25*(1), 461. DOI: 10.1186/s12879-025-10831-8 PMID: 40181265

Knight, L., & Schatz, E. (2022). Social support for improved ART adherence and retention in care among older people living with HIV in urban South Africa: A complex balance between disclosure and stigma. *International Journal of Environmental Research and Public Health*, *19*(18), 11473. DOI: 10.3390/ijerph191811473 PMID: 36141746

Krüsi, A., & Shannon, K. (2022). The Intersecting Social and Structural Contexts of Navigating HIV Risk and Access to Care among Women. *WOMEN'S HEALTH IN CANADA*, 331. https://utppublishing.com/doi/abs/10.3138/9781442628472#page=346

Kumar, P., Sangal, B., Ramanathan, S., Ammassari, S., & Venkatesh, S. R. (2018). Unsafe injecting practices, sexual risk behaviours and determinants of HIV among men who inject drugs: Results from Integrated Biological and Behavioural Surveillance in India. *International Journal of STD & AIDS, 29*(11), 1066–1075. DOI: 10.1177/095646241876980 PMID: 29747557

Laymouna, M. A. (2023). *Informing the Development of a Chatbot for Pharmacist Needs in HIV Care*. McGill University.

Li, L., Wu, S., Wu, Z., Sun, S., Cui, H., & Jia, M. (2006). Understanding family support for people living with HIV/AIDS in Yunnan, China. *AIDS and Behavior, 10*, 509–517. DOI: 10.1007/s10461-006-9071-0 PMID: 16741672

Masila, H. M. (2024). *Using asset-based community development approaches to combat the spread of HIV/AIDS in Mombasa county, Kenya* (Master's thesis, VID Specialized University. Stavanger).

Miller, R. L., Rutledge, J., & Ayala, G. (2021). Breaking down barriers to HIV care for gay and bisexual men and transgender women: The Advocacy and Other Community Tactics (ACT) Project. *AIDS and Behavior, 25*(8), 2551–2567. DOI: 10.1007/s10461-021-03216-w PMID: 33730253

Monroe-Wise, A., Barr-DiChiara, M., Mozalevskis, A., Msimanga, B., de Mello, M. B., Senya, K., & Baggaley, R. (2025). Can network-based testing services have an impact beyond testing for HIV? *Sexual Health, 22*(2). Advance online publication. DOI: 10.1071/SH24027 PMID: 40193579

Mugerwa, M. (2023). *Prevalence, Associated Factors, Barriers and Facilitators of Disclosure of HIV status to sexual partners among Young People Living with HIV/AIDS in care at an Urban HIV Clinic, Kampala, Uganda* (Doctoral dissertation, Makerere University). http://makir.mak.ac.ug/handle/10570/12752

Muwonge, C. M., Kembabazi, A., Nakalema, G., Ekatushabe, M., Kwarikunda, D., Kibedi, H., & Ssenyonga, J. (2022). Psychological Well-Being Among Young People Living with HIV: Role of Social Support, Self-Esteem and Socio-Demographic Variables. In *Embracing Well-Being in Diverse African Contexts: Research Perspectives* (pp. 171–194). Springer International Publishing., DOI: 10.1007/978-3-030-85924-4_8

Mwabenga, B. K. (2019). *Effectiveness of HIV and AIDS Social Support Coping Skill to PLWHA in Kinondoni Municipality, Dar es Salaam: A Case Study of Mwananyamala Hospital* (Doctoral dissertation, The Open University of Tanzania). http://repository.out.ac.tz/2994/

Ndashimye, E., & Arts, E. J. (2019). The urgent need for more potent antiretroviral therapy in low-income countries to achieve UNAIDS 90-90-90 and complete eradication of AIDS by 2030. *Infectious Diseases of Poverty*, *8*(04), 67–74. DOI: 10.1186/s40249-019-0573-1 PMID: 31370888

Nsanzimana, S., Rwibasira, G. N., Malamba, S. S., Musengimana, G., Kayirangwa, E., Jonnalagadda, S., Rezende, E. F., Eaton, J. W., Mugisha, V., Remera, E., Muhamed, S., Mulindabigwi, A., Omolo, J., Weisner, L., Moore, C., Patel, H., & Justman, J. E. (2022). HIV incidence and prevalence among adults aged 15-64 years in Rwanda: Results from the Rwanda Population-based HIV Impact Assessment (RPHIA) and District-level Modeling, 2019. *International Journal of Infectious Diseases*, *116*, 245–254. DOI: 10.1016/j.ijid.2022.01.032 PMID: 35066161

Ntiboneka, A. (2015). *Reduction Of HIV/AIDS Impacts Through PLHIV Clubs' Income Generating Projects: The case of Upendo Club People living with HIV in Mungonya Ward, Kigoma District Council* (Doctoral dissertation, The Open University Of Tanzania). http://repository.out.ac.tz/1124/

Nwosu, C. M. (2024). Level of education and comprehensive knowledge about HIV/AIDS among women aged 15-49 years in Southern Nigeria: A cross-sectional study. https://www.diva-portal.org/smash/record.jsf?pid=diva2%3A1875833&dswid=-7116

Obeagu, E. I., Igwe, M. C., & Obeagu, G. U. (2024). The Power of Unity: Collective Efforts in Confronting HIV Stigma. *Elite Journal of Public Health*, *2*(3), 22–36.

Obeagu, E. I., & Obeagu, G. U. (2024). Moving forward together: Collaborative strategies in HIV prevention across Africa–a narrative review. *Annals of Medicine and Surgery (London)*, *•••*, 10–1097. DOI: 10.1097/MS9.0000000000002961 PMID: 40852004

Obeagu, E. I., & Obeagu, G. U. (2024). Unmasking the Truth: Addressing Stigma in the Fight Against HIV. *Elite Journal of Public Health, 2*(1), 8-22. https://kiu.ac.ug/assets/publications/1415_unmasking-the-truth-addressing-stigma-in-the-fight-against-hiv.pdf

Pagkas-Bather, J., Young, L. E., Chen, Y. T., & Schneider, J. A. (2020). Social network interventions for HIV transmission elimination. *Current HIV/AIDS Reports*, *17*, 450–457. DOI: 10.1007/s11904-020-00524-z PMID: 32720253

Payagala, S., & Pozniak, A. (2024). The global burden of HIV. *Clinics in Dermatology*, *42*(2), 119–127. DOI: 10.1016/j.clindermatol.2024.02.001 PMID: 38387533

Pontes-Pereira, P. S., Antonini, M., Fedocci, E. M. M., Costa, C. R. B., Esquivel-Rubio, A. I., Botelho, E. P., Gir, E., & Reis, R. K. (2023). Prevalence of chronic non-communicable diseases in people living with HIV. *Acta Paulista de Enfermagem, 36*, eAPE01132. Advance online publication. DOI: 10.37689/acta-ape/2023AO011322

Ridgeway, K. (2024). *Psychosocial factors and HIV care engagement among adolescents and young adults living with HIV in Akwa Ibom and Cross River states, Nigeria* (Doctoral dissertation, Johns Hopkins University). https://jscholarship.library.jhu.edu/items/83e491f2-61be-45d3-9e92-5215c747e907

Salmen, C. R., Hickey, M. D., Fiorella, K. J., Omollo, D., Ouma, G., Zoughbie, D., Salmen, M. R., Magerenge, R., Tessler, R., Campbe, H., Geng, E., Gandhi, M., Bukusi, E. A., & Cohen, C. R. (2015). "Wan Kanyakla"(We are together): Community transformations in Kenya following a social network intervention for HIV care. *Social Science & Medicine, 147*, 332–340. DOI: 10.1016/j.socscimed.2015.11.021 PMID: 26638145

Shelton, R. C., Lee, M., Brotzman, L. E., Crookes, D. M., Jandorf, L., Erwin, D., & Gage-Bouchard, E. A. (2019). Use of social network analysis in the development, dissemination, implementation, and sustainability of health behavior interventions for adults: A systematic review. *Social Science & Medicine, 220*, 81–101. DOI: 10.1016/j.socscimed.2018.10.013 PMID: 30412922

Sivaram, S., Johnson, S., Bentley, M. E., Srikrishnan, A. K., Latkin, C. A., Go, V. F., Solomon, S., & Celentano, D. D. (2007). Exploring "wine shops" as a venue for HIV prevention interventions in urban India. *Journal of Urban Health, 84*, 563–576. DOI: 10.1007/s11524-007-9196-0 PMID: 17486455

Sivaram, S., Zelaya, C., Srikrishnan, A. K., Latkin, C., Go, V. F., Solomon, S., & Celentano, D. (2009). Associations between social capital and HIV stigma in Chennai, India: Considerations for prevention intervention design. *AIDS Education and Prevention, 21*(3), 233–250. DOI: 10.1521/aeap.2009.21.3.233 PMID: 19519238

Stojanovski, K., Naja-Riese, G., King, E. J., & Fuchs, J. D. (2021). A systematic review of the social network strategy to optimize HIV testing in key populations to end the epidemic in the United States. *AIDS and Behavior, 25*, 2680–2698. DOI: 10.1007/s10461-021-03259-z PMID: 33871730

Teixeira da Silva, D., Bouris, A., Voisin, D., Hotton, A., Brewer, R., & Schneider, J. (2020). Social networks moderate the syndemic effect of psychosocial and structural factors on HIV risk among young Black transgender women and men who have sex with men. *AIDS and Behavior, 24*(1), 192–205. DOI: 10.1007/s10461-019-02575-9 PMID: 31289985

Thirumalai, D. (2017). *Association between intimate partner violence and HIV infection among married Indian women in Theni District, Tamil Nadu, India*. University of California., https://www.proquest.com/openview/f183d8cb585715b3ca0cc12a54f5f791/1?cbl=18750&pq-origsite=gscholar

Threats, M., & Bond, K. (2021). HIV information acquisition and use among young black men who have sex with men who use the internet: Mixed methods study. *Journal of Medical Internet Research, 23*(5), e22986. DOI: 10.2196/22986 PMID: 33960953

Treves-Kagan, S., Steward, W. T., Ntswane, L., Haller, R., Gilvydis, J. M., Gulati, H., Barnhart, S., & Lippman, S. A. (2015). Why increasing availability of ART is not enough: A rapid, community-based study on how HIV-related stigma impacts engagement to care in rural South Africa. *BMC Public Health, 16*, 1–13. DOI: 10.1186/s12889-016-2753-2 PMID: 26823077

Tso, L. S., Tang, W., Li, H., Yan, H. Y., & Tucker, J. D. (2016). Social media interventions to prevent HIV: A review of interventions and methodological considerations. *Current Opinion in Psychology, 9*, 6–10. DOI: 10.1016/j.copsyc.2015.09.019 PMID: 26516632

Veenstra, R., Dijkstra, J. K., Steglich, C., & Van Zalk, M. H. (2013). Network–behavior dynamics. *Journal of Research on Adolescence, 23*(3), 399–412. DOI: 10.1111/jora.12070

Veinot, T. C. (2009). Interactive acquisition and sharing: Understanding the dynamics of HIV/AIDS information networks. *Journal of the American Society for Information Science and Technology, 60*(11), 2313–2332. DOI: 10.1002/asi.21151

Wambaire, M. N. (2019). *Determinants of Social Network Site Preferences for Accessing Reproductive Health Information among Students in Public Universities in Nairobi, Kenya* (Doctoral dissertation, JKUAT-COHRED). http://ir.jkuat.ac.ke/handle/123456789/5041

Ward, P. R., & Fauk, N. K. (2025). Structural conditions, social networks, and the HIV vulnerability among Indonesian male labour migrants and motorbike taxi drivers. *International Journal for Equity in Health, 24*(1), 61. DOI: 10.1186/s12939-025-02420-7 PMID: 40033297

Waterfield, K. C., Shah, G. H., Etheredge, G. D., & Ikhile, O. (2021). Consequences of COVID-19 crisis for persons with HIV: The impact of social determinants of health. *BMC Public Health, 21*, 1–7. DOI: 10.1186/s12889-021-10296-9 PMID: 33546659

West, B. S. (2019). Social networks of substance-using populations: Key issues and promising new approaches for HIV. *Current HIV/AIDS Reports*, *16*, 48–56. DOI: 10.1007/s11904-019-00425-w PMID: 30659477

Wolf, P. J. (2022). American Young Adults' Self-Perception of Interpersonal Communication with Family and Friends Online through Social Media and In-Person. https://digitalcommons.liberty.edu/doctoral/3754/

World Health Organization. (2021). *Consolidated guidelines on HIV prevention, testing, treatment, service delivery and monitoring: recommendations for a public health approach*. World Health Organization.

Yang, X., Fang, T., Mobarak, S. A., Wang, J., Wang, C., Huang, S., Jiang, L., Chen, Xi., Li, H., Chang, W., Zhang, L., Mo, J., & Ning, C. (2020). Social network strategy as a promising intervention to better reach key populations for promoting HIV prevention: A systematic review and meta-analysis. *Sexually Transmitted Infections*, *96*(7), 485–491. DOI: 10.1136/sextrans-2019-054349 PMID: 32209639

Zhang, B., Wang, Y., Vasilakos, A. V., & Ma, J. (2013). Mobile social networking: Reconnect virtual community with physical space. *Telecommunication Systems*, *54*, 91–110. DOI: 10.1007/s11235-013-9718-x

Zhang, L., Ni, Z., Liu, Y., & Chen, H. (2023). The effectiveness of e-health on reducing stigma, improving social support and quality of life among people living with HIV: A systematic review and meta-analysis of randomized controlled trials. *International Journal of Nursing Studies*, *148*, 104606. DOI: 10.1016/j.ijnurstu.2023.104606 PMID: 37801937

APPENDIX

Abbreviations

Acquired immunodeficiency syndrome - AIDS
Antiretroviral Therapy - ART
Global Fund to Fight AIDS, Tuberculosis and Malaria - GFATM
Human Immunodeficiency Virus - HIV
Integrated Counseling Testing Center - ICTC
Injecting Drug Usage - IDU
Men sex with Men - MSM
Non-Governmental Organization - NGO
National Institute of Mental Health - NIMH
People Living with HIV - PLHIV
Randomized controlled for the trials - RCTs
Sexual Transmission Diseases - STD
Social Support Networks - SSNs

Chapter 8
Ethical AI in HIV Treatment:
Balancing Innovation, Privacy, and Equity

S. Ida Evangeline
https://orcid.org/0000-0003-2997-7897
Government College of Engineering, Tirunelveli, India

ABSTRACT

The integration of artificial intelligence (AI) into HIV treatment is reshaping clinical and public health approaches through personalized care, predictive analytics, and automated decision-making. While these innovations promise improved patient outcomes and more efficient healthcare delivery, they also raise pressing ethical concerns that must be addressed to ensure equitable and responsible implementation. This chapter explores the ethical dimensions of AI in HIV care, focusing on issues such as data privacy, algorithmic bias, informed consent, explainability, and global health equity. We examine how AI tools—ranging from risk prediction models and drug discovery platforms to wearable health monitors and epidemic forecasting systems—transform the management of HIV while introducing new vulnerabilities related to sensitive data and structural inequities. Through a critical analysis of emerging technologies and real-world case studies, we propose a framework for ethical AI development rooted in fairness-aware machine learning, and privacy-preserving methodologies.

DOI: 10.4018/979-8-3373-2863-8.ch008

1. INTRODUCTION

The integration of artificial intelligence into HIV treatment marks a transformative shift in the medical field, fundamentally altering how healthcare professionals approach diagnosis, disease progression monitoring, personalized therapy, and the broader management of public health initiatives. AI technologies—spanning machine learning algorithms, natural language processing, computer vision, and real-time data analytics from smart devices—offer the potential to not only enhance the precision of clinical decisions but also to automate and scale interventions in ways previously unimaginable (Olaboye et al. 2024). Using vast and varied datasets, AI can recognize fine grained patterns in viral load trajectories, fine tune antiretroviral therapy protocols, and even predict regional outbreaks before they burgeon. Early detection, continuous monitoring, and individualized treatment are critical for improving the quality of life and the length of life of the patient in HIV care, where this digital evolution is particularly promising (Senel & Beka, 2025).

However, these advancements also bring to the forefront an array of complex ethical challenges. The deployment of AI in healthcare intersects directly with the core principles of biomedical ethics—autonomy, beneficence, non-maleficence, and justice—and failure to adequately address these principles risks undermining the very populations these innovations intend to help. Concerns over data privacy and surveillance loom large, especially considering the sensitive and often stigmatized nature of HIV-related information (Rahsepar Meadi et al. 2025). Another critical issue is algorithmic bias, where AI models trained on insufficient or skewed datasets can make inaccurate or discriminatory recommendations that disproportionately affect marginalized groups like LGBTQ+ people, people of color, and residents of low income or rural areas. Many AI systems are opaque, which makes informed consent a problematic tenet because patients and even providers don't know how decisions are being made. Furthermore, the digital divide may further increase existing gaps in global HIV care, as underdeveloped regions may be left out of the AI revolution in HIV care due to infrastructure or technology limitations (Garett et al. 2024).

Given these intersecting concerns, this chapter offers a comprehensive exploration of the ethical dimensions of AI in HIV treatment. We begin by outlining the most impactful AI applications currently shaping HIV care, from predictive modeling to AI-enhanced drug discovery. The discussion then moves to the ethical terrain, examining how issues such as data security, algorithmic fairness, explainability, and global accessibility must be navigated to ensure equitable innovation. The chapter draws on interdisciplinary perspectives, real-world case studies, and contemporary regulatory frameworks to offer critical insights into how ethical AI can be responsibly developed and deployed across various healthcare settings. We aim not just to expose ethical pitfalls, but also to lay out forward thinking options to allow AI to be a tool for empowerment, not exclusion. Finally, we call for a human centered, ethically grounded approach to AI innovation for HIV care that prioritizes transparency, inclusivity, and the dignity and rights of all patients.

Figure 1 illustrates the layered ethical foundations required for responsible AI deployment in HIV care. It integrates biomedical ethics principles, design strategies like fairness-aware learning and privacy safeguards, and cross-cutting enablers such as informed consent, contextual sensitivity, and global data governance.

Figure 1. Ethical AI framework for HIV care

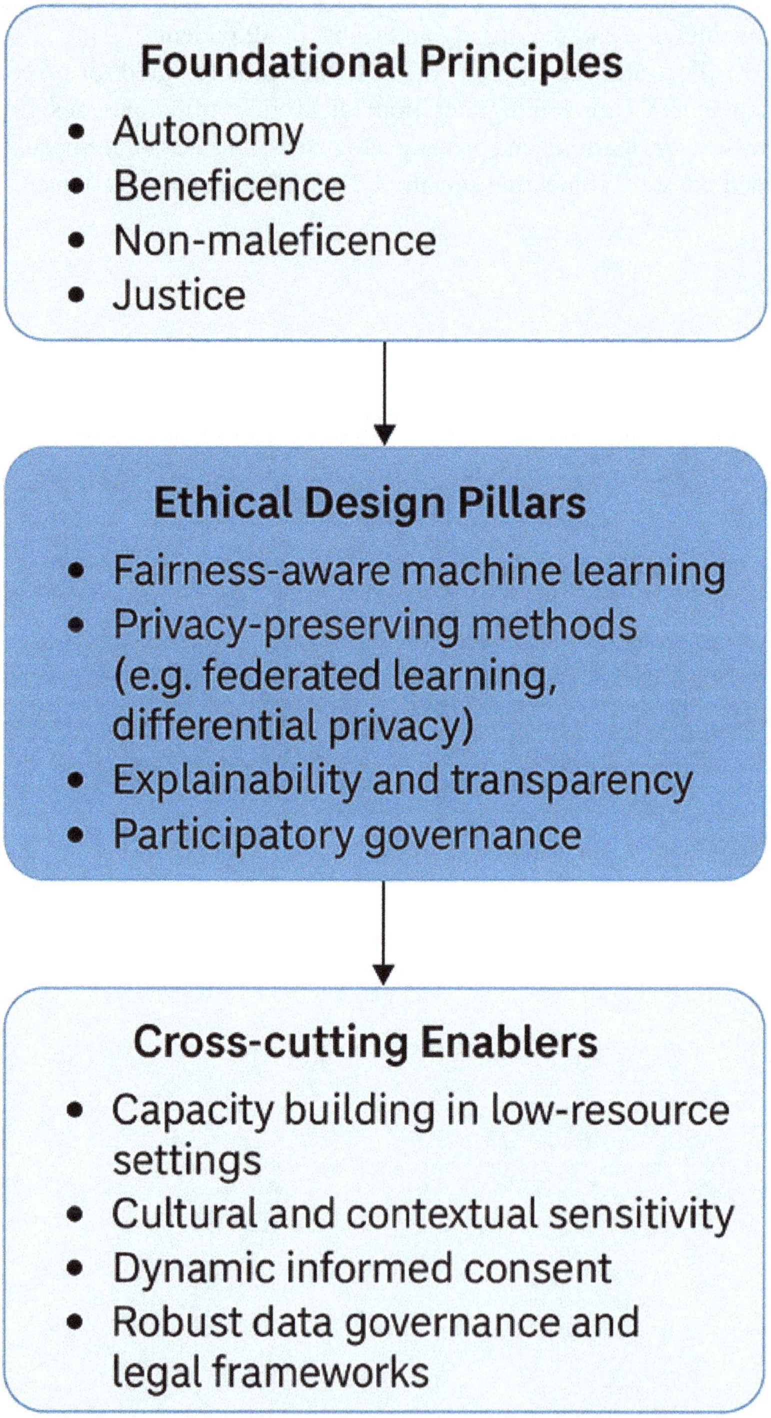

2. AI APPLICATIONS IN HIV TREATMENT

AI technologies are fundamentally transforming the landscape of HIV treatment by facilitating more precise, proactive, and patient-centric care strategies. Among the most impactful tools are machine learning models, which are increasingly utilized to forecast disease trajectories, assess individual patient risk, and optimize antiretroviral therapy (ART) regimens based on granular clinical data such as CD4 counts, viral load trends, co-morbidities, and adherence history. The predictive analytics help healthcare providers identify patients who are at increased risk of virologic failure or opportunistic infections and provide earlier and more targeted interventions, leading to better treatment outcomes and resource utilization. In the pharmaceutical domain, AI is also central to expedite the drug discovery process by means of computational methods, like deep learning based virtual screening and molecular docking simulations. In silico approaches are highly efficient in terms of time and cost to find new compounds or re position existing drugs for HIV treatment, particularly in the era of emerging resistance to first line therapy (Jin & Zhang, 2025).

Beyond the clinic and laboratory, AI is driving innovations in digital health through the integration of wearable devices and mobile applications. These tools enable real-time monitoring of physiological indicators such as heart rate, sleep patterns, and medication adherence, offering continuous, passive data collection that informs dynamic treatment adjustments. This data is processed by AI algorithms to identify anomalies or behavioral trends to support interventions based on individual lifestyles and challenges. In public health, AI epidemiological models, powered by AI, integrate data from various sources, ranging from mobility patterns to climate data to social networks, to forecast outbreak hotspots, inform vaccination or testing campaigns, and allocate healthcare resources with unprecedented accuracy. Care delivery is further augmented by natural language processing, to mine unstructured clinical notes, electronic health records, and patient reported outcomes to discover insights that inform clinical decision making, reduce administrative burden, and highlight high risk cases for review (Koh et al. 2024).

In addition, AI is capable of integrating such heterogeneous data as genomics and proteomics, as well as social determinants of health, to give a holistic view of HIV pathogenesis and treatment response. This systems understanding can be used to develop truly personalized medicine approaches that match care to each patient's unique biological and socio-environmental profile. Additionally, community based interventions are being facilitated by AI driven platforms including chatbot assisted counseling and AI curated educational resources that engage patients in a culturally sensitive and scalable way (Roche et al. 2024). Figure 2 illustrates how diverse data sources—ranging from clinical biomarkers to social determinants—feed into AI tools for risk prediction, drug discovery, diagnostics, and public health interventions. It also highlights the downstream effects on health system outcomes and the essential layer of ethical oversight.

Figure 2. HIV–AI ecosystem

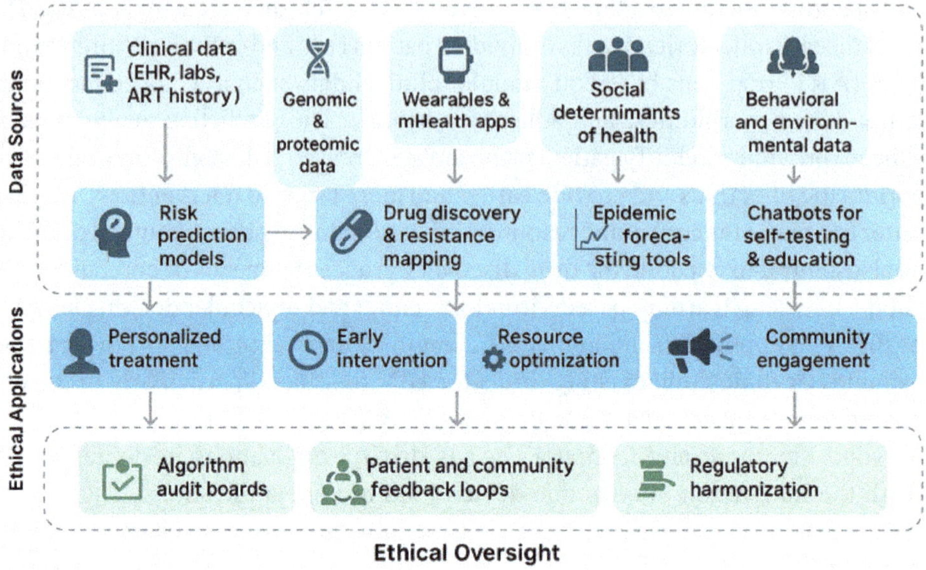

These applications have, however, tremendous potential to transform the lives of individuals and communities, and their success relies on the availability of diverse, high quality datasets that accurately reflect the populations being served, a dependence which raises numerous ethical, technical and logistical challenges that are addressed in subsequent sections. However, AI is a potent enabler of anticipatory and equitable HIV care that can fill current diagnostic, treatment, and prevention gaps across the spectrum of healthcare contexts.

3. DATA PRIVACY AND SECURITY IN AI-DRIVEN HIV CARE

As AI-driven HIV care continues to evolve, its foundation on the integration and analysis of large-scale, sensitive datasets underscores the critical need to prioritize data privacy and security. These datasets often include electronic health records, genomic sequences, mobile health data from apps and wearable sensors, demographic identifiers, and behavioral information use patterns. These data points are not simply clinical metrics when it comes to HIV, a condition still highly stigmatized in many parts of the world, and if exposed, can lead to discrimination, social ostracization, loss of job or legal persecution, particularly in jurisdictions where HIV transmission or homosexuality is criminalized (Garett et al. 2024).

The reliance of AI on comprehensive, granular data amplifies these risks. AI models require large volumes of diverse data for effective training and validation, often involving complex data flows across institutions, borders, and cloud environments. Many AI systems are also opaque — often described as 'black boxes' — meaning that it can be difficult to see how data is processed and how conclusions are drawn, which can make it hard for patients or even providers to understand what information is being used and why. In such contexts, the traditional notions of patient confidentiality and consent are insufficient. Therefore, such effective safeguards must include advanced technical solutions like end-to-end encryption during data transmission and storage, secure multi-party computation which allows joint data analysis without data sharing, and differential privacy techniques that obscure individual identities in the aggregate datasets but preserve data utility (Adeniyi et al. 2024).

Blockchain technology also offers promising solutions by creating tamper-proof, decentralized health records where access permissions are governed by the patient, enabling fine-grained control and transparent audit trails. However, such technologies must be implemented with strong data governance frameworks that clearly articulate the purposes of data collection, limits to usage, retention policies and procedures for breach notification. The development of these frameworks should involve active stakeholder engagement to establish ethical alignment and public trust (Rahman, 2024).

In addition, informed consent processes need to be reimagined to reflect the subtleties of AI driven care. Consent should be dynamic and continuous, and should be presented in a clear and accessible way so that individuals understand how an AI system works, what data it needs, what risks it entails and how to opt out or revoke consent. This is particularly important in communities that do not have a high digital literacy, where misunderstandings could mean unintended exposure or coercion. In cross border collaborations and data sharing initiatives, the challenge becomes even more complex given that there are discrepancies between the regulatory regimes (the GDPR in the EU, HIPAA in the US and the lack of defined protections elsewhere), which can lead to compliance and enforcement concerns (Pantanowitz et al., 2024).

Finally, it is important to focus on building a culture of ethical responsibility and accountability beyond technical and legal measures. AI developers, healthcare providers and institutions must embrace ethical data stewardship, transparency and public engagement. For the treatment of HIV, where mistrust and marginalization have a long history, protecting data privacy is not only a legal obligation, but the right thing to do. The failure to uphold this trust may discourage individuals from interacting with AI driven tools or participating in crucial research, thus limiting the power and reach of the technologies. AI will only be able to fully realize its potential in HIV treatment if privacy and security are built into every layer of the digital healthcare ecosystem (Ayari & Ammar, 2024).

4. ALGORITHMIC BIAS AND HEALTH EQUITY

Algorithmic bias in AI systems used for HIV treatment presents a profound and multifaceted ethical challenge, particularly as these technologies increasingly influence diagnostic processes, risk stratification, treatment planning, and public health interventions. Usually, this bias comes from the data used to train these models, which may not represent certain populations or reflect historical inequities present in the healthcare system. If datasets are mainly data from Western, urban, male, or high income populations, the AI models that are derived can miss the subtleties of the needs, biological differences, and healthcare experiences of other groups, such as women, ethnic minorities, rural inhabitants, and low income individuals. Algorithmic bias can exacerbate health disparities in HIV care, where marginalized communities (LGBTQ+ individuals, people who inject drugs, sex workers, or people living in socioeconomically disadvantaged regions) already face systemic barriers to care and where inaccurate risk predictions, misdiagnoses, or suboptimal treatment recommendations may result (Ratwani et al. 2024).

For example, an AI system trained predominantly on data from high-income urban clinics may not recognize atypical disease progression patterns common in undernourished populations or individuals co-infected with tuberculosis, leading to delayed interventions. Likewise, language models that do not support a variety of linguistic expressions or dialects may miss out on important self reported symptoms or behavioral risk factors in patient interactions. Bias is not just a function of data, but also design choices such as which features are prioritized, how outcomes are weighted, and what thresholds determine risk categories, all of which may represent implicit values and assumptions of the developers. In addition, AI performance metrics are not disaggregated by demographics, so differential accuracy rates across population subgroups are hidden and harm is obscured (Flores et al. 2024).

Addressing these challenges requires a multipronged approach. Fairness-aware machine learning techniques should be employed from the outset to identify and mitigate disparate impacts through strategies like reweighting, adversarial debiasing, or post-processing adjustments. The curation of diverse and inclusive dataset is essential and requires deliberate efforts to collect and integrate data from underrepresented populations, including the social determinants of health, and culturally relevant contextual variables that affect HIV risk and treatment outcomes. In addition, all AI models used in a clinical or public health setting should be subjected to rigorous fairness evaluation with transparent reporting of performance across subgroups by gender, race, socioeconomic status, and geographic location. The AI lifecycle should have continuous bias audits built in with mechanisms for retraining and recalibration as new data becomes available (Jaiteh et al. 2024).

Governance is also equally important in promoting equity. Bias testing and equity impact assessments must be mandated as prerequisites for approval and deployment of AI in healthcare by regulatory frameworks. The perspectives of those most at risk of harm should be institutionalized through ethical review boards and community advisory panels in the development and oversight of AI. Further, capacity building initiatives are required to enable stakeholders in low resource settings to participate in the development, evaluation and adaptation of AI tools appropriate to their context (Tao et al. 2025).

If not intentionally designed for equity, AI systems can continue the same problems they aim to solve. To avoid this, equity needs to be baked into not only what the AI is trying to generate, but also into the values, practices and accountability mechanisms that drive how it is designed, deployed, and continues to evolve. To be instruments of justice in the global fight against HIV, these technologies can only function by confronting bias at every stage of the AI pipeline.

5. EXPLAINABILITY, TRUST, AND INFORMED CONSENT

As AI systems assume increasingly critical roles in HIV treatment—from algorithmic triage and risk prediction to autonomous diagnostic support and therapy optimization—the demand for explainability becomes not only a technical requirement but an ethical imperative. The term explainable AI refers to the design of systems that can be explained in terms of their outputs that are understandable and interpretable to both clinicians and patients. In the context of HIV care, which is complex and deeply personal, with clinical decisions made in the context of sensitive trade-offs and large psychosocial impacts, explainability encourages transparency and reinforces clinical accountability. In order for healthcare professionals to validate the relevance of an AI generated treatment recommendation or risk assessment, detect anomalies, and communicate findings to patients, the rationale of the AI recommendation must be traceable. The lack of interpretability not only erodes the clinicians' confidence in using these tools but also erodes the patient trust, which may drive patient disengagement of care or incorrect decisions made based on misunderstood outputs (Sun et al. 2025).

The reliability, fairness and alignment of AI with human values are inextricably linked to trust in AI. When patients understand how AI tools work, feel they're being used ethically and are empowered in the decision making process, they're more likely to accept and benefit from AI driven interventions. In HIV treatment, for example, patients may already be dealing with stigma, misinformation and medical mistrust based on historical discrimination. Therefore, trust needs to be intentionally designed for, and features that promote interpretability, like visual explanations, patient facing summaries, and scenario based decision pathways which make explicit how different inputs impact AI recommendations (Ma et al. 2025).

In AI powered healthcare, informed consent must go beyond forms to be signed or verbal explanations. It should be dynamic, iterative and context aware, giving people easy to access, culturally sensitive information about what the role of AI is in their care. For example, this can include explaining the types of data collected (clinical biomarkers, behavioral indicators, location data), what data is used for, potential risks of algorithmic bias or technical failure, and whether human oversight exists. Communicating with populations with low digital literacy is especially important as they may not understand abstract AI concepts or distinguish between human and machine decision making. Multimodal communication tools such as infographics, storytelling, and multilingual resources should be used by ethical AI systems to bridge these knowledge gaps and provide actual understanding (Guo & Chen, 2025).

Furthermore, AI enhanced HIV care should be built on the principles of shared decision-making. Clinicians should partner with patients, instead of treating AI as a silent, infallible authority, by discussing AI generated recommendations, inviting patient values and preferences, and collaboratively deciding what is best for the patient. The model also improves autonomy, diminishes paternalism, and aids in mitigating power imbalances that arise from more complex technologies (Reid et al. 2025).

Regulatory bodies and institutional review boards will need to update ethical standards to institutionalize these practices to reflect the unique challenges of AI. This entails requiring transparency in algorithmic design and performance metrics, requiring clear documentation of informed consent procedures pertaining to AI applications and ensuring oversight mechanisms for auditing AI systems in practice. Moreover, the legal protections should also adapt to the harms of opaque and unexplainable AI decisions and provide avenues for redress to the affected individuals (Yigit et al. 2025).

Finally, the ethical integration of AI into HIV care necessitates the need for more than technical efficacy; it requires a change in clinical workflows, patient communication and regulatory oversight to be transparent, interpretable and trustworthy. The human elements that are essential to compassionate, equitable healthcare can be supported—not supplanted—by AI when we prioritize explainability and consent.

6. GOVERNANCE, REGULATION, AND GLOBAL ETHICS

The ethical deployment of AI in HIV treatment hinges on the establishment of robust governance structures and regulatory frameworks that not only facilitate innovation but also uphold accountability, protect patient rights, and promote global health equity (Jin & Zhang, 2025). Because AI systems are becoming key drivers of clinical and public health decisions, their regulation must adapt to the specific risks they present, especially in areas where the stakes are especially high, including HIV care, where historical stigma, social discrimination, and data vulnerability all play a role. However, existing global frameworks are essential because they institutionalize important principles such as data minimization, the right to explanation, and explicit informed consent. The World Health Organization's ethical guidelines for AI in health place the same emphasis on inclusiveness, transparency, human oversight and sustainability. While these frameworks describe important values, they do not lay out clear operational pathways for how to achieve these principles across a range of healthcare settings, particularly those with large HIV burdens and weak digital governance infrastructure (Kamulegeya et al. 2025).

The second most important challenge relates to the asymmetry of regulatory maturity across countries. While high income countries may have strong data protection laws, regulatory bodies, and technological safeguards, low and middle income countries may not have the legal, institutional or technical capacity to effectively regulate AI (Gandhi et al. 2025). Not only is this disparity an ethical issue of data sovereignty and digital colonialism, but it also creates settings in which AI tools may be deployed with insufficient oversight, and can even exacerbate rather than mitigate health inequities. These issues are further compounded by the digital divide, which leads to stark inequalities in internet access, cloud computing infrastructure and AI literacy that exclude many communities from participating in, or benefiting from, AI enabled HIV care. If we do not strive to democratize access to digital health infrastructure, AI will exacerbate global health inequity (Gera et al. 2025).

Effective governance must therefore be more than compliance driven checklists and instead include, participatory and context sensitive frameworks. There is a need for community engagement in order to ensure that patients, advocates and local health workers are involved in the shaping of AI policies and identifying risks as well as co design interventions that reflect lived realities. To monitor the deployment and impact of AI systems, including those used in high stakes clinical decisions and public health surveillance, ethical oversight mechanisms such as interdisciplinary ethics committees, independent algorithm review boards, and public accountability panels should be institutionalized. Further, clear lines of responsibility must be drawn throughout the AI lifecycle, assigning responsibility for data quality, algorithmic performance, unintended consequences, and redress mechanisms for harm (Hou et al. 2025).

Equally important is multilateral cooperation to harmonize standards and promote equitable innovation. International organizations, regional alliances, and global health initiatives must work together to establish interoperable regulatory models, encourage responsible data sharing agreements with built in ethical safeguards, and strengthen capacity building programs in low resource settings. Moreover, views from the Global South should be incorporated into global governance with the aim that ethical norms are not imposed by high income countries alone but are instead reflective of a plurality of cultural, legal, and health system contexts (Afzal et al. 2025). Human rights, fairness, accountability, and sustainability can therefore be embedded into AI governance frameworks through which stakeholders can ensure that technological progress in HIV care is not made at the expense of ethical compromise. Rather, it can be used as a tool for promoting justice, improving health systems, and promoting global solidarity in the struggle against HIV.

7. FUTURE DIRECTIONS IN ETHICAL AI FOR HIV

As artificial intelligence continues to redefine the boundaries of medical innovation, the future of ethical AI in HIV treatment must emphasize designing systems that are not only technologically advanced but fundamentally aligned with principles of human dignity, equity, and trust. Despite the promise of AI in transforming HIV care, its real-world deployment faces several practical challenges in low-resource settings. These include limited digital infrastructure (such as unreliable internet or lack of cloud access), shortage of trained personnel to manage AI systems, low levels of digital literacy among both healthcare providers and patients, and inconsistent access to electricity or smartphones. Furthermore, the absence of regulatory frameworks and data protection laws may hinder ethical and secure implementation. These barriers not only restrict adoption but may also introduce risks of algorithmic misuse or community mistrust if not addressed with context-specific strategies and sustained investment. Federated learning is one of the most promising advancements that allows AI models to be collaboratively trained across various institutions or geographies without the need for centralizing sensitive data. However, in the case of HIV care, where privacy concerns are especially heightened due to stigma and risk of discrimination, this decentralized approach maintains privacy while still benefiting from the wealth of global health data. In addition to preventing data monopolies, federated learning promotes local data sovereignty and enables health systems in low- and middle-income countries to participate in and reap the rewards of AI innovation while maintaining control of patient information (Li et al. 2025).

Another transformative frontier lies in the development of AI-powered HIV self-testing platforms that integrate ethical safeguards from the ground up. They are equipped with intelligent symptom checkers, real time digital counseling, and adaptive feedback systems, which can greatly increase access to early diagnosis and linkage to care in remote or underserved areas. But their deployment must be voluntary, anonymous for the user, and culturally appropriate. Interfaces should be multilingual; accessible to those with different levels of literacy; and designed in collaboration with community stakeholders in a manner that reflects social norms and reduces fear of testing. These tools should have equity aware algorithms, i.e., algorithms that are sensitive to local contexts and do not inadvertently marginalize high risk population (Frade et al. 2025).

AI also has the potential to be used for public health intervention applications like epidemic forecasting, outbreak hotspot detection, and behavioral nudging for ART adherence. However, they need to be governed by transparency and community engagement in order to prevent surveillance like overreach or ethical violations. For instance, while an AI system predicting risk in certain neighborhoods should not profile or stigmatize these communities, it should enable support to flow through inclusive and empowering interventions (Khan et al. 2025).

Interdisciplinary collaboration emerges as central to these future pathways. The development of ethical AI should be a co-creation among data scientists and engineers; clinicians; ethicists; social scientists; patient advocates; and policymakers. In this way, these diverse perspectives ensure that the AI tools represent real world complexities, uphold patient agency, and align with the broader public health goals. For this to be possible, there needs to be systems in place to document decision logic, monitor for adverse outcomes, and institutional learning through audit trails. In addition, embedding explainability by design will help demystify AI processes, increase trust, and increase meaningful patient-clinician interactions (Mukherjee et al. 2025).

In the future, capacity building in low resource settings is essential to democratizing the benefits of AI. That includes funding digital infrastructure, training local health professionals in AI literacy and ethics, and creating governance mechanisms that are attuned to community needs. International support is needed to back equitable innovation with cross border knowledge exchange and solidarity in developing ethical, context appropriate technologies (Siyamayambo et al. 2025).

The next generation of AI systems for HIV care must be designed to do more than maximize clinical performance, but must uphold a higher ethical vision—to protect the most vulnerable, to respect cultural difference, and to be a step toward a more just and inclusive healthcare system in every advance. Incorporating fairness, transparency, and respect for human rights into the values of innovation will help ensure that AI improves, rather than erodes, the integrity of HIV care.

8. CONCLUSION

As artificial intelligence becomes increasingly embedded in the fabric of HIV treatment, it heralds a new era in the way we approach the disease—redefining how we detect infections, tailor treatments, monitor progress, and manage public health responses. AI stands to dramatically improve patient outcomes, streamline healthcare delivery, and strengthen the responsiveness of global health systems by allowing more precise diagnostics, predictive modeling, and personalized therapy regimens. But this power to transform is a profound ethical responsibility. While AI integration into HIV care must ultimately lead to clinical and operational efficiency, it should also be a means to advance equity, protect rights, and uphold dignity of all stakeholders in the HIV response.

Throughout this chapter, we have examined the multifaceted ethical challenges that accompany AI deployment in HIV care—from the risk of algorithmic bias and privacy breaches to the complexities of informed consent and the digital divide. These issues are central to innovation and not ancillary to it. If AI systems are built without sufficient consideration for fairness, transparency, and inclusivity, they can serve to perpetuate existing health disparities, erode patient trust, and marginalize vulnerable populations from the promise of technological progress. On the other hand, when guided by strong ethical frameworks, community participation, and regulatory oversight, AI can be a force for health justice.

The path forward requires a deliberate and coordinated effort to embed ethics at every stage of the AI lifecycle—from data collection and model design to deployment, evaluation, and governance. Machine learning must become fairness aware, privacy preserving (e.g. federated learning), explainable AI and user centered design, the norm rather than the exception. There should also be continued investment in capacity building for low resource settings and international collaboration to harmonize regulations and ensure equitable access to AI technologies. Collaboration is key with multiple stakeholders, including technologists, clinicians, ethicists, patients and policymakers, to co create AI solutions that are contextually relevant and socially responsible.

The future of ethical AI in HIV treatment is not a technological challenge, but a moral imperative. It asks us to rethink innovation through the eyes of empathy, inclusion, and justice. Anchoring AI in these values allows us to be sure that the next generation of digital health tools will revolutionize HIV care, and do so in a way that is humane, equitable and deserving of the trust of the community that it serves. By doing this, AI can be not only a catalyst of progress but also a symbol of ethical leadership in the global battle against HIV.

REFERENCES

Adeniyi, A. O., Arowoogun, J. O., Okolo, C. A., Chidi, R., & Babawarun, O. (2024). Ethical considerations in healthcare IT: A review of data privacy and patient consent issues. *World Journal of Advanced Research and Reviews*, *21*(2), 1660–1668.

Afzal, M., Agarwal, S., Elshaikh, R. H., Babker, A. M., Osman, E. A. I., Choudhary, R. K., & Sah, A. K. (2025). Innovative Diagnostic Approaches and Challenges in the Management of HIV: Bridging Basic Science and Clinical Practice. *Life (Chicago, Ill.)*, *15*(2), 209. PMID: 40003618

Ayari, A., & Ammar, A. (2024). AI Accountability, Ethics, and Human Resource Implications. In *Ethical Challenges for the Future of Neurosurgery* (pp. 47–56). Springer Nature Switzerland.

Flores, L., Kim, S., & Young, S. D. (2024). Addressing bias in artificial intelligence for public health surveillance. *Journal of Medical Ethics*, *50*(3), 190–194. PMID: 37130756

Frade, S., Mendonca, R., Cooper, S., Morris, S., Lee, H., Gupta, K., & Rech, D. (2025). HealthPulse AI: Enhancing Diagnostic Trust and Accessibility in Under-Resourced Settings through AI. *VeriXiv*, *2*, 54.

Gandhi, R. T., Landovitz, R. J., Sax, P. E., Smith, D. M., Springer, S. A., Günthard, H. F., & Saag, M. S. (2025). Antiretroviral drugs for treatment and prevention of HIV in adults: 2024 recommendations of the International Antiviral Society–USA Panel. *Journal of the American Medical Association*, *333*(7), 609–628. PMID: 39616604

Garett, R., Kim, S., & Young, S. D. (2024). Ethical Considerations for Artificial Intelligence Applications for HIV. *AI*, *5*(2), 594–601.

Gera, A., Dhull, A., Singh, A., & Singh, K. K. (2025). Legal and regulatory issues related to AI in healthcare. In *Responsible and Explainable Artificial Intelligence in Healthcare* (pp. 259–283). Academic Press.

Guo, W., & Chen, Y. (2025). Investigating Whether AI Will Replace Human Physicians and Understanding the Interplay of the Source of Consultation, Health-Related Stigma, and Explanations of Diagnoses on Patients' Evaluations of Medical Consultations: Randomized Factorial Experiment. *Journal of Medical Internet Research*, *27*, e66760. PMID: 40053785

Hou, C., Wei, J., Zhang, H., & Li, H. (2025). Evolving strategies in the diagnosis and treatment of HIV-associated neurocognitive disorders. *Reviews in the Neurosciences*, (0).

Jaiteh, M., Phalane, E., Shiferaw, Y. A., Voet, K. A., & Phaswana-Mafuya, R. N. (2024). Utilization of machine learning algorithms for the strengthening of HIV testing: A systematic review. *Algorithms, 17*(8), 362.

Jin, R., & Zhang, L. (2025). AI applications in HIV research: Advances and future directions. *Frontiers in Microbiology, 16*, 1541942. PMID: 40051479

Kamulegeya, L. H., Kagolo, I., Kabakaari, B., Atuhaire, J., Nasamula, R., & Bwanika, J. M. (2025). Technology-Assisted Interventions in the Delivery of HIV Prevention, Care, and Treatment Services in Sub-Saharan Africa: Scoping Review. *Journal of Medical Internet Research, 27*, e68352. PMID: 40233346

Khan, H., Alzabut, J., Almutairi, D. K., & Alqurashi, W. K. (2025). The Use of Artificial Intelligence in Data Analysis with Error Recognitions in Liver Transplantation in HIV-AIDS Patients Using Modified ABC Fractional Order Operators. *Fractal and Fractional, 9*(1).

Koh, M. C. Y., Ngiam, J. N., Yong, J., Tambyah, P. A., & Archuleta, S. (2024). The role of an artificial intelligence model in antiretroviral therapy counselling and advice for people living with HIV. *HIV Medicine, 25*(4), 504–508. PMID: 38169077

Li, N., Lewin, A., Ning, S., Waito, M., Zeller, M. P., & Tinmouth, A.Canadian Transfusion Trials Group. (2025). Privacy-preserving federated data access and federated learning: Improved data sharing and AI model development in transfusion medicine. *Transfusion, 65*(1), 22–28. PMID: 39610333

Ma, Y., Achiche, S., Tu, G., Vicente, S., Lessard, D., Engler, K., & Lebouché, B. (2025). The first AI-based Chatbot to promote HIV self-management: A mixed methods usability study. *HIV Medicine, 26*(2), 184–206. PMID: 39390632

Mukherjee, A., Mukherjee, T., & Roy, M. M. (2025). A Study of AI Application Through Integrated and Systematic Moral Cognitive Therapy in the Healthcare Sector. *Design and Forecasting Models for Disease Management*, 47-76.

Olaboye, J. A., Maha, C. C., Kolawole, T. O., & Abdul, S. (2024). Artificial intelligence in monitoring HIV treatment adherence: A conceptual exploration. *International Medical Science Research Journal, 4*(6), 681–692.

Pantanowitz, L., Hanna, M., Pantanowitz, J., Lennerz, J., Henricks, W. H., Shen, P., & Rashidi, H. H. (2024). Regulatory aspects of AI-ML. *Modern Pathology*, •••, 100609. PMID: 39260776

Rahman, M. M. (2024). Ethical and Technological Convergence: AI and Blockchain in Halal Healthcare. *Artificial Intelligence-Enabled Blockchain Technology and Digital Twin for Smart Hospitals*, 451-466.

Rahsepar Meadi, M., Sillekens, T., Metselaar, S., van Balkom, A., Bernstein, J., & Batelaan, N. (2025). Exploring the Ethical Challenges of Conversational AI in Mental Health Care: Scoping Review. *JMIR Mental Health*, *12*, e60432. PMID: 39983102

Ratwani, R. M., Sutton, K., & Galarraga, J. E. (2024). Addressing AI algorithmic bias in health care. *Journal of the American Medical Association*, *332*(13), 1051–1052. PMID: 39230911

Reid, M. J., Otieno, B. A., van Heerden, A., Sikazwe, I., Baptiste, S. L., Mendonca, R., & Sundaram, M. (2025). Announcing the Lancet Global Health Commission on artificial intelligence (AI) and HIV: Leveraging AI for equitable and sustainable impact. *The Lancet. Global Health*, *13*(4), e611–e612. PMID: 40155096

Roche, S. D., Ekwunife, O. I., Mendonca, R., Kwach, B., Omollo, V., Zhang, S., & Ortblad, K. F. (2024). Measuring the performance of computer vision artificial intelligence to interpret images of HIV self-testing results. *Frontiers in Public Health*, *12*, 1334881. PMID: 38384878

Senel, B., & Beka, H. (2025). Artificial Intelligence in HIV Diagnosis and Treatment: A Comprehensive Review. *Cumhuriyet Medical Journal*, *47*(1), 10–21.

Siyamayambo, C., Phalane, E., & Phaswana-Mafuya, R. N. (2025). Diagnosis and Management of Sexually Transmitted Infections Using Artificial Intelligence Applications Among Key and General Populations in Sub-Saharan Africa: A Systematic Review and Meta-Analysis. *Algorithms*, *18*(3), 151.

Sun, Q., Akman, A., & Schuller, B. W. (2025). Explainable artificial intelligence for medical applications: A review. *ACM Transactions on Computing for Healthcare*, *6*(2), 1–31.

Tao, J., Maguire-Wilkerson, A., Rusley, J., Wray, T., & Chan, P. A. (2025). Implementing conversational artificial intelligence technology for the prevention of HIV and other sexually transmitted infections in real-world settings. *AIDS*, *39*(3), 324–327. PMID: 39878675

Yigit, I., Wilson, T. E., Taylor, T. N., Kassaye, S. G., Weiser, S. D., Cohen, M. H., & Turan, B. (2025). Association of Experienced Stigma in Healthcare Settings with Health outcomes among Black women living with HIV: Mediating roles of internalized stigma, anticipated Stigma, and trust in HIV Care. *Social Science & Medicine*, *366*, 117699. PMID: 39823813

Compilation of References

Abrahim, S. A., Girma, M., Habteselassie, A., Gezahegn, N., Feleke, A., Berheto, T. M., Demissie, M., Belete, W., & Deressa, T. (2019). Diagnostic accuracy of HIV test kits, Genscreen Ultra and Bioelisa. *HIV/AIDS (Auckland, N.Z.)*, *11*, 17–22. DOI: 10.2147/HIV.S184603 PMID: 30804685

Achwoka, D. E. (2021). *Non-communicable Diseases (NCDS) Burden Among People Living With HIV/AIDS (PLHIV) in Kenya* (Doctoral dissertation, University of Nairobi). https://erepository.uonbi.ac.ke/handle/11295/157294

Adeniyi, A. O., Arowoogun, J. O., Okolo, C. A., Chidi, R., & Babawarun, O. (2024). Ethical considerations in healthcare IT: A review of data privacy and patient consent issues. *World Journal of Advanced Research and Reviews*, *21*(2), 1660–1668.

Adeyemo, J. O., & Subramaniam, P. R. (2024). A review on data analytical techniques for predicting HIV treatment outcome using selected biomarkers. In *2024 International Conference on Science, Engineering and Business for Driving Sustainable Development Goals (SEB4SDG)* (pp. 1–9). IEEE. https://doi.org/ (replace with actual DOI if available)DOI: 10.1109/SEB4SDG.2024.example

Afzal, M., Agarwal, S., Elshaikh, R. H., Babker, A. M., Osman, E. A. I., Choudhary, R. K., & Sah, A. K. (2025). Innovative Diagnostic Approaches and Challenges in the Management of HIV: Bridging Basic Science and Clinical Practice. *Life (Chicago, Ill.)*, *15*(2), 209. PMID: 40003618

Aidoo-Frimpong, G. A., Adekunle, T., Abu'Baare, G. R., & Adu, C. (2025). Community-Driven Recommendations for Developing Culturally Aligned Messaging to Improve Pre-Exposure Prophylaxis Acceptability and Uptake Among US-Based African Immigrants. *AIDS Patient Care and STDs*. Advance online publication. DOI: 10.1089/apc.2025.0020 PMID: 40106264

Airhihenbuwa, C. O., Ford, C. L., & Iwelunmor, J. I. (2014). Why culture matters in health interventions: Lessons from HIV/AIDS stigma and NCDs. *Health Education & Behavior*, *41*(1), 78–84. DOI: 10.1177/1090198113487199 PMID: 23685666

Ajuna, N., Tumusiime, B., Amanya, J., Awori, S., Rukundo, G. Z., & Asiimwe, J. B. (2021). Social networks and barriers to ART adherence among young adults (18–24 years) living with HIV at selected primary health facilities of South-Western Uganda: A Qualitative Study. *HIV/AIDS (Auckland, N.Z.)*, •••, 939–958. PMID: 34675686

Al-Khayat, Z. A. Y., Agha, N. F. S., Majeed, P. D., Alharmni, K. I. F., & Agha, D. N. F. (2021). Prevalence of HIV among newly diagnosed tuberculosis patients in Erbil Governorate, Iraq. *Journal of Contemporary Medical Sciences*, *7*(2), 102–107. DOI: 10.22317/jcms.v7i2.955

Altuntaş-Aydın, Ö., Gündüz, A., İnan, A., Kumbasar-Karaosmanoğlu, H., Mete, B., Tekin, S., Yıldız, D. S., & Tabak, F. (2022). Initiation of rapid antiretroviral therapsy in HIV infection. *Klimik Dergisi*, *35*(1), 1–5. DOI: 10.36519/kd.2022.3699

Al-Worafi, Y. M. (2024). Medical and Health Sciences in Developing Countries: Sample Size Calculations and Sampling Techniques. In *Handbook of Medical and Health Sciences in Developing Countries: Education, Practice, and Research* (pp. 1–10). Springer International Publishing.

Amadhila, E. M., & Shawapala, T. (2022). Are social protection grants alleviating poverty among vulnerable groups in Namibia?–The case of older persons and persons with disabilities. *African Review of Economics and Finance*, *14*(2), 119–141. https://journals.co.za/doi/abs/10.10520/ejc-aref_v14_n2_a8

Amiri, F., Roshanaei, G., Olfati Far, M., Najafi, R., & Poorolajal, J. (2021). Survival analysis of the human immunodeficiency virus in iranian patients: A multistate model. *Journal of Arak University of Medical Sciences*, *24*(2), 180–195. DOI: 10.32598/jams.24.2.5530.2

Amirkhanian, Y. A. (2014). Social networks, sexual networks and HIV risk in men who have sex with men. *Current HIV/AIDS Reports*, *11*, 81–92. DOI: 10.1007/s11904-013-0194-4 PMID: 24384832

Andigema, A. S., Cyrielle, N. T., Koudoum, P. L., & Vladimir, A. J. (2023). Ai in the management of hiv: Case study cameroon. International. *Journal of Virology and Aids*, *10*(1). Advance online publication. DOI: 10.23937/2469-567x/1510089

Anjum, A., Rehman, A. U., Siddique, H., Rabaan, A. A., Alhumaid, S., Garout, M., Almuthree, S. A., Halwani, M. A., Turkistani, S. A., Qutob, H., Albayat, H., Aljeldah, M., Shammari, B. R. A., Alshahrani, F. S., Alghamdi, A. S., Alduwaihi, S. M., Alibraheem, A. A., Zeb, S., & Zeshan, B. (2022). Evaluation of Hematological, Biochemical Profiles and Molecular Detection of Envelope Gene (gp-41) in Human Immunodeficiency Virus (HIV) among Newly Diagnosed Patients. *Medicina (Kaunas, Lithuania)*, *59*(1), 93. DOI: 10.3390/medicina59010093 PMID: 36676716

Antoine, D., Chupikova, I., Jalodia, R., Singh, P. K., & Roy, S. (2024). Chronic Morphine Treatment and Antiretroviral Therapy Exacerbate HIV-Distal Sensory Peripheral Neuropathy and Induce Distinct Microbial Alterations in the HIV Tg26 Mouse Model. *International Journal of Molecular Sciences*, *25*(3). Advance online publication. DOI: 10.3390/ijms25031569 PMID: 38338849

Areri, H. A., Marshall, A., & Harvey, G. (2020). Interventions to improve self-management of adults living with HIV on antiretroviral therapy: A systematic review. *PLoS One*, *15*(5), e0232709. DOI: 10.1371/journal.pone.0232709 PMID: 32392245

Armstead, A. B., Wilkerson, J. M., Gemeinhardt, G., Nyitray, A., & Collins, D. M. (2021). Antiretroviral therapy adherence, functional independence, and falls among people with HIV. *Occupational Therapy in Health Care*, *35*(3), 318–335. DOI: 10.1080/07380577.2021.1938337 PMID: 34137654

Assembly, U. G. (2021). Political declaration on HIV and AIDS: ending inequalities and getting on track to end AIDS by 2030. In *74th Plenary Meeting* (Vol. 8). https://www.unaids.org/sites/default/files/media_asset/2021_political-declaration-on-hiv-and-aids_en.pdf

Aunon, F. M. (2020). *Development and evaluation of a theory-informed mHealth intervention to promote viral suppression among women living with HIV who engage in sex work in Mombasa, Kenya: the role of text messaging, social support and stigma*. University of Washington.

Ayari, A., & Ammar, A. (2024). AI Accountability, Ethics, and Human Resource Implications. In *Ethical Challenges for the Future of Neurosurgery* (pp. 47–56). Springer Nature Switzerland.

Ayieko, P., Kisanga, E., Mshana, G., Nkosi, S., Hansen, C. H., Parry, C. D. H., Weiss, H. A., Grosskurth, H., Hayes, R. J., Morojele, N. K., & Kapiga, S. (2024). Epidemiology of alcohol use and alcohol use disorders among people living with HIV on antiretroviral therapy in Northwest Tanzania: Implications for ART adherence and case management. *AIDS Care*, *36*(5). Advance online publication. DOI: 10.1080/09540121.2023.2299324 PMID: 38295268

Ayiigah, J. L. Y., Domapielle, M. K., & Sumankuuro, J. (2024). Stigma toward people living with Human Immunodeficiency Virus: Insights from Anti-Retroviral Therapy clients in north-eastern Ghana. *Social Sciences & Humanities Open*, *9*. Advance online publication. DOI: 10.1016/j.ssaho.2024.100860

Balsamo, A. (2021). Study of deferiprone-induced agranulocytosis in β-thalassemic patients through a metabolomics approach. https://iris.unica.it/handle/11584/316317

Balzer, L. B., Havlir, D. V., Kamya, M. R., Chamie, G., Charlebois, E. D., Clark, T. D., Koss, C. A., Kwarisiima, D., Ayieko, J., Sang, N., Kabami, J., Atukunda, M., Jain, V., Camlin, C. S., Cohen, C. R., Bukusi, E. A., Van Der Laan, M., & Petersen, M. L. (2020). Machine Learning to Identify Persons at High-Risk of Human Immunodeficiency Virus Acquisition in Rural Kenya and Uganda. *Clinical Infectious Diseases*, *71*(9), 2326–2333. DOI: 10.1093/cid/ciz1096 PMID: 31697383

Banda, J. H. (2024). *Achieving the 2030 Goal of Ending HIV: An Advanced Analysis of Strategic Intervetnitions*. Socio Economic Challenges, and Biomedical Progress., DOI: 10.61784/wjbs3013

Barmania, F., & Pepper, M. S. (2013). CC chemokine receptor type five (CCR5): An emerging target for the control of HIV infection. *Applied & Translational Genomics*, *2*, 3–16. DOI: 10.1016/j.atg.2013.05.004 PMID: 27942440

Beecroft, A., Vaikla, O., & Pant Pai, N. (2024). Digital HIV self-testing as an exemplar: A perspective on benefits, challenges, and opportunities. *Expert Review of Molecular Diagnostics*, *24*(10), 913–925. DOI: 10.1080/14737159.2024.2406974 PMID: 39323182

Bekker, L. G., Beyrer, C., Mgodi, N., Lewin, S. R., Delany-Moretlwe, S., Taiwo, B., & Lazarus, J. V. (2023). HIV infection. *Nature Reviews. Disease Primers*, *9*(1), 42. PMID: 37591865

Bella, R., Kaminski, R., Mancuso, P., Young, W. B., Chen, C., Sariyer, R., Fischer, T., Amini, S., Ferrante, P., Jacobson, J. M., Kashanchi, F., & Khalili, K. (2018). Removal of HIV DNA by CRISPR from Patient Blood Engrafts in Humanized Mice. *Molecular Therapy. Nucleic Acids*, *12*, 275–282. DOI: 10.1016/j.omtn.2018.05.021 PMID: 30195766

Belus, J. M., Msimango, L. I., van Heerden, A., Magidson, J. F., Bradley, V. D., Mdakane, Y., van Rooyen, H., & Barnabas, R. V. (2024). Barriers, Facilitators, and Strategies to Improve Participation of a Couple-Based Intervention to Address Women's Antiretroviral Therapy Adherence in KwaZulu-Natal, South Africa. *International Journal of Behavioral Medicine*, *31*(1). Advance online publication. DOI: 10.1007/s12529-023-10160-7 PMID: 36854871

Bennin, L. (2024). *Mental Health And Psychological Well-Being Assessment Of People Living With Hiv/Aids In Cape Coast Teaching Hospital* (Doctoral dissertation, University of Cape Coast). https://ir.ucc.edu.gh/xmlui/handle/123456789/11632

Berger, A., Muenchhoff, M., Hourfar, K., Kortenbusch, M., Ambiel, I., Stegmann, L., Heim, A., Sarrazin, C., Ehret, R., Daniel, V., Wasner, M., Plantier, J. C., Eberle, J., Gürtler, L., Haberl, A. E., Stürmer, M., & Keppler, O. T. (2020). Severe under-quantification of HIV-1 group O isolates by major commercial PCR-based assays. *Clinical microbiology and infection: the official publication of the European Society of Clinical Microbiology and Infectious Diseases, 26*(12), 1688.e1–1688.e7. DOI: 10.1016/j.cmi.2020.03.004

Berg, R. C., Page, S., & Øgård-Repål, A. (2021). The effectiveness of peer-support for people living with HIV: A systematic review and meta-analysis. *PLoS One*, *16*(6), e0252623. DOI: 10.1371/journal.pone.0252623 PMID: 34138897

Bhardwaj, K., Soryan, I., Saxena, D., Gandhi, D., & Viswas, S. (2024). Breaking Down Barriers: How Cloud Computing Drives Interoperability in Health Care. In *International Conference on Information and Communication Technology for Intelligent Systems* (pp. 101-111). Singapore: Springer Nature Singapore. doi:DOI: 10.1007/978-981-97-6678-9_9

Birore, C. M., Wu, L., Abrefa-Gyan, T., & Lewis, M. W. (2022). Social support and quality of life among people living with HIV/AIDS (PLWHA) in Ghana. *Journal of Family Issues*, *43*(8), 2159–2180. DOI: 10.1177/0192513X21103004

Bloom, D. E., & Cadarette, D. (2019). Infectious disease threats in the twenty-first century: Strengthening the global response. *Frontiers in Immunology*, *10*, 549. DOI: 10.3389/fimmu.2019.00549 PMID: 30984169

Board on Population Health, Public Health Practice, Committee on HIV Screening, & Access to Care. (2011). *HIV Screening and Access to Care: Exploring the Impact of Policies on Access to and Provision of HIV Care.*

Board, N. L., Yuan, Z., Wu, F., Moskovljevic, M., Ravi, M., Sengupta, S., Mun, S. S., Simonetti, F. R., Lai, J., Tebas, P., Lynn, K., Hoh, R., Deeks, S. G., Siliciano, J. D., Montaner, L. J., & Siliciano, R. F. (2024). Bispecific antibodies promote natural killer cell-mediated elimination of HIV-1 reservoir cells. *Nature Immunology*, *25*(3). Advance online publication. DOI: 10.1038/s41590-023-01741-5 PMID: 38278966

Brandner, L. O. U. (2021). The social capital of creative freelancers. Networking practices in digital and urban spheres. https://iris.uniroma1.it/handle/11573/1568978

Bristow, C. C., Leon, S. R., Huang, E., Ramos, L. B., Vargas, S. K., Flores, J. A., Konda, K. A., Caceres, C. F., & Klausner, J. D. (2016). Field Evaluation of a Dual Rapid Immunodiagnostic Test for HIV and Syphilis Infection in Peru. *Sexually Transmitted Diseases*, *43*(1), 57–60. DOI: 10.1097/OLQ.0000000000000387 PMID: 26650998

Broadhead, R. S., Heckathorn, D. D., Altice, F. L., Van Hulst, Y., Carbone, M., Friedland, G. H., O'Connor, P. G., & Selwyn, P. A. (2002). Increasing drug users' adherence to HIV treatment: Results of a peer-driven intervention feasibility study. *Social Science & Medicine*, *55*(2), 235–246. DOI: 10.1016/S0277-9536(01)00167-8 PMID: 12144138

Castro, J. G., & Alcaide, M. L. (2016). High rates of sexually transmitted infections in HIV-infected patients attending an STI clinic. *Southern Medical Journal*, *109*(1), 1. DOI: 10.14423/SMJ.0000000000000389 PMID: 26741862

Cederbaum, J. A., Rice, E., Craddock, J., Pimentel, V., & Beaver, P. (2017). Social networks of HIV-positive women and their association with social support and depression symptoms. *Women & Health*, *57*(2), 268–282. DOI: 10.1080/03630242.2016.1157126 PMID: 26910637

Challacombe, S. J. (2020). Global inequalities in HIV infection. *Oral Diseases*, *26*(S1), 16–21. DOI: 10.1111/odi.13386 PMID: 32862524

Chan, H. P., Hadjiiski, L. M., & Samala, R. K. (2020). Computer-aided diagnosis in the era of deep learning. *Medical Physics*, *47*(5), e218–e227. DOI: 10.1002/mp.14146 PMID: 32418340

Chaudhary, J. K., Sharma, H., Tadiboina, S. N., Singh, R., Khan, M. S., & Garg, A. (2023). Applications of machine learning in viral disease diagnosis. In *2023 10th International Conference on Computing for Sustainable Global Development (INDIACom)* (pp. 1167–1172). IEEE.

Chauhan, R., Goel, A., Alankar, B., & Kaur, H. (2024). Predictive modeling and web-based tool for cervical cancer risk assessment: A comparative study of machine learning models. *MethodsX*, *12*, 102653. Advance online publication. DOI: 10.1016/j.mex.2024.102653 PMID: 38524310

Chellaiyan, V. G., Raut, D. K., & Khokhar, A. (2018). Integrated counseling and HIV testing centers of Delhi: An evaluation. *Journal of Family Medicine and Primary Care*, *7*(4), 791–795. DOI: 10.4103/jfmpc.jfmpc_128_17 PMID: 30234055

Chen, C., Chen, H., Wu, L., Gong, Q., & He, J. (2024). Factors influencing rapid antiretroviral therapy initiation in Jiulongpo, Chongqing, China: A retrospective cohort from 2018 to 2022. *AIDS Research and Therapy*, *21*(1). Advance online publication. DOI: 10.1186/s12981-024-00601-y PMID: 38494484

Chen, F., Wang, J., Ma, J., Song, L., Yan, H., Wang, F., Yang, Z., & Li, F. (2024). Novel DNA Biosensing Platform for Detecting HIV Integrase for Highly Sensitive and Quantitative HIV Detection, Diagnosis, and Therapeutic Monitoring. *ACS Omega*, *9*(23), 25042–25053. DOI: 10.1021/acsomega.4c02229 PMID: 38882085

Chen, L., & Shi, J. (2015). Social support exchanges in a social media community for people living with HIV/AIDS in China. *AIDS Care*, *27*(6), 693–696. DOI: 10.1080/09540121.2014.991678 PMID: 25532704

Chen, Y., Yu, W., Cai, L., Liu, B., & Guo, F. (2024). Enhancing HIV/STI decision-making: Challenges and opportunities in leveraging predictive models for individuals, healthcare providers, and policymakers. *Journal of Translational Medicine*, *22*(1), 886. Advance online publication. DOI: 10.1186/s12967-024-05678-9 PMID: 39354498

Chen, Z., Si, T., Ying, L., Guiying, C., Píng, X. J., & Wang, M. (2024). A case of multiple ART intolerance responds to Albuvirtide and Dolutegravir: Case report and literature review. *Heliyon*, *10*(6). Advance online publication. DOI: 10.1016/j.heliyon.2024.e27219 PMID: 38524593

Chesson, H. W., Mayaud, P., & Aral, S. O. (2017). *Sexually transmitted infections: impact and cost-effectiveness of prevention*. The International Bank for Reconstruction and Development.

Chien, I., Deliu, N., & Turner, R.. (2022). Multi-disciplinary fairness considerations in machine learning for clinical trials. In *Proceedings of the 2022 ACM Conference on Fairness, Accountability, and Transparency (FAccT '22)* (pp. 906–924). Association for Computing Machinery. https://doi.org/DOI: 10.1145/3531146.3533157

Chilundo, S., Gaspar, I., Keating, R., Fortmann, J., Filimão, D., Nguimfack, A., Pereira, I., Alfredo, C., Gudo, P. S., Langa, A., Dirlikov, E., Greenberg, S., Pathmanathan, I., & Couto, A. (2024). HIV Antiretroviral Therapy Scale-Up in Mozambique and Estimated Averted HIV Infections and Related Deaths, 2004–2023. *medRxiv*. DOI: 10.1101/2024.11.19.24317542

Chinyandura, C., Jiyane, A., Tsalong, X., Struthers, H. E., McIntyre, J. A., & Rees, K. (2022). Supporting retention in HIV care through a holistic, patient-centred approach: A qualitative evaluation. *BMC Psychology*, *10*(1), 17. DOI: 10.1186/s40359-022-00722-x PMID: 35093165

Chiou, P. Y., Hung, C. C., & Chen, C. Y. (2022). Sexual partner referral for HIV testing through social networking platforms: Cross-sectional study. *JMIR Public Health and Surveillance*, *8*(4), e32156. DOI: 10.2196/32156 PMID: 35380540

Chun, H. M., Dirlikov, E., Cox, M. H., Sherlock, M. W., Obeng-Aduasare, Y., Sato, K., Voetsch, A. C., Ater, A. D., Romano, E. R., Tomlinson, H., Modi, S., Achrekar, A., & Nkengasong, J.CDC Global HIV Working Group. (2023). Vital Signs: Progress Toward Eliminating HIV as a Global Public Health Threat Through Scale-Up of Antiretroviral Therapy and Health System Strengthening Supported by the U.S. President's Emergency Plan for AIDS Relief - Worldwide, 2004-2022. *MMWR. Morbidity and Mortality Weekly Report*, *72*(12), 317–324. DOI: 10.15585/mmwr.mm7212e1 PMID: 36952290

Cihlar, T., & Fordyce, M. (2016). Current status and prospects of HIV treatment. *Current Opinion in Virology*, *18*, 50–56. DOI: 10.1016/j.coviro.2016.03.004 PMID: 27023283

Clumeck, N., Pozniak, A., & Raffi, F. (2008). European AIDS Clinical Society (EACS) guidelines for the clinical management and treatment of HIV-infected adults. *HIV Medicine*, *9*(2), 65–71. DOI: 10.1111/j.1468-1293.2007.00533.x PMID: 18257769

Comfort, A. B., Asiimwe, S., Amaniyre, G., Orrell, C., Moody, J., Musinguzi, N., Bwana, M. B., Bangsberg, D. R., Haberer, J. E., Tsai, A. C., Ware, N., & Tumwesigye, E. (2024). Social networks and HIV treatment adherence among people with HIV initiating treatment in rural Uganda and peri-urban South Africa. *SSM - Population Health*, *25*. Advance online publication. DOI: 10.1016/j.ssmph.2023.101593 PMID: 38292051

Conyers, L. M., Richardson, L. A., Datti, P. A., Koch, L. C., & Misrok, M. (2017). A critical review of health, social, and prevention outcomes associated with employment for people living with HIV. *AIDS Education and Prevention*, *29*(5), 475–490. DOI: 10.1521/aeap.2017.29.5.475 PMID: 29068719

Cornman, H., Grimm, C. D., & Rana, S. (2005). Engaging Local Non-Governmental Organizations (NGOs) in the Response to HIV/AIDS. https://scholars.unh.edu/anth_facpub/2/

Corona, D., Pérez-Valero, I., Camacho, A., Gutiérrez Liarte, Á., Montero-Alonso, M., Alemán, M. R., Ruiz-Seco, P., Pérez González, A., Riera, M., Jarrin, I., Rivero-Juárez, A., & Rivero, A. (2024). Effectiveness and safety of bictegravir/emtricitabine/tenofovir alafenamide in HIV late presenters. *International Journal of Antimicrobial Agents*, *63*(1). Advance online publication. DOI: 10.1016/j.ijantimicag.2023.107016 PMID: 37890734

Cox, L. E., & Brennan-Ing, M. (2017). Medical, social and supportive services for older adults with HIV. *Interdisciplinary Topics in Gerontology and Geriatrics*, *42*, 204–221. DOI: 10.1159/000448563 PMID: 27875834

Craddock, J. B., Franke, N. D., & Kingori, C. (2022). Associations of social network- and individual-level factors with HIV testing, condom use, and interest in PrEP among young black women. *Archives of Sexual Behavior*, *51*(5), 2473–2483. DOI: 10.1007/s10508-022-02306-7 PMID: 35676567

Cuadros, D. F., Huang, Q., Mathenjwa, T., Gareta, D., Devi, C., & Musuka, G. (2024). Unlocking the potential of telehealth in Africa for HIV: Opportunities, challenges, and pathways to equitable healthcare delivery. *Frontiers in Digital Health*, *6*, 1278223. DOI: 10.3389/fdgth.2024.1278223 PMID: 38500968

Dagnaw, L. (2024). *Prevalence and Associated Risk Factors of Tuberculosis (Tb) Among Adult Human Immunodeficiency Virus (Hiv)/Acquired Immunodeficiency Syndrome (Aids) Patients Attending Health Facilities of South Achefer District Northwestern Ethiopia* (Doctoral dissertation). http://ir.bdu.edu.et/bitstream/handle/123456789/16079/Dagnaw.pdf?sequence=1

Dandri, M., Murray, J. M., Lutgehetmann, M., Volz, T., Lohse, A. W., & Petersen, J. (2008). Virion half-life in chronic hepatitis B infection is strongly correlated with levels of viremia. *Hepatology (Baltimore, Md.)*, *48*(4), 1079–1086. https://aasldpubs.onlinelibrary.wiley.com/doi/pdf/10.1002/hep.22469 PMID: 18697217

Darvishi, S., Rahmani, K., Sey, S., Khazaei, S., Homayonnezhad, S., & Hamidi, O. (2020). The survival rate and its predictors in hiv-infected patients of kurdistan province, iran: a retrospective cohort study. DOI: 10.21203/rs.3.rs-39398/v1

Dash, P. K., Kaminski, R., Bella, R., Su, H., Mathews, S., Ahooyi, T. M., Chen, C., Mancuso, P., Sariyer, R., Ferrante, P., Donadoni, M., Robinson, J. A., Sillman, B., Lin, Z., Hilaire, J. R., Banoub, M., Elango, M., Gautam, N., Mosley, R. L., & Gendelman, H. E. (2019). Sequential LASER ART and CRISPR Treatments Eliminate HIV-1 in a Subset of Infected Humanized Mice. *Nature Communications*, *10*(1), 2753. DOI: 10.1038/s41467-019-10366-y PMID: 31266936

De Andrade, S. L. E., Moreira Freire, M. E., Collet, N., Brandão, G. C. G., Souza, M. H. D. N., & Nogueira, J. D. A. (2022). Structure of social networks of people living with HIV and AIDS. *Revista da Escola de Enfermagem da USP*, *56*, e20210525. DOI: 10.1590/1980-220X-REEUSP-2021-0525 PMID: 35201256

De Cock, K. M., & Weiss, H. A. (2000). The global epidemiology of HIV/AIDS. *Tropical Medicine & International Health*, *5*(7). Advance online publication. DOI: 10.1046/j.1365-3156.2000.00590.x PMID: 10964276

Degenhardt, L., Webb, P., Colledge-Frisby, S., Ireland, J., Wheeler, A., Ottaviano, S., Willing, A., Kairouz, A., Cunningham, E. B., Hajarizadeh, B., Leung, J., Tran, L. T., Price, O., Peacock, A., Vickerman, P., Farrell, M., Dore, G. J., Hickman, M., & Grebely, J. (2023). Epidemiology of injecting drug use, prevalence of injecting-related harm, and exposure to behavioural and environmental risks among people who inject drugs: A systematic review. *The Lancet. Global Health*, *11*(5), e659–e672. https://www.thelancet.com/journals/langlo/article/PIIS2214-109X(23)00057-8/fulltext PMID: 36996857

Değer, S. U., & Can, H. (2025). A predictive study on HCV using automated machine learning models. *Computers in Biology and Medicine*, *188*, 109897. Advance online publication. DOI: 10.1016/j.compbiomed.2024.109897 PMID: 39983359

Demir, T., Yıldıran, D., & Kılıç, S. (2021). Experience of the National HIV-AIDS Reference Center of Turkey, in the Transition to the New HIV Diagnostic Algorithm; Comparative Analysis of Line-Immunoassay Test and Bio-Rad Geenius™ HIV-1/2 Antibody Confirmatory Assay. *Mikrobiyoloji Bulteni*, *55*(1), 17–29. DOI: 10.5578/mb.20028 PMID: 33590978

Dennis, A. M., Frost, S. D. W., Enders, K., Cressman, A. E., Volz, E., Adams, N., Miller, W. C., Cohen, M. S., Mobley, V., Samoff, E., & Eron, J. J. (2021). HIV-1 Transmission linkages among persons with incident infection to inform public health surveillance. *EClinicalMedicine*, *37*, 100968. DOI: 10.1016/j.eclinm.2021.100968 PMID: 34195581

Derkinderen, N. (2017). *Knowledge Attitude and Practice towards HIV/AIDS Prevention among Myanmar Female Sex Workers in Maesot District, Tak.* Province., DOI: 10.58837/CHULA.THE.2017.484

Devy, S. R. (2020). Community Health Worker-Based Empowerment Against Stigmatization of People Living with HIV/AIDS: A Meta-Synthesis. *Systematic Reviews in Pharmacy*, *11*(5).

Di Teodoro, G. (2024). Toward personalized medicine and transparent decision-making with machine learning models for complex diseases: A focus on HIV-1 and type 2 diabetes. *[Journal Name not provided—please insert correct journal title].*

Didi, N. P. (2014). *Predictors of HIV Self Disclosure to Sexual Partners by Sero-Positive Adults in Informal Settlements: A Case of Central Division, Nairobi County, Kenya* (Doctoral dissertation, Kenyatta University).

Douglas-Jones, I. M. (2014). *The willingness of tavern and shebeen owners in Gqebera, Port Elizabeth to implement or strengthen existing HIV prevention efforts and measures in their establishments* (Doctoral dissertation, Stellenbosch: Stellenbosch University). https://scholar.sun.ac.za/items/28fa9e67-9ac5-472c-afd5-1dcf07246b85

Drain, P. K., Dorward, J., Bender, A., Lillis, L., Marinucci, F., Sacks, J., Bershteyn, A., Boyle, D. S., Posner, J. D., & Garrett, N. (2019). Point-of-care HIV viral load testing: An essential tool for a sustainable global HIV/AIDS response. *Clinical Microbiology Reviews, 32*(3), 10–1128. DOI: 10.1128/cmr.00097-18 PMID: 31092508

Dulli, L., Ridgeway, K., Packer, C., Murray, K. R., Mumuni, T., Plourde, K. F., Chen, M., Olumide, A., Ojengbede, O., & McCarraher, D. R. (2020). A social media–based support group for youth living with HIV in Nigeria (SMART Connections): Randomized controlled trial. *Journal of Medical Internet Research, 22*(6), e18343. DOI: 10.2196/18343 PMID: 32484444

Duncan, D., Duncan, J., Kramer, B., Nilsson, A. Y., Haile, B., Butcher, A., Chugh, S., Baum, P., Aldrovandi, G. M., Young, S., Avery, A. K., Tashima, K., Valsamakis, A., Yao, J. D., Chang, M., & Coombs, R. W. (2021). An HIV Diagnostic Testing Algorithm Using the cobas HIV-1/HIV-2 Qualitative Assay for HIV Type Differentiation and Confirmation. *Journal of Clinical Microbiology, 59*(7), e0303020. DOI: 10.1128/JCM.03030-20 PMID: 33853869

Dunn Navarra, A. M., Gormley, M., Liang, E., Loughran, C., Vorderstrasse, A., Garcia, D. R., Rosenberg, M. G., Fletcher, J., & Goldsamt, L. A. (2024). Developing and testing a web-based platform for antiretroviral therapy (ART) adherence support among adolescents and young adults (AYA) living with HIV. *PEC Innovation, 4*. Advance online publication. DOI: 10.1016/j.pecinn.2024.100263 PMID: 38463238

Duthe, J. C., Bouzille, G., Sylvestre, E., Chazard, E., Arvieux, C., & Cuggia, M. (2021). How to identify potential candidates for HIV pre-exposure prophylaxis: An AI algorithm reusing real-world hospital data. In *Public Health and Informatics* (pp. 714–718). IOS Press.

Dzinamarira, T., Mbunge, E., & Chingombe, I.. (2024). Using machine learning models to plan HIV services: Emerging opportunities in design, implementation and evaluation. *SAMJ: South African Medical Journal, 114*(6b), 86–90. PMID: 39041524

Ehrenkranz, P., Grimsrud, A., Holmes, C. B., Preko, P., & Rabkin, M. (2021). Expanding the vision for differentiated service delivery: a call for more inclusive and truly patient-centered care for people living with HIV. *JAIDS Journal of Acquired Immune Deficiency Syndromes, 86*(2), 147 152. doi: DOI: 10.1097/QAI.0000000000002549

Eissa, M. E. (2025). A BRIEF OVERVIEW OF HIV TREATMENT STRATEGIES: A FOCUSED LOOK AT CHALLENGES AND OPPORTUNITIES. *Universal Journal of Pharmaceutical Research.*

Eissa, N. M. E. (2025). A BRIEF OVERVIEW OF HIV TREATMENT STRATEGIES: a FOCUSED LOOK AT CHALLENGES AND OPPORTUNITIES. *Universal Journal of Pharmaceutical Research.* https://doi.org/DOI: 10.22270/ujpr.v10i1.1273

Erdinç, F. Ş., Tülek, N., Ataman Hatipoğlu, Ç., Gürkaynak, P., Aya Kılıç, E. K., Kınıklı, S., & Ertem, G. (2018). Evaluation of the surgeons' approach to hiv infection. *Flora the Journal of Infectious Diseases and Clinical Microbiology, 23*(4), 167–171. DOI: 10.5578/flora.67359

Esra, R., Mmelesi, M., Ketlogetswe, A. T., Wolock, T. M., Howes, A., Nong, T., Matlhaga, M. T., Ratladi, S., Ramaabya, D., & Imai-Eaton, J. W. (2024). Improved Indicators for Subnational Unmet Antiretroviral Therapy Need in the Health System: Updates to the Naomi Model in 2023. *Journal of Acquired Immune Deficiency Syndromes, 95*(1). Advance online publication. DOI: 10.1097/QAI.0000000000003324 PMID: 38180736

Eze, C. E., Igwama, G. T., Nwankwo, E. I., & Victor, E. (2024). AI-driven health data analytics for early detection of infectious diseases: A conceptual exploration of US public health strategies.

Ezenwaji, C. O., Alum, E. U., & Ugwu, O. P. C. (2025). Bridging the gap: Telemedicine as a solution for HIV care inequities in rural and vulnerable communities. *International Journal for Equity in Health, 24*(1), 205. DOI: 10.1186/s12939-025-02584-2 PMID: 40660269

Fahad Naim, Awais Naeem, Fahim Shah, Umair-ul-Islam, Sohail Adnan, & Muhammad Hamid. (2024). Assessment of Non-HIV Comorbidities Among HIV-Infected Patients on Anti-Retroviral therapy (ART) in a Teaching Hospital Kohat, Pakistan. *Annals of PIMS-Shaheed Zulfiqar Ali Bhutto Medical University, 13*(4). https://doi .org/DOI: 10.48036/apims.v13i4.974

Fasakin, K. A., Ajayi, O. D., Ibijola, A. A., Adeniyi, A. A., Ajetunmobi, W. A., Ajetunmobi, O. A., Adewara, O. E., Bakare, A., & Oyegue, B. E. (2024). Hiv diagnostic algorithms in a resource-limited setting: A comparative study. *Journal of Advances in Medical and Pharmaceutical Sciences, 26*(7), 79–94. DOI: 10.9734/jamps/2024/v26i7703

Fassinou, L. C., Songwa Nkeunang, D., Delvaux, T., Nagot, N., & Kirakoya-Samadoulougou, F. (2024). Adherence to option B + antiretroviral therapy and associated factors in pregnant and breastfeeding women in Sub-Saharan Africa: A systematic review and meta-analysis. *BMC Public Health*, *24*(1). Advance online publication. DOI: 10.1186/s12889-023-17004-9 PMID: 38183014

Fedr, R., Kahounová, Z., Remšík, J., Reiterová, M., Kalina, T., & Souček, K. (2023). Variability of fluorescence intensity distribution measured by flow cytometry is influenced by cell size and cell cycle progression. *Scientific Reports*, *13*(1), 4889. DOI: 10.1038/s41598-023-31990-1 PMID: 36966193

Février, M., Dorgham, K., & Rebollo, A. (2011). CD4+ T cell depletion in human immunodeficiency virus (HIV) infection: Role of apoptosis. *Viruses*, *3*(5), 586. DOI: 10.3390/v3050586 PMID: 21994747

Fieggen, J., Smith, E., Arora, L., & Segal, B. (2022). The role of machine learning in HIV risk prediction. *Frontiers in Reproductive Health*, *4*. Advance online publication. DOI: 10.3389/frph.2022.1062387 PMID: 36619681

Flores, L., Kim, S., & Young, S. D. (2024). Addressing bias in artificial intelligence for public health surveillance. *Journal of Medical Ethics*, *50*(3), 190–194. PMID: 37130756

Fox, M. P., Pascoe, S., Huber, A. N., Murphy, J., Phokojoe, M., Gorgens, M., Rosen, S., Wilson, D., Pillay, Y., & Fraser-Hurt, N. (2019). Adherence clubs and decentralized medication delivery to support patient retention and sustained viral suppression in care: Results from a cluster-randomized evaluation of differentiated ART delivery models in South Africa. *PLoS Medicine*, *16*(7), e1002874. DOI: 10.1371/journal.pmed.1002874 PMID: 31335865

Frade, S., Mendonca, R., Cooper, S., Morris, S., Lee, H., Gupta, K., & Rech, D. (2025). HealthPulse AI: Enhancing Diagnostic Trust and Accessibility in Under-Resourced Settings through AI. *VeriXiv*, *2*, 54.

Frescura, L., Godfrey-Faussett, P., Feizzadeh, A., El-Sadr, W., Syarif, O., & Ghys, P. D. (2025). Testing Treatment Target Working Group. (2022). Achieving the 95 95 95 targets for all: A pathway to ending AIDS. *PLoS One*, *17*(8), e0272405. DOI: 10.1371/journal.pone.0272405 PMID: 35925943

Gandhi, R. T., Landovitz, R. J., Sax, P. E., Smith, D. M., Springer, S. A., Günthard, H. F., & Saag, M. S. (2025). Antiretroviral drugs for treatment and prevention of HIV in adults: 2024 recommendations of the International Antiviral Society–USA Panel. *Journal of the American Medical Association*, *333*(7), 609–628. PMID: 39616604

Garett, R., Kim, S., & Young, S. D. (2024). Ethical Considerations for Artificial Intelligence Applications for HIV. *AI*, *5*(2), 594–601.

Gashu, K. D. (2024). The Digital Ecosystem and Major Public Health Informatics Initiatives in Resource-Limited Settings. In *Public Health Informatics: Implementation and Governance in Resource-Limited Settings* (pp. 97-140). Cham: Springer Nature Switzerland. doi:DOI: 10.1007/978-3-031-71118-3_4

Gatechompol, S., Kerr, S. J., Cardoso, S. W., Samaneka, W., Tripathy, S., Godbole, S., Ghate, M., Kanyama, C., Nyirenda, M., Sugandhavesa, P., Machado, A., Van Leth, F., Campbell, T. B., Swindlells, S., Avihingsanon, A., & Cobelens, F. (2024). Monocyte to lymphocyte ratio and hemoglobin level to predict tuberculosis after antiretroviral therapy initiation. *AIDS*, *38*(1). Advance online publication. DOI: 10.1097/QAD.0000000000003713 PMID: 37696248

Gautheret-Dejean, A., Bocobza, J., Brunet, S., Damond, F., Plantier, J. C., & Barin, F. (2015). Performance of rapid tests for discrimination between HIV-1 and/or HIV-2 infections. *Journal of Medical Virology*, *87*(12), 2061–2066. DOI: 10.1002/jmv.24282 PMID: 26081750

Gebremedhin, K., & Haye, T. (2019). Factors associated with anemia among people living with hiv/aids taking art in ethiopia. *Advances in Hematology*, ●●●, 1–8. DOI: 10.1155/2019/9614205 PMID: 30941180

George, G., Chaturvedi, S., Corbishley, C., & Atun, R. (2024). Relational coordination and stigma at work: How frontline employees compensate for failures in public health systems. *Journal of Management Studies*, *61*(3), 752–784. DOI: 10.1111/joms.12813

Gera, A., Dhull, A., Singh, A., & Singh, K. K. (2025). Legal and regulatory issues related to AI in healthcare. In *Responsible and Explainable Artificial Intelligence in Healthcare* (pp. 259–283). Academic Press.

German Advisory Committee Blood (Arbeitskreis Blut), Subgroup 'Assessment of Pathogens Transmissible by Blood. (2016). Human immunodeficiency virus (HIV). *Transfusion Medicine and Hemotherapy; Offizielles Organ der Deutschen Gesellschaft für Transfusionsmedizin und Immunhämatologie*, *43*(3), 203–222. DOI: 10.1159/000445852 PMID: 27403093

Ghazvinian, A., Feng, B., & Feng, J. (2025). Enhancing efficiency in the healthcare sector through multi-objective optimization of freight cost and delivery time in the HIV drug supply chain using machine learning. *Systems*, *13*(2), 91. Advance online publication. DOI: 10.3390/systems13020091

Grace, D., Steinberg, M., Kwag, M., Chown, S. A., Doupe, G., Trussler, T., Rekart, M., & Gilbert, M. (2014). Diagnostic technologies in practice. *Qualitative Health Research*, *25*(2), 205–217. DOI: 10.1177/1049732314549813 PMID: 25201583

Gray, E. R., Turbé, V., Lawson, V. E., Page, R. H., Cook, Z. C., Ferns, R. B., Nastouli, E., Pillay, D., Yatsuda, H., Athey, D., & McKendry, R. A. (2018). Ultra-rapid, sensitive and specific digital diagnosis of hiv with a dual-channel saw biosensor in a pilot clinical study. *NPJ Digital Medicine*, 1(1)., s. DOI: 10.1038/s41746-018-0041-5

Greifinger, R., & Dick, B. (2011). Provision of psychosocial support for young people living with HIV: Voices from the field. *SAHARA J : Journal of Social Aspects of HIV/AIDS Research Alliance*, *8*(1), 33–41. DOI: 10.1080/17290376.2011.9724982 PMID: 23237644

Guiraud, V., Ciczora, Y., Cardona, M., Defer, C., Gréaume, S., Nogues, D., & Gautheret-Dejean, A. (2024). Sensitivity and specificity of the new Bio-Rad HIV screening test, Access HIV combo V2. *Journal of Clinical Microbiology*, *62*(5), e0009524. DOI: 10.1128/jcm.00095-24 PMID: 38534108

Guo, W., & Chen, Y. (2025). Investigating Whether AI Will Replace Human Physicians and Understanding the Interplay of the Source of Consultation, Health-Related Stigma, and Explanations of Diagnoses on Patients' Evaluations of Medical Consultations: Randomized Factorial Experiment. *Journal of Medical Internet Research*, *27*, e66760. PMID: 40053785

Gupta, I., & Barman, K. (2021). Health, development, and HIV in India. In *Oxford Research Encyclopedia of Asian History*. DOI:DOI: 10.1093/acrefore/9780190277727.013.424

Gupta, M., Kumar, A., Kumar, A., & Mathur, V. (2024). Reversible blindness in cryptococcal meningitis with human immunodeficiency virus infection. *International Journal of Research in Medical Sciences*, *12*(3). Advance online publication. DOI: 10.18203/2320-6012.ijrms20240553

Halasa-Rappel, Y. A., Gaumer, G., Khatri, D., Hurley, C. L., Jordan, M., & Nandakumer, A. K. (2021). The tale of two epidemics: Hiv/aids in ghana and namibia. *The Open AIDS Journal*, *15*(1), 63–72. DOI: 10.2174/1874613602115010063

Haleyur Giri Setty, M. K., Lee, S., Lathrop, J., & Hewlett, I. K. (2020). Biotin Interference in Point of Care HIV Immunoassay. *BioResearch Open Access*, *9*(1), 243–246. DOI: 10.1089/biores.2020.0038 PMID: 33269113

Hamid, O., Tapak, M., Poorolajal, J., Amini, P., & Tapak, L. (2017). Application of random survival forest for competing risks in prediction of cumulative incidence function for progression to AIDS. *Epidemiology, Biostatistics, and Public Health, 14*(4). Advance online publication. DOI: 10.2427/12663

Han, J., Wang, Y., Wang, B., & Tong, H. (2023). Diagnostic efficacy of photostimulated chemiluminescence assay for detecting anti-hiv antibodies: A retrospective study. *Polish Journal of Microbiology, 72*(4), 461–466. DOI: 10.33073/pjm-2023-043 PMID: 38095515

Harichund, C., Karim, Q. A., Kunene, P., Simelane, S., & Moshabela, M. (2019). HIV self-testing as part of a differentiated HIV testing approach: Exploring urban and rural adult experiences from KwaZulu-Natal, South Africa using a cross-over study design. *BMC Public Health, 19*(1), 53. DOI: 10.1186/s12889-018-6366-9 PMID: 30634943

Haris, M., & Abbas, R. (2024). Four decades of HIV: Global trends, testing assays, treatment, and challenges. *Zoonoses, 4*(1), 997. DOI: 10.15212/ZOONOSES-2023-0039

Harkness, A., Morales, V., Defreitas, W., Atuluru, P., Jaramillo, J., Weinstein, E. R., Feaster, D. J., Safren, S., & Balise, R. (2022). Impact of COVID-19 on HIV service delivery in Miami-Dade County: A mixed methods study. *BMC Health Services Research, 22*(1), 1476. DOI: 10.1186/s12913-022-08849-8 PMID: 36463177

Hawkins, D., Blott, M., Clayden, P., De Ruiter, A., Foster, G., Gilling-Smith, C., Layall, G. H., Mercey, D., Newell, M. L., O'Shea, S., Smith, R., Sunderland, J., Wood, C., & Taylor, G. (2005). Guidelines for the management of HIV infection in pregnant women and the prevention of mother-to-child transmission of HIV. *Virology Papers*, 151.

Heidt, B., Siqueira, W. F., Eersels, K., Diliën, H., van Grinsven, B., Fujiwara, R. T., & Cleij, T. J. (2020). Point of care diagnostics in resource-limited settings: A review of the present and future of PoC in its most needed environment. *Biosensors (Basel), 10*(10), 133. DOI: 10.3390/bios10100133 PMID: 32987809

He, J., Zhong, S., Qin, C., Nong, A., Lin, Z., Liang, H., Zhang, F., Jiang, J., Pan, P., Wei, W., Liu, J., Liu, D., Ye, L., Liang, H., & Liang, B. (2024). The trend, prevalence and potential risk factors of secondary HIV transmission among HIV/AIDS individuals receiving ART in Guangxi, China: A longitudinal cross-sectional study. *Emerging Microbes & Infections, 13*(1), 2429622. DOI: 10.1080/22221751.2024.2429622 PMID: 39552513

Herman, T. (2021). *Impact of Integrating Directly Observed Therapy with Care Coordination in Improving Anti-Retroviral Therapy Adherence for Patients Who Are HIV Positive and Non-Suppressed* (Doctoral dissertation, D'Youville College).

Hermann, K., Van Damme, W., Pariyo, G. W., Schouten, E., Assefa, Y., Cirera, A., & Massavon, W. (2009). Community health workers for ART in sub-Saharan Africa: Learning from experience–capitalizing on new opportunities. *Human Resources for Health*, *7*, 1–11. DOI: 10.1186/1478-4491-7-31 PMID: 19358701

Hernandez, C., Gorska, A. M., & Eugenin, E. (2024). Mechanisms of HIV-mediated blood-brain barrier compromise and leukocyte transmigration under the current antiretroviral era. *iScience*, *27*(3). Advance online publication. DOI: 10.1016/j.isci.2024.109236 PMID: 38487019

Hess, K. L., Crepaz, N., Rose, C., Purcell, D., & Paz-Bailey, G. (2017). Trends in sexual behavior among men who have sex with men (MSM) in high-income countries, 1990–2013: A systematic review. *AIDS and Behavior*, *21*, 2811–2834. DOI: 10.1007/s10461-017-1799-1 PMID: 28555317

Hill, M. (2019). *Characterizing the Social Networks & Art Adherence Behaviors of Trans Women Living with HIV* (Doctoral dissertation, University of Georgia).

Hilty, D. M., Gentry, M. T., McKean, A. J., Cowan, K. E., Lim, R. F., & Lu, F. G. (2020). Telehealth for rural diverse populations: Telebehavioral and cultural competencies, clinical outcomes and administrative approaches. *mHealth*, *6*, 20. DOI: 10.21037/mhealth.2019.10.04 PMID: 32270012

Hiremath, R. N. (2021). *A Prospective Study To Assess The Factors Affecting Nutritional Status Of People Living With Hiv/Aids (Plha) Receiving Anti-Retroviral Therapy (Art)* (Doctoral dissertation, BLDE (Deemed to be University)). https://digitallibrary.bldedu.ac.in/handle/123456789/4166

Hlaing, M. M. (2024). *The Effect of Social Support on HIV-related Stigma among People Living with HIV/AIDS (Case Study of Myeik Township)(Mi Mi Hlaing, 2024)* (Doctoral dissertation, MERAL Portal).

Hoffmann, C. J., Gonzalez, C. J., & Stein, D. K. (2023). Second-line ART after treatment failure or for regimen simplification. *Medical Care*, *2*, 2–25.

Holman, A. G., & Gabuzda, D. (2012). A machine learning approach for identifying amino acid signatures in the HIV env gene predictive of dementia. *PLoS One*, *7*(11), e49538. Advance online publication. DOI: 10.1371/journal.pone.0049538 PMID: 23166702

Hosaka, K. R., Kang, E., Huff, J., Shaw, S., & Duomai, S. (2021). Livelihood intervention and mental well-being among women living with HIV in Delhi. *AIDS Care*, *33*(8), 1037–1043. DOI: 10.1080/09540121.2020.1837336 PMID: 33103920

Hou, C., Wei, J., Zhang, H., & Li, H. (2025). Evolving strategies in the diagnosis and treatment of HIV-associated neurocognitive disorders. *Reviews in the Neurosciences*, (0).

Hourfar, K., Eberle, J., Müller, M., Micha Nübling, C., Chudy, M., Kress, J., Gürtler, L., Mayr-Wohlfart, U., Schrezenmeier, H., Hellmann, I., Luhm, J., Kraas, S., Ringwald, J., Gubbe, K., Frank, K., Karl, A., Tonn, T., Jaeger, M., Sireis, W., & Schmidt, M. (2018). Human immunodeficiency virus 1 dual-target nucleic acid technology improves blood safety: 5 years of experience of the German Red Cross blood donor service Baden-Württemberg-Hessen. *Transfusion*, *58*(12), 2886–2893. DOI: 10.1111/trf.14919 PMID: 30325043

Hu, S., Jing, F., Fan, C., Dai, Y., Xie, Y., Zhou, Y., Lv, H., He, X., Wu, D., Tucker, J. D., & Tang, W. (2024). Social network strategies to distribute HIV self-testing kits: A global systematic review and network meta-analysis. *Journal of the International AIDS Society*, *27*(7), e26342. DOI: 10.1002/jia2.26342 PMID: 39048927

Ibrahim, K., Kahle, E. M., Christiani, Y., & Suryani, S. (2024). Utilization of social media for the prevention and control of HIV/AIDS: A scoping review. *Journal of Multidisciplinary Healthcare*, •••, 2443–2458. https://www.tandfonline.com/doi/full/10.2147/JMDH.S465905#references-Section PMID: 38799010

Iedema, R., Allen, S., Britton, K., & Gallagher, T. H. (2012). What do patients and relatives know about problems and failures in care? *BMJ Quality & Safety*, *21*(3), 198–205. DOI: 10.1136/bmjqs-2011-000100 PMID: 22178930

Ingold, H., Mwerinde, O., Ross, A. L., Leach, R., Corbett, E. L., Hatzold, K., Johnson, C. C., Ncube, G., Nyirenda, R., & Baggaley, R. C. (2019). The Self-Testing AfRica (STAR) Initiative: accelerating global access and scale-up of HIV self-testing. *Journal of the International AIDS Society, 22 Suppl 1*(Suppl Suppl 1), e25249. DOI: 10.1002/jia2.25249

Ingole, N., Sarkate, P., Paranjpe, S. M., Sarode, R., Shinde, S., & Mehta, P. R. (2014). HIV Diagnosis in Resource Constrained Setting: How Good Is the Current Algorithm? *World Journal of AIDS*, *4*, 45–51. DOI: 10.4236/wja.2014.41006

Jaiteh, M., Phalane, E., Shiferaw, Y. A., Voet, K. A., & Phaswana-Mafuya, R. N. (2024). Utilization of machine learning algorithms for the strengthening of HIV testing: A systematic review. *Algorithms*, *17*(8), 362. Advance online publication. DOI: 10.3390/a17080362

Jaspal, R., Eriksson, P., & Nynäs, P. (2021). Identity, threat and coping among gay men living with HIV in Finland. *Cogent Psychology*, *8*(1), 1878980. DOI: 10.1080/23311908.2021.1878980

Jewell, B. L., Mudimu, E., Stover, J., Ten Brink, D., Phillips, A. N., Smith, J. A., Martin-Hughes, R., Teng, Y., Glaubius, R., Mahiane, S. G., Bansi-Matharu, L., Taramusi, I., Chagoma, N., Morrison, M., Doherty, M., Marsh, K., Bershteyn, A., Hallett, T. B., & Kelly, S. L.HIV Modelling Consortium. (2020). Potential effects of disruption to HIV programmes in sub-Saharan Africa caused by COVID-19: Results from multiple mathematical models. *The Lancet. HIV*, *7*(9), e629–e640. DOI: 10.1016/S2352-3018(20)30211-3 PMID: 32771089

Ji, H. (2007). Association of interferon regulatory factor-1 polymorphisms with resistance to infection by HIV-1 in Kenyan female sex workers.

Jia, X. C., Xia, Z. H., Shi, N., Wang, Y. P., Luo, Z. X., Yang, Y. L., & Shi, X. Z. (2020). The factors associated with natural disease progression from HIV to AIDS in the absence of ART, a propensity score matching analysis. *Epidemiology and Infection*, *148*, e57. DOI: 10.1017/S0950268820000540 PMID: 32089142

Jin, R., & Zhang, L. (2025). AI applications in HIV research: Advances and future directions. *Frontiers in Microbiology*, *16*, 1541942. Advance online publication. DOI: 10.3389/fmicb.2025.1541942 PMID: 40051479

Johansson, E., Nazziwa, J., Freyhult, E., Hong, M., Neptin, M., Karlson, S., Rezeli, M., da Silva, Z. J., Biague, A. J., Lindman, J., Palm, A., Medstrand, P., Månsson, F., Norrgren, H., Jansson, M., & Esbjörnsson, J.SWEGUB CORE group. (2024). Distinct plasma protein profiles distinguish faster from slower disease progression in hiv-1 and hiv-2 infections. DOI: 10.1101/2024.07.23.24310457

Jones-Esan, L., Somasiri, N., & Lorne, K. (2024). Enhancing healthcare delivery through digital health interventions: a systematic review on telemedicine and mobile health applications in Low and Middle-Income Countries (LMICs). *Research Square*. doi: DOI: 10.21203/rs.3.rs-5189203/v1

Kalemeera, F., Ndevahoma, S., Mubita, M., & Godman, B. (2022). Evaluation of Namibia's antiretroviral therapy guidelines' recommendations for switching from first-line to second-line, using predictors of first-line treatment failure: An exploratory study. *Expert Review of Anti-Infective Therapy*, *20*(6), 915–921. DOI: 10.1080/14787210.2022.2015325 PMID: 34878350

Kamal, S., Urata, J., Cavassini, M., Liu, H., Kouyos, R., Bugnon, O., & Schneider, M. P. (2021). Random forest machine learning algorithm predicts virologic outcomes among HIV infected adults in Lausanne, Switzerland using electronically monitored combined antiretroviral treatment adherence. *AIDS Care*, *33*(4), 530–536. PMID: 32266825

Kamau, S. G., Akatusasira, R., Namatovu, A., Kibet, E., Ssekitto, J. M., Mamun, M. A., & Kaggwa, M. M. (2024). The level of antiretroviral therapy (ART) adherence among orphan children and adolescents living with HIV/AIDS: A systematic review and meta-analysis. *PLoS ONE, 19*(2 February). https://doi.org/DOI: 10.1371/journal.pone.0295227

Kamulegeya, L. H., Kagolo, I., Kabakaari, B., Atuhaire, J., Nasamula, R., & Bwanika, J. M. (2025). Technology-Assisted Interventions in the Delivery of HIV Prevention, Care, and Treatment Services in Sub-Saharan Africa: Scoping Review. *Journal of Medical Internet Research*, *27*, e68352. PMID: 40233346

Kanise, H., van Oosterhout, J. J., Bisani, P., Songo, J., Matola, B. W., Chipungu, C., Simon, K., Cox, C., Hosseinipour, M. C., Sagno, J. B., Hoffman, R. M., Wallrauch, C., Phiri, S., Steegen, K., Jahn, A., Nyirenda, R., & Heller, T. (2024). Virological Findings and Treatment Outcomes of Cases That Developed Dolutegravir Resistance in Malawi's National HIV Treatment Program. *Viruses*, *16*(1). Advance online publication. DOI: 10.3390/v16010029 PMID: 38257730

Kaufman, M. R., Cornish, F., Zimmerman, R. S., & Johnson, B. T. (2014). Health behavior change models for HIV prevention and AIDS care: Practical recommendations for a multi-level approach. *JAIDS Journal of Acquired Immune Deficiency Syndromes*, *66*, S250–S258. DOI: 10.1097/QAI.0000000000000236 PMID: 25007194

Kawichai, S., Nelson, K. E., Natpratan, C., Celentano, D. D., Khamboonruang, C., Natpratan, P., & Beyrer, C. (2005). Personal history of voluntary HIV counseling and testing (VCT) among adults aged 19–35 years living in peri-urban communities, Chiang Mai, northern Thailand. *AIDS and Behavior*, *9*, 233–242. DOI: 10.1007/s10461-005-3904-0 PMID: 15933842

Keddem, S., Agha, A., Morawej, S., Buck, A., Cronholm, P., Sonalkar, S., & Kearney, M. (2023). Characterizing Twitter Content about HIV Pre-exposure Prophylaxis (PrEP) for women: Qualitative content analysis. *Journal of Medical Internet Research*, *25*, e43596. PMID: 37166954

Keter, G. (2023). *The Impact of Demographic Factors on Adverse Drug Reactions and Survival Rates Among Hiv Patients in Nairobi County From 2015 to 2021* (Doctoral dissertation, University of Nairobi). https://erepository.uonbi.ac.ke/handle/11295/164239

Khan, H., Alzabut, J., Almutairi, D. K., & Alqurashi, W. K. (2025). The Use of Artificial Intelligence in Data Analysis with Error Recognitions in Liver Transplantation in HIV-AIDS Patients Using Modified ABC Fractional Order Operators. *Fractal and Fractional*, *9*(1).

Kibibi, W. H. (2024). Harnessing artificial intelligence for HIV drug resistance prediction and personalized treatment. *NEWPORT INTERNATIONAL JOURNAL OF RESEARCH IN MEDICAL SCIENCES*, *5*(3), 59–64. DOI: 10.59298/nijrms/2024/5.3.5964

Kigongo, V. J., Nankabirwa, J. I., Kitutu, F. E., Ssenyonga, R., Mutebi, R. K., Kazibwe, A., Kiguba, R., Kambugu, A. D., & Castelnuovo, B. (2024). Dyslipidemia among adult people living with HIV on dolutegravir – based antiretroviral therapy at a private tertiary hospital in Kampala, Uganda: Burden and determinants. *BMC Infectious Diseases*, *24*(1). Advance online publication. DOI: 10.1186/s12879-023-08892-8 PMID: 38183002

Kiirya, Y., Kitaka, S., Kalyango, J., Rujumba, J., Obeng-Amoako, G. A. O., & Amollo, M., Nan gendo, J., Karamagi, C., Musooke, P., & Katahoire, A. (2025). Acceptability of an online peer support group as a strategy to improve antiretroviral therapy adherence among young people in Kampala district, Uganda: Qualitative findings. *BMC Infectious Diseases*, *25*(1), 461. DOI: 10.1186/s12879-025-10831-8 PMID: 40181265

Kileel, E. M., Zheng, A., Bor, J., Fox, M. P., Crowther, N. J., George, J. A., Khoza, S., Rosen, S., Venter, W. D. F., Raal, F., Hibberd, P., & Brennan, A. T. (2024). Does Engagement in HIV Care Affect Screening, Diagnosis, and Control of Noncommunicable Diseases in Sub-Saharan Africa? A Systematic Review and Meta-analysis. *AIDS and Behavior*, *28*(2). Advance online publication. DOI: 10.1007/s10461-023-04248-0 PMID: 38300475

Klinnert, S., Freitag, P. C., Plückthun, A., & Metzner, K. J. (2023). Targeting hiv-1 with crispr/cas9 delivered by retargeted adenoviruses effectively suppresses viral replication. DOI: 10.1101/2023.12.18.572146

Knight, L., & Schatz, E. (2022). Social support for improved ART adherence and retention in care among older people living with HIV in urban South Africa: A complex balance between disclosure and stigma. *International Journal of Environmental Research and Public Health, 19*(18), 11473. DOI: 10.3390/ijerph191811473 PMID: 36141746

Koh, M. C. Y., Ngiam, J. N., Yong, J., Tambyah, P. A., & Archuleta, S. (2024). The role of an artificial intelligence model in antiretroviral therapy counselling and advice for people living with HIV. *HIV Medicine*, *25*(4). Advance online publication. DOI: 10.1111/hiv.13604 PMID: 38169077

Kolluri, V. (2016). An innovative study exploring revolutionizing healthcare with AI: personalized medicine: predictive diagnostic techniques and individualized treatment. *Journal of Emerging Technologies and Innovative Research, 218*, •••. https://www.researchgate.net/publication/380730035

Kondo, M., Sudo, K., Sano, T., Kawahata, T., Itoda, I., Iwamuro, S., Yoshimura, Y., Tachikawa, N., Kojima, Y., Mori, H., Fujiwara, H., Hasegawa, N., & Kato, S. (2018). Comparative evaluation of the Geenius HIV 1/2 Confirmatory Assay and the HIV-1 and HIV-2 Western blots in the Japanese population. *PLoS One*, *13*(10), e0198924. DOI: 10.1371/journal.pone.0198924 PMID: 30379808

Konishi, K., Nakagawa, H., Asaoka, T., Kasamatsu, Y., Goto, T., & Shirano, M. (2024). Brief communication: Body composition and hidden obesity in people living with HIV on antiretroviral therapy. *AIDS Research and Therapy*, *21*(1). Advance online publication. DOI: 10.1186/s12981-024-00599-3 PMID: 38429716

Korenromp, E. L., Williams, B. G., Schmid, G. P., & Dye, C. (2009). Clinical prognostic value of RNA viral load and CD4 cell counts during untreated HIV-1 infection—A quantitative review. *PLoS One*, *4*(6), e5950. DOI: 10.1371/journal.pone.0005950 PMID: 19536329

Koss, C. A., Charlebois, E. D., Ayieko, J., Kwarisiima, D., Kabami, J., Balzer, L. B., Atukunda, M., Mwangwa, F., Peng, J., Mwinike, Y., Owaraganise, A., Chamie, G., Jain, V., Sang, N., Olilo, W., Brown, L. B., Marquez, C., Zhang, K., Ruel, T. D., & Havlir, D. V. (2020). Uptake, engagement, and adherence to pre-exposure prophylaxis offered after population HIV testing in rural Kenya and Uganda: 72-week interim analysis of observational data from the SEARCH study. *The Lancet. HIV*, *7*(4), e249–e261. https://www.thelancet.com/journals/lanhiv/article/PIIS2352-3018(19)30433-3/fulltext PMID: 32087152

Krüsi, A., & Shannon, K. (2022). The Intersecting Social and Structural Contexts of Navigating HIV Risk and Access to Care among Women. *WOMEN'S HEALTH IN CANADA*, 331. https://utppublishing.com/doi/abs/10.3138/9781442628472#page=346

Kumar, K., Kumar, P., Deb, D., Unguresan, M.-L., & Muresan, V. (2023). Artificial intelligence and machine learning based intervention in medical infrastructure: A review and future trends. *Health Care*, *11*(2), 207. Advance online publication. DOI: 10.3390/healthcare11020207 PMID: 36673575

Kumar, P., Sangal, B., Ramanathan, S., Ammassari, S., & Venkatesh, S. R. (2018). Unsafe injecting practices, sexual risk behaviours and determinants of HIV among men who inject drugs: Results from Integrated Biological and Behavioural Surveillance in India. *International Journal of STD & AIDS*, *29*(11), 1066–1075. DOI: 10.1177/095646241876980 PMID: 29747557

Kumar, Y., Koul, A., Singla, R., & Ijaz, M. F. (2023). Artificial intelligence in disease diagnosis: A systematic literature review, synthesizing framework and future research agenda. *Journal of Ambient Intelligence and Humanized Computing*, *14*(7), 8459–8486. DOI: 10.1007/s12652-021-03612-z PMID: 35039756

Kumbale, C. M., & Voit, E. O. (2021). Toward personalized medicine for HIV/AIDS. *Journal of AIDS and HIV treatment, 3*(2), 37.

Laar, A. (2022). Access to Life-Saving Public Health Goods by Persons Infected with or Affected by HIV. In *Balancing the Socio-political and Medico-ethical Dimensions of HIV: A Social Public Health Approach* (pp. 51–63). Springer International Publishing., DOI: 10.1007/978-3-031-09191-9_4

Lai, J. (2023). Developing a predictive information system for determining the prognosis of HIV and tuberculosis co-infection in incarcerated individuals. *International Journal for Applied Information Management*, *3*(2), 101–110.

Lainjo, B. (2024). Artificial intelligence with machine learning and the enigmatic discovery of HIV cure. *Journal of Autonomous Intelligence*, *7*(2).

Lainjo, B. (2024). Original Research Article Artificial intelligence with machine learning and the enigmatic discovery of HIV cure. *Journal of Autonomous Intelligence*, *7*(2).

Lakshmanan, K., & Liu, B. M. (2025). Impact of point-of-care testing on diagnosis, treatment, and surveillance of vaccine-preventable viral infections. *Diagnostics (Basel)*, *15*(2), 123. DOI: 10.3390/diagnostics15020123 PMID: 39857007

Land, H. (2015). Diverse people affected by HIV/AIDS. *Transformative Social Work Practice, 25.*

Laymouna, M. A. (2023). *Informing the Development of a Chatbot for Pharmacist Needs in HIV Care*. McGill University.

Lee, Y. H., Bang, J. H., Park, S. M., Kang, C. R., Cho, S. I., Oh, M. D., & Lee, J. K. (2018). Cost-Effectiveness of Voluntary HIV Testing Strategies in a Very Low-Prevalence Country, the Republic of Korea. *Journal of Korean Medical Science, 33*(46), e304. DOI: 10.3346/jkms.2018.33.e304 PMID: 30416412

Liang, X., Alam, N., Sultana, T., Bandara, E., & Shetty, S. (2024). Designing A Blockchain-Empowered Telehealth Artifact for Decentralized Identity Management and Trustworthy Communication: Interdisciplinary Approach. *Journal of Medical Internet Research, 26*, e46556. DOI: 10.2196/46556 PMID: 39320943

Li, L., Feng, X., Zhao, F., Yuan, D., An, X., Tian, X., Wu, H., Su, B., Zhang, T., & Liu, L. (2024). Real-world performance of hiv low viral load values in diagnosing acute hiv infection in a tertiary care hospital in beijing, china. *BMC Infectious Diseases*, *24*(1). Advance online publication. DOI: 10.1186/s12879-024-09486-8 PMID: 38879487

Li, L., Wu, S., Wu, Z., Sun, S., Cui, H., & Jia, M. (2006). Understanding family support for people living with HIV/AIDS in Yunnan, China. *AIDS and Behavior, 10*, 509–517. DOI: 10.1007/s10461-006-9071-0 PMID: 16741672

Lim, S. Y., Lee, J., Osuna, C. E., Vikhe, P., Schalk, D. R., Chen, E., Fray, E., Kumar, M., Schultz-Darken, N., Rakasz, E., Capuano, S., Ladd, R. A., Gil, H. M., Evans, D. T., Jeng, E. K., Seaman, M., Martin, M., Van Dorp, C., Perelson, A. S., & Whitney, J. B. (2024). Induction of durable remission by dual immunotherapy in SHIV-infected ART-suppressed macaques. *Science, 383*(6687). Advance online publication. DOI: 10.1126/science.adf7966 PMID: 38422185

Li, N., Lewin, A., Ning, S., Waito, M., Zeller, M. P., & Tinmouth, A.Canadian Transfusion Trials Group. (2025). Privacy-preserving federated data access and federated learning: Improved data sharing and AI model development in transfusion medicine. *Transfusion*, *65*(1), 22–28. PMID: 39610333

Li, R., Duffee, D., & Gbadamosi-Akindele, M. F. (2023). CD4 count. In *StatPearls* [Internet]. StatPearls Publishing., https://www.ncbi.nlm.nih.gov/sites/books/NBK470231/

Liu, A. Y., Laborde, N. D., Coleman, K., Vittinghoff, E., Gonzalez, R., Wilde, G., & Buchbinder, S. (2021). DOT diary: Developing a novel mobile app using artificial intelligence and an electronic sexual diary to measure and support PrEP adherence among young men who have sex with men. *AIDS and Behavior*, *25*, 1001–1012. PMID: 33044687

Li, Z., Uno, N., Ding, X., Avery, L., Banach, D., & Liu, C. (2023). Bioinspired CRISPR-Mediated Cascade Reaction Biosensor for Molecular Detection of HIV Using a Glucose Meter. *ACS Nano*, *17*(4), 3966–3975. DOI: 10.1021/acsnano.2c12754 PMID: 36762838

Long, E. (2011). Hiv screening via fourth-generation immunoassay or nucleic acid amplification test in the united states: A cost-effectiveness analysis. *PLoS One*, *6*(11), e27625. DOI: 10.1371/journal.pone.0027625 PMID: 22110698

Macchia, E., Sarcina, L., Picca, R. A., Manoli, K., Di Franco, C., Scamarcio, G., & Torsi, L. (2019). Ultra-low hiv-1 p24 detection limits with a bioelectronic sensor. *Analytical and Bioanalytical Chemistry*, *412*(4), 811–818. DOI: 10.1007/s00216-019 PMID: 31865415

Madapuji Srinivasan, M. (2024). *Molecular Mechanisms and Host Factors Involved in HIV-1 Latency* (Doctoral dissertation, Université d'Ottawa/University of Ottawa). https://ruor.uottawa.ca/server/api/core/bitstreams/1aa1292f-c82e-4cbe-88ed-ebc6e9a450ce/content

Mahlalela, N. B., Manne-Goehler, J., Ohene-Kwofie, D. B., Adams, L., Montana, L., Kahn, K., Rohr, J. K., Bärnighausen, T., & Gómez-Olivé, F. X. (2024). The Association Between HIV-Related Stigma and the Uptake of HIV Testing and ART Among Older Adults in Rural South Africa: Findings from the HAALSI Cohort Study. *AIDS and Behavior*, *28*(3). Advance online publication. DOI: 10.1007/s10461-023-04222-w PMID: 38286975

Manjate, A., Nilsson, C., Axelsson, M., Lindroth, S., Sirbu, D., Sacarlal, J., Andersson, S., & Unemo, M. (2024). Laboratory-based evaluation of the 4th-generation AlereTM HIV Combo rapid point-of-care test. *PLoS One*, *19*(2), e0298912. DOI: 10.1371/journal.pone.0298912 PMID: 38394120

Manoto, S. L., Lugongolo, M., Govender, U., & Mthunzi-Kufa, P. (2018). Point of Care Diagnostics for HIV in Resource Limited Settings: An Overview. *Medicina (Kaunas, Lithuania)*, *54*(1), 3. DOI: 10.3390/medicina54010003 PMID: 30344234

Mantell, J. E., Khalifa, A., Christian, S. N., Romo, M. L., Mwai, E., George, G., Strauss, M., Govender, K., & Kelvin, E. A. (2022). Preferences, beliefs, and attitudes about oral fluid and blood-based HIV self-testing among truck drivers in Kenya choosing not to test for HIV. *Frontiers in Public Health*, *10*, 911932. DOI: 10.3389/fpubh.2022.911932 PMID: 36438254

Marcus, J. L., Sewell, W. C., Balzer, L. B., & Krakower, D. S. (2020). Artificial intelligence and machine learning for HIV prevention: Emerging approaches to ending the epidemic. *Current HIV/AIDS Reports*, *17*, 171–179. PMID: 32347446

Marsh, K., Eaton, J. W., Mahy, M., Sabin, K., Autenrieth, C. S., Wanyeki, I., Daher, J., & Ghys, P. D. (2019). Global, regional and country-level 90-90-90 estimates for 2018: assessing progress towards the 2020 target. *AIDS (London, England)*, *33 Suppl 3*(Suppl 3), S213–S226. DOI: 10.1097/QAD.0000000000002355

Masila, H. M. (2024). *Using asset-based community development approaches to combat the spread of HIV/AIDS in Mombasa county, Kenya* (Master's thesis, VID Specialized University. Stavanger).

Maskew, M., Sharpey-Schafer, K., De Voux, L., Crompton, T., Bor, J., Rennick, M., & Pisa, P. (2022). Applying machine learning and predictive modeling to retention and viral suppression in South African HIV treatment cohorts. *Scientific Reports*, *12*(1), 12715. PMID: 35882962

Masur, P. B. H., Kaplan, J. E., & Holmes, K. K. (2002). Guidelines for preventing opportunistic infections among HIV-infected persons—2002: Recommendations of the US Public Health Service and the Infectious Diseases Society of America. *Annals of Internal Medicine*, *137*(5_Part_2), 435–478. DOI: 10.7326/0003-4819-137-5_Part_2-200209031-00002 PMID: 12617574

Ma, Y., Achiche, S., Tu, G., Vicente, S., Lessard, D., Engler, K., & Lebouché, B. (2025). The first AI-based Chatbot to promote HIV self-management: A mixed methods usability study. *HIV Medicine*, *26*(2), 184–206. PMID: 39390632

Mayasi Ngongo, N., Kamangu Ntambwe, E., Situakibanza Nani-Tuma, H., Mbula Mambimbi, M., Mandina Ndona, M., Longokolo Mashi, M., Bepouka Izizag, B., Lukiana, T., Odio Ossam, J., Mangala Sonzi, D., Maes, N., Moutschen, M., El Moussaoui, M., & Darcis, G. (2023). Human Immunodeficiency Virus Viral Load Monitoring and Rate of Virologic Suppression Among Patients Receiving Antiretroviral Therapy in Democratic Republic of the Congo, 2013-2020. *Open Forum Infectious Diseases*, *10*(6), ofad242. Advance online publication. DOI: 10.1093/ofid/ofad242 PMID: 37363052

McIntyre, A. (2024). *The role of CD4+ help in promoting CD8+ T cell function following allogeneic haematopoietic stem cell transplantation* (Doctoral dissertation, UCL (University College London)). https://discovery.ucl.ac.uk/id/eprint/10188958/

McIntyre, J. (2005). Maternal health and HIV. *Reproductive Health Matters, 13*(25), 129–135. DOI: 10.1016/S0968-8080(05)25184-4 PMID: 16035606

Mekonnen, Z. A. (2024). Public Health Informatics: An Overview. *Public Health Informatics: Implementation and Governance in Resource-Limited Settings*, 27-61. doi:DOI: 10.1007/978-3-031-71118-3_2

Mereu, A., Liori, A., Fadda, L., Puddu, M., Chessa, L., Contu, P., & Sardu, C. (2022). What do young people know about HIV? Results of a cross sectional study on 18-24-year-old students. *Journal of Preventive Medicine and Hygiene, 63*(4), E541. PMID: 36891004

Meya, D. B., Kiragga, A. N., Nalintya, E., Banturaki, G., Akullo, J., Kalyesubula, P., Sessazi, P., Bitakalamire, H., Kabanda, J., Kalamya, J. N., Namale, A., Bateganya, M., Kagaayi, J., Gutreuter, S., Adler, M. R., & Mitruka, K. (2022). Impact of an intensive facility-community case management intervention on 6-month HIV outcomes among select key and priority populations in Uganda. *AIDS Research and Therapy, 19*(1), 62. DOI: 10.1186/s12981-022-00486-9 PMID: 36471321

Mhlanga, D. (2022). The role of artificial intelligence and machine learning amid the COVID-19 pandemic: What lessons are we learning on 4IR and the sustainable development goals. *International Journal of Environmental Research and Public Health, 19*(3), 1879. Advance online publication. DOI: 10.3390/ijerph19031879 PMID: 35162901

Miller, R. L., Rutledge, J., & Ayala, G. (2021). Breaking down barriers to HIV care for gay and bisexual men and transgender women: The Advocacy and Other Community Tactics (ACT) Project. *AIDS and Behavior, 25*(8), 2551–2567. DOI: 10.1007/s10461-021-03216-w PMID: 33730253

Miriti, D., Marwa, I., & Muriuki, J. (2025). Clinical factors Associated with Viral Load Suppression Among HIV and AIDS-Positive Children (0–14 Years) Attending Meru County Referral Hospital, Meru County, Kenya.

Mlambo, N. (2021). *A Non-Governmental Organistion's Psycho-Social and Educational Support for Orphans and Vulnerable Children in Soweto*. University of Johannesburg., https://www.proquest.com/openview/16788e444b4dbe9be04a69d4144ab366/1?cbl=2026366&diss=y&pq-origsite=gscholar

Mody, A., Sohn, A. H., Iwuji, C., Tan, R. K., Venter, F., & Geng, E. H. (2024). HIV epidemiology, prevention, treatment, and implementation strategies for public health. *Lancet*, *403*(10425), 471–492. PMID: 38043552

Monroe-Wise, A., Barr-DiChiara, M., Mozalevskis, A., Msimanga, B., de Mello, M. B., Senya, K., & Baggaley, R. (2025). Can network-based testing services have an impact beyond testing for HIV? *Sexual Health*, *22*(2). Advance online publication. DOI: 10.1071/SH24027 PMID: 40193579

Mornah, L. N., Saaka, M., & Pireh, D. (2024). Magnitude and Predictors of Dietary Diversity among HIV-Infected Adults on Antiretroviral Therapy: The Case of North-Western, Ghana. *AIDS Research and Treatment*, *2024*. Advance online publication. DOI: 10.1155/2024/2777908 PMID: 38328798

Morvan, M. G., Teque, F. C., Locher, C. P., & Levy, J. A. (2021). The CD8+ T Cell noncytotoxic antiviral responses. *Microbiology and Molecular Biology Reviews : MMBR*, *85*(2), 10–1128. DOI: 10.1128/mmbr.00155-20 PMID: 33980586

Moscona, R., Wagner, T., Geva, M., Bucris, E., Erster, O., Zuckerman, N. S., & Mor, O. (2024). Novel amplicons based method for near-full-length genome (NFLG) sequencing of HIV-1 group M recombinant forms. DOI: 10.1101/2024.08.04.606545

Moya, Z. R., Pillay, S., & Magula, N. (2024). Assessing index CD4 and associated outcomes at 1-year in a tertiary HIV clinic, KwaZulu-Natal. *South African Family Practice*, *66*(1). Advance online publication. DOI: 10.4102/safp.v66i1.5803 PMID: 38299523

Msafiri, F., Manjate, A., & Lindroth, S. (2022). Vaccine-induced seroreactivity impacts the accuracy of hiv testing algorithms in sub-saharan africa: An exploratory study. *Vaccines*, *10*(7), 1062. DOI: 10.3390/vaccines10071062 PMID: 35891226

Mudrick, N. R., Breslin, M. L., Nielsen, K. A., & Swager, L. C. (2020). Can disability accommodation needs stored in electronic health records help providers prepare for patient visits? A qualitative study. *BMC Health Services Research*, *20*, 1–18. DOI: 10.1186/s12913-020-05808-z PMID: 33066788

Mugerwa, M. (2023). *Prevalence, Associated Factors, Barriers and Facilitators of Disclosure of HIV status to sexual partners among Young People Living with HIV/AIDS in care at an Urban HIV Clinic, Kampala, Uganda* (Doctoral dissertation, Makerere University). http://makir.mak.ac.ug/handle/10570/12752

Mukherjee, A., Mukherjee, T., & Roy, M. M. (2025). A Study of AI Application Through Integrated and Systematic Moral Cognitive Therapy in the Healthcare Sector. *Design and Forecasting Models for Disease Management*, 47-76.

Mukuna, D. M., Decroo, T., & Nyapokoto, C. M. (2024). Effect of dolutegravir-based versus efavirenz-based antiretroviral therapy on excessive weight gain in adult treatment-naïve HIV patients at Matsanjeni health center, Eswatini: A retrospective cohort study. *AIDS Research and Therapy*, *21*(1). Advance online publication. DOI: 10.1186/s12981-023-00591-3 PMID: 38185696

Mulumba, E. M., Kayembe, M. F., Chewe, W. C., Chanda, C., Dube, N., Chituta, C., Hamooya, B. M., Kasweka, F. T., Matabishi, M., & Assani, M. B. (2025). Performance of the VISITECT® CD4 Test for Rapid Identification of Advanced HIV Disease at AHF-Supported Sites in Zambia: A Diagnostic Accuracy Analysis in a Zambian Population. medRxiv, 2025-01. doi:DOI: 10.1101/2025.01.06.25320078

Musab, A., Gobir, I. Y., Zakari, Y., Kabuga, A. I., & Rogo, L. D. (2022). Plasma levels of secretory calreticulin among hiv infected patients in bauchi state. *J AIDS HIV Treat*, *5*(1), 1–8. DOI: 10.33696/aids.5.040

Mutabazi, J. C., Zarowsky, C., & Trottier, H. (2017). The impact of programs for prevention of mother-to-child transmission of HIV on health care services and systems in sub-Saharan Africa-A review. *Public Health Reviews*, *38*, 1–27. DOI: 10.1186/s40985-017-0072-5 PMID: 29450099

Muwonge, C. M., Kembabazi, A., Nakalema, G., Ekatushabe, M., Kwarikunda, D., Kibedi, H., & Ssenyonga, J. (2022). Psychological Well-Being Among Young People Living with HIV: Role of Social Support, Self-Esteem and Socio-Demographic Variables. In *Embracing Well-Being in Diverse African Contexts: Research Perspectives* (pp. 171–194). Springer International Publishing., DOI: 10.1007/978-3-030-85924-4_8

Mwabenga, B. K. (2019). *Effectiveness of HIV and AIDS Social Support Coping Skill to PLWHA in Kinondoni Municipality, Dar es Salaam: A Case Study of Mwananyamala Hospital* (Doctoral dissertation, The Open University of Tanzania). http://repository.out.ac.tz/2994/

Nalwanga, D., & Musiime, V. (2022). Children living with HIV: A narrative review of recent advances in pediatric HIV research and their implications for clinical practice. *Therapeutic Advances in Infectious Disease*, *9*, 20499361221077544. DOI: 10.1177/20499361221077544 PMID: 35186289

Naranjo, O., Torices, S., Clifford, P. R., Rodriguez, T., Osborne, O. M., Tiburcio, D., Fattakhov, N., Park, M., Stevenson, M., & Toborek, M. (2024). AKT signaling modulates latent viral reservoir viability in HIV-1-infected blood–brain barrier pericytes. *The Journal of Biological Chemistry*, *300*(1). Advance online publication. DOI: 10.1016/j.jbc.2023.105526 PMID: 38043797

Nasri, E., Fakhim, H., & Jafari-Sales, A. (2022). Prevalence of human t-lymphotropic virus type 1 in brain-dead organ donors. *Archives of Clinical Infectious Diseases, 17*(1). Advance online publication. DOI: 10.5812/archcid-116005

Nasrullah, M., Ethridge, S. F., Delaney, K. P., Wesolowski, L. G., Granade, T. C., Schwendemann, J., Boromisa, R. D., Heffelfinger, J. D., Owen, S. M., & Branson, B. M. (2011). Comparison of alternative interpretive criteria for the HIV-1 Western blot and results of the Multispot HIV-1/HIV-2 Rapid Test for classifying HIV-1 and HIV-2 infections. *Journal of clinical virology: the official publication of the Pan American Society for Clinical Virology, 52 Suppl 1*, S23–S27. DOI: 10.1016/j.jcv.2011.09.020

Ndashimye, E., & Arts, E. J. (2019). The urgent need for more potent antiretroviral therapy in low-income countries to achieve UNAIDS 90-90-90 and complete eradication of AIDS by 2030. *Infectious Diseases of Poverty*, *8*(04), 67–74. DOI: 10.1186/s40249-019-0573-1 PMID: 31370888

Nichol, A. A., Bendavid, E., Mutenherwa, F., Patel, C., & Cho, M. K. (2021). Diverse experts' perspectives on ethical issues of using machine learning to predict HIV/AIDS risk in sub-Saharan Africa: A modified Delphi study. *BMJ Open*, *11*(7), e052287. PMID: 34321310

Nikolopoulos, G. K., & Tsantes, A. G. (2022). Recent HIV infection: Diagnosis and public health implications. *Diagnostics (Basel)*, *12*(11), 2657. DOI: 10.3390/diagnostics12112657 PMID: 36359500

Njuba, L., Gómez-Morantes, J. E., Herrera, A., & Camacho, S. (2024). Health information systems in extreme contexts: Using mobile phones to fight AIDS in Uganda. *The Electronic Journal on Information Systems in Developing Countries, 90*(3). Advance online publication. DOI: 10.1002/isd2.12314

Nkambule, B. S. (2022). *Factors Associated With Access to HIV Care in East and Southern Africa* (Doctoral dissertation, National Yang Ming Chiao Tung University).

Nsanzimana, S., Rwibasira, G. N., Malamba, S. S., Musengimana, G., Kayirangwa, E., Jonnalagadda, S., Rezende, E. F., Eaton, J. W., Mugisha, V., Remera, E., Muhamed, S., Mulindabigwi, A., Omolo, J., Weisner, L., Moore, C., Patel, H., & Justman, J. E. (2022). HIV incidence and prevalence among adults aged 15-64 years in Rwanda: Results from the Rwanda Population-based HIV Impact Assessment (RPHIA) and District-level Modeling, 2019. *International Journal of Infectious Diseases, 116*, 245–254. DOI: 10.1016/j.ijid.2022.01.032 PMID: 35066161

Ntiboneka, A. (2015). *Reduction Of HIV/AIDS Impacts Through PLHIV Clubs' Income Generating Projects: The case of Upendo Club People living with HIV in Mungonya Ward, Kigoma District Council* (Doctoral dissertation, The Open University Of Tanzania). http://repository.out.ac.tz/1124/

Nursalam, N., Sukartini, T., Misutarno, M., & Priyantini, D. (2024). Adherence to antiretroviral therapy, CD4 count, viral load and opportunistic infections in people with HIV/AIDS: A cross-sectional study. *Jurnal Ners*, *19*(1). Advance online publication. DOI: 10.20473/jn.v19i1.49958

Nwosu, C. M. (2024). Level of education and comprehensive knowledge about HIV/AIDS among women aged 15-49 years in Southern Nigeria: A cross-sectional study. https://www.diva-portal.org/smash/record.jsf?pid=diva2%3A1875833&dswid=-7116

Nyamboga, T. O., & Obeagu, E. I. (2024). Sustainable Solutions: Strategic Management for Long-Term HIV Care in At-Risk Populations. *Elite Journal of Public Health*, *2*(7), 63-74. https://kiu.ac.ug/assets/publications/3245_sustainable-solutions-strategic-management-for-long-term-hiv-care-in-at-risk-populations.pdf

Obeagu, E. I., & Obeagu, G. U. (2024). Unmasking the Truth: Addressing Stigma in the Fight Against HIV. *Elite Journal of Public Health, 2*(1), 8-22. https://kiu.ac.ug/assets/publications/1415_unmasking-the-truth-addressing-stigma-in-the-fight-against-hiv.pdf

Obeagu, E. I. (2024). Reducing Viral Load Impact: Blood Transfusions as a Complementary Approach in HIV Treatment. *International Journal of Medical Sciences and Pharma Research*, *10*(3), 56–62. DOI: 10.22270/ijmspr.v10i3.115

Obeagu, E. I., Igwe, M. C., & Obeagu, G. U. (2024). The Power of Unity: Collective Efforts in Confronting HIV Stigma. *Elite Journal of Public Health*, *2*(3), 22–36.

Obeagu, E. I., & Obeagu, G. U. (2024). Mental Health and Psychosocial Effects of natural disaster on HIV Patients. *The Sciences*, *4*(1), 38–44. https://kiu.ac.ug/assets/publications/1401_mental-health-and-psychosocial-effects-of-natural-disaster-on-hiv-p-atients.pdf

Obeagu, E. I., & Obeagu, G. U. (2024). Moving forward together: Collaborative strategies in HIV prevention across Africa–a narrative review. *Annals of Medicine and Surgery (London)*, •••, 10–1097. DOI: 10.1097/MS9.0000000000002961 PMID: 40852004

Obeagu, E. I., Ubosi, N. I., Obeagu, G. U., & Akram, M. (2024). Early Infant Diagnosis: Key to Breaking the Chain of HIV Transmission. *Elite Journal of Public Health, 2*(1), 52–61.

Odame-Takyi, K. T. (2016). *Implementation of HIV/AIDS policy in the Gauteng Department of Roads and Transport*. University of the Witwatersrand., https://www.proquest.com/openview/3204e91daeae914b9d16279f7ca8e739/1?cbl=2026366&diss=y&pq-origsite=gscholar

OG, A. (2024). Investigating the Relationship between Medication Adherence Behaviors and the Achievement of Sustained Viral Load Suppression among People Living with HIV (PLHIV) on Antiretroviral Therapy (ART) in Akwa Ibom State, from 2018 - 2022. *Public Health Open Access, 8*(1). Advance online publication. DOI: 10.23880/phoa-16000270

Okere, N. E., Sambu, V., Ndungile, Y., van Praag, E., Hermans, S., Naniche, D., de Wit, T. F. R., Maokola, W., & Gomez, G. B. (2021). The Shinyanga Patient: A Patient's Journey through HIV Treatment Cascade in Rural Tanzania. *International Journal of Environmental Research and Public Health, 18*(16), 8418. DOI: 10.3390/ijerph18168418 PMID: 34444166

Olaboye, N. J. A., Maha, N. C. C., Kolawole, N. T. O., & Abdul, N. S. (2024). Artificial intelligence in monitoring HIV treatment adherence: A conceptual exploration. *International Journal of Multidisciplinary Research Updates, 7*(2), 068–082. https://doi.org/DOI: 10.53430/ijmru.2024.7.2.0036

Olaboye, J. A., Maha, C. C., Kolawole, T. O., & Abdul, S. (2024). Artificial intelligence in monitoring HIV treatment adherence: A conceptual exploration. *International Medical Science Research Journal, 4*(6), 681–692.

Olaleye, S. A., Sanusi, I. T., Salo, J., & Olaleye, E. O. (2023). Home care and mobile health services provision for rural dwellers: a conceptual framework of poverty alleviation and rural development. https://aisel.aisnet.org/iceb2023/34/

Olaya, F., Brin, M., Caraballo, P. B., Halpern, M., Jia, H., Ramírez, S. O., Padilla, J. J., Stonbraker, S., & Schnall, R. (2024). A randomized controlled trial of the dissemination of an mHealth intervention for improving health outcomes: The WiseApp for Spanish-speakers living with HIV study protocol. *BMC Public Health, 24*(1). Advance online publication. DOI: 10.1186/s12889-023-17538-y PMID: 38233908

Omondi, F. H., Sudderuddin, H., Shahid, A., Kinloch, N. N., Jones, B. R., Miller, R. L., & Brumme, Z. L. (2021). HIV proviral burden, genetic diversity, and dynamics in viremic controllers who subsequently initiated suppressive antiretroviral therapy. *mBio, 12*(6), e02490–e21. PMID: 34781741

Ophinni, Y., Inoue, M., Kotaki, T., & Kameoka, M. (2018). CRISPR/Cas9 system targeting regulatory genes of HIV-1 inhibits viral replication in infected T-cell cultures. *Scientific Reports*, *8*(1), 7784. DOI: 10.1038/s41598-018-26190-1 PMID: 29773895

Ortblad, K. F., Chanda, M. M., Musoke, D. K., Ngabirano, T., Mwale, M., Nakitende, A., Chongo, S., Kamungoma, N., Kanchele, C., Bärnighausen, T., & Oldenburg, C. E. (2018). Acceptability of HIV self-testing to support pre-exposure prophylaxis among female sex workers in Uganda and Zambia: Results from two randomized controlled trials. *BMC Infectious Diseases*, *18*(1), 503. DOI: 10.1186/s12879-018-3415-z PMID: 30286737

Otange, B., Birech, Z., Rop, R., & Oyugi, J. (2019). Estimation of hiv-1 viral load in plasma of hiv-1-infected people based on the associated raman spectroscopic peaks. *Journal of Raman Spectroscopy : JRS*, *50*(5), 620–628. DOI: 10.1002/jrs.5557

Oturu, K., O'Brien, O., & Ozo-Eson, P. I. (2024). Barriers and enabling structural forces affecting access to antiretroviral therapy in Nigeria. *BMC Public Health*, *24*(1). Advance online publication. DOI: 10.1186/s12889-023-17271-6 PMID: 38184516

Oyedele, O., & Ntusi, N. (2021). A multinomial modelling of the factors that impact viral load levels in adults on anti-retroviral therapy in namibia. *ISTJN*, *14*, 73–82. DOI: 10.32642/istjn.v14i.1569

Padhi, A., Agarwal, A., Saxena, S. K., & Katoch, C. D. S. (2023). Transforming clinical virology with AI, machine learning and deep learning: A comprehensive review and outlook. *Virusdisease*, *34*(3), 345–355. DOI: 10.1007/s13337-023-00843-6 PMID: 37780897

Pagkas-Bather, J., Young, L. E., Chen, Y. T., & Schneider, J. A. (2020). Social network interventions for HIV transmission elimination. *Current HIV/AIDS Reports*, *17*, 450–457. DOI: 10.1007/s11904-020-00524-z PMID: 32720253

Pantanowitz, L., Hanna, M., Pantanowitz, J., Lennerz, J., Henricks, W. H., Shen, P., & Rashidi, H. H. (2024). Regulatory aspects of AI-ML. *Modern Pathology*, *•••*, 100609. PMID: 39260776

Parekh, B. S., Ou, C. Y., Fonjungo, P. N., Kalou, M. B., Rottinghaus, E., Puren, A., Alexander, H., Hurlston Cox, M., & Nkengasong, J. N. (2018). Diagnosis of Human Immunodeficiency Virus Infection. *Clinical Microbiology Reviews*, *32*(1), e00064–e18. DOI: 10.1128/CMR.00064-18 PMID: 30487166

Parker, J., Carrasco, A.F., & Chen, J. (2019). BioRad BioPlex® HIV Ag-Ab assay: Incidence of false positivity in a low-prevalence population and its effects on the current HIV testing algorithm. *Journal of clinical virology: the official publication of the Pan American Society for Clinical Virology, 116*, 1–3. DOI: 10.1016/j.jcv.2019.04.002

Pattanapanyasat, K., & Thakar, M. R. (2005). CD4+ T cell count as a tool to monitor HIV progression & anti-retroviral therapy. *The Indian Journal of Medical Research, 121*(4), 539–549. PMID: 15817962

Payagala, S., & Pozniak, A. (2024). The global burden of HIV. *Clinics in Dermatology, 42*(2), 119–127. DOI: 10.1016/j.clindermatol.2024.02.001 PMID: 38387533

Peeriga, R., & Manubolu, K. (2025). Pioneering Technologies to Revolutionize Antiviral Treatment. In *Global Perspectives on Antiviral Drug Development* (pp. 175–216). IGI Global Scientific Publishing., DOI: 10.4018/979-8-3693-9276-8.ch005

Pelaez-Prestel, H., Mozas-Gutierrez, J., Lafuente, E. M., & Reche, P. A. (2024). Hiv-1 protein coding sequences are present in relevant bacteria. DOI: 10.1101/2024.12.04.626764

Periáñez, Á., Schmitz, K., Makhupula, L., Hassan, M., Moleko, M., del Río, A. F., . . . Tang, D. (2024). Optimizing HIV Patient Engagement with Reinforcement Learning in Resource-Limited Settings. *arXiv preprint arXiv:2408.07629.*

Pertiwi, R., Woelansari, E., & Puspitasari, A. (2023). Correlation between hiv rapid test and hiv viral load in hiv patients at haji hospital in surabaya. *International Journal of Advanced Health Science and Technology, 3*(4), 223–228. DOI: 10.35882/ijahst.v3i4.290

Peter, T., Ellenberger, D., Kim, A. A., Boeras, D., Messele, T., Roberts, T., Stevens, W., Jani, I., Abimiku, A., Ford, N., Katz, Z., & Nkengasong, J. N. (2017). Early antiretroviral therapy initiation: Access and equity of viral load testing for HIV treatment monitoring. *The Lancet. Infectious Diseases, 17*(1), e26–e29. DOI: 10.1016/S1473-3099(16)30212-2 PMID: 27773596

Pham, M. D., Nguyen, H. V., Anderson, D., Crowe, S., & Luchters, S. (2022). Viral load monitoring for people living with HIV in the era of test and treat: Progress made and challenges ahead–a systematic review. *BMC Public Health, 22*(1), 1203. DOI: 10.1186/s12889-022-13504-2 PMID: 35710413

Pham, M. D., Romero, L., Parnell, B., Anderson, D. A., Crowe, S. M., & Luchters, S. (2017). Feasibility of antiretroviral treatment monitoring in the era of decentralized HIV care: A systematic review. *AIDS Research and Therapy*, *14*, 1–18. DOI: 10.1186/s12981-017-0131-5 PMID: 28103895

Pilcher, C. D., Louie, B., Facente, S., Keating, S., Hackett, J.Jr, Vallari, A., Hall, C., Dowling, T., Busch, M. P., Klausner, J. D., Hecht, F. M., Liska, S., & Pandori, M. W. (2013). Performance of rapid point-of-care and laboratory tests for acute and established HIV infection in San Francisco. *PLoS One*, *8*(12), e80629. DOI: 10.1371/journal.pone.0080629 PMID: 24349007

Plebani, M., Nichols, J. H., Luppa, P. B., Greene, D., Sciacovelli, L., Shaw, J., Khan, A. I., Carrar, P., Freckmann, G., Dimech, W., Zaninotto, M., Spannagl, M., Huggett, J., Kost, G. J., Trenti, T., Padoan, A., Thomas, A., Banfi, G., & Lippi, G. (2025). Point-of-care testing: State-of-the art and perspectives. [CCLM]. *Clinical Chemistry and Laboratory Medicine*, *63*(1), 35–51. PMID: 38880779

Poindexter, C. C. (2010). *Handbook of HIV and social work: Principles, practice, and populations*. John Wiley & Sons., https://books.google.co.in/books?hl=en&lr=&id=w4M2vh_0Cs4C&oi=fnd&pg=PT24&dq=The+case+management+of+HIV-affected+patients,+when+handled+by+healthcare+workers,+follows+certain+strategies+to+reduce+unwanted+outcome&ots=-FpQcofbLl&sig=pec_J_Rgvoa5B-jZQiZWzkKbcRg&redir_esc=y#v=onepage&q&f=false

Pontes-Pereira, P. S., Antonini, M., Fedocci, E. M. M., Costa, C. R. B., Esquivel-Rubio, A. I., Botelho, E. P., Gir, E., & Reis, R. K. (2023). Prevalence of chronic non-communicable diseases in people living with HIV. *Acta Paulista de Enfermagem*, *36*, eAPE01132. Advance online publication. DOI: 10.37689/acta-ape/2023AO011322

Posse, J. L., Dios, P. D., & Scully, C. (2017). Viral diseases transmissible by kissing. *Saliva Protection and Transmissible Diseases*, *53*. Advance online publication. DOI: 10.1016/B978-0-12-813681-2.00004-4

Qayyum, S. F., Khan, H., & Rukh, G. (2024). Incidence of Opportunistic Infections in HIV Patients at Anti-Retroviral Therapy (ART) Adherence Unit, Islamabad Pakistan. *Journal of Health and Rehabilitation Research*, *4*(1). Advance online publication. DOI: 10.61919/jhrr.v4i1.542

Quaker, A. S., Shirima, L. J., & Msuya, S. E. (2024). Trend and factors associated with non-suppression of viral load among adolescents on ART in Tanzania: 2018–2021. *Frontiers in Reproductive Health*, *6*. Advance online publication. DOI: 10.3389/frph.2024.1309740 PMID: 38292142

Rahman, M. M. (2024). Ethical and Technological Convergence: AI and Blockchain in Halal Healthcare. *Artificial Intelligence-Enabled Blockchain Technology and Digital Twin for Smart Hospitals*, 451-466.

Rahsepar Meadi, M., Sillekens, T., Metselaar, S., van Balkom, A., Bernstein, J., & Batelaan, N. (2025). Exploring the Ethical Challenges of Conversational AI in Mental Health Care: Scoping Review. *JMIR Mental Health, 12*, e60432. PMID: 39983102

Ratwani, R. M., Sutton, K., & Galarraga, J. E. (2024). Addressing AI algorithmic bias in health care. *Journal of the American Medical Association, 332*(13), 1051–1052. PMID: 39230911

Reid, M. J., Otieno, B. A., van Heerden, A., Sikazwe, I., Baptiste, S. L., Mendonca, R., & Sundaram, M. (2025). Announcing the Lancet Global Health Commission on artificial intelligence (AI) and HIV: Leveraging AI for equitable and sustainable impact. *The Lancet. Global Health, 13*(4), e611–e612. PMID: 40155096

Ridgeway, K. (2024). *Psychosocial factors and HIV care engagement among adolescents and young adults living with HIV in Akwa Ibom and Cross River states, Nigeria* (Doctoral dissertation, Johns Hopkins University). https://jscholarship.library.jhu.edu/items/83e491f2-61be-45d3-9e92-5215c747e907

Rietveld, C. A., & Patel, P. C. (2024). Antiretroviral Therapy Coverage, Entrepreneurship, and Development in Low- and Middle-Income Countries. *Business & Society*. Advance online publication. DOI: 10.1177/00076503241232070

Roberts, T., Cohn, J., Bonner, K., & Hargreaves, S. (2016). Scale-up of Routine Viral Load Testing in Resource-Poor Settings: Current and Future Implementation Challenges. *Clinical Infectious Diseases, 62*(8), 1043–1048. DOI: 10.1093/cid/ciw001 PMID: 26743094

Rocca, S., Zangari, P., Cotugno, N., De Rossi, A., Ferns, B., Petricone, D., Rinaldi, S., Giaquinto, C., Bernardi, S., Rojo, P., Rossi, P., Pahwa, S., Nastouli, E., & Palma, P.EPIICAL Consortium. (2019). Human Immunodeficiency Virus (HIV)-Antibody Repertoire Estimates Reservoir Size and Time of Antiretroviral Therapy Initiation in Virally Suppressed Perinatally HIV-Infected Children. *Journal of the Pediatric Infectious Diseases Society, 8*(5), 433–438. DOI: 10.1093/jpids/piy080 PMID: 30169837

Roche, S. D., Ekwunife, O. I., Mendonca, R., Kwach, B., Omollo, V., Zhang, S., Ongwen, P., Hattery, D., Smedinghoff, S., Morris, S., Were, D., Rech, D., Bukusi, E. A., & Ortblad, K. F. (2024). Measuring the performance of computer vision artificial intelligence to interpret images of HIV self-testing results. *Frontiers in Public Health, 12*, 1334881. DOI: 10.3389/fpubh.2024.1334881 PMID: 38384878

Rosen, J. G., Ddaaki, W. G., Nakyanjo, N., Chang, L. W., Vo, A. V., Zhao, T., & Galiwango, R. M. (2024). The potential promise and pitfalls of point-of-care viral load monitoring to expedite HIV treatment decision-making in rural Uganda: A qualitative study. *BMC Health Services Research, 24*(1), 1265. DOI: 10.1186/s12913-024-11747-w PMID: 39434090

Rufu, A., Chitindingu, K., Chinofunga, S., Dupwa, B., & Mugurungi, O. (2022). Designing, Developing, pilot implementation and evaluation of a mobile android based tool to improve health outcomes in adolescents and young adults living with HIV: An Agile model Human-Centered Design Science three-phase Methodology. doi:DOI: 10.21203/rs.3.rs-1914197/v1

Sadiq, E., Katzew, S., Nel, J., Tade, G., Woodiwiss, A., Norton, G., & Modi, G. (2024). Stroke, HIV and the Immune Reconstitution Inflammatory Syndrome in the absence of opportunistic infections. *Journal of the Neurological Sciences, 457*. Advance online publication. DOI: 10.1016/j.jns.2024.122880 PMID: 38219384

Sah, A. K., Elshaikh, R. H., Shalabi, M. G., Abbas, A. M., Prabhakar, P. K., Babker, A. M. A., Choudhary, R. K., Gaur, V., Choudhary, A. S., & Agarwal, S. (2025). Role of artificial intelligence and personalized medicine in enhancing HIV management and treatment outcomes. *Life (Chicago, Ill.), 15*(5), 745. DOI: 10.3390/life15050745 PMID: 40430173

Sah, A. K., Elshaikh, R. H., Shalabi, M. G., Abbas, A. M., Prabhakar, P. K., Babker, A. M., & Agarwal, S. (2025). Role of Artificial Intelligence and Personalized Medicine in Enhancing HIV Management and Treatment Outcomes. *Life (Chicago, Ill.), 15*(5), 745. PMID: 40430173

Saha, R., Malviya, L., Jadhav, A., & Dangi, R. (2024). Early stage HIV diagnosis using optimized ensemble learning technique. *Biomedical Signal Processing and Control, 89*, 105787. Advance online publication. DOI: 10.1016/j.bspc.2023.105787

Saleh, R. A. A., Ghaleb, M., & Shafik, W., & ERTUNÇ, H. M. (2024). Efficient white blood cell identification with hybrid inception-xception network. *The Journal of Supercomputing, 80*(17), 25155–25187.

Salmen, C. R., Hickey, M. D., Fiorella, K. J., Omollo, D., Ouma, G., Zoughbie, D., Salmen, M. R., Magerenge, R., Tessler, R., Campbe, H., Geng, E., Gandhi, M., Bukusi, E. A., & Cohen, C. R. (2015). "Wan Kanyakla"(We are together): Community transformations in Kenya following a social network intervention for HIV care. *Social Science & Medicine, 147*, 332–340. DOI: 10.1016/j.socscimed.2015.11.021 PMID: 26638145

Saltini, P., Tassis, B., Ronchi, A., Tagliabue, C., Di Pietro, G., Dellepiane, R. M., Muscatello, A., Giacomelli, A., Pugni, L., Ferrazzi, E., Bandera, A., & Bozzi, G. (2024). Preventing HIV mother-to-child transmission in a vertically infected pregnant woman with multiclass drug resistance, role of bis-in-die dolutegravir and neonatal AZT prophylaxis: A case report. *Heliyon, 10*(1). Advance online publication. DOI: 10.1016/j.heliyon.2023.e23072 PMID: 38163123

Samuel, K. (n.d.). *Stepping into the AI-driven future of HIV prevention and care.* Aidsmap.com. Retrieved October 18, 2025, from https://www.aidsmap.com/news/jul-2025/stepping-ai-driven-future-hiv-prevention-and-care

Sande, M. G., Rodrigues, J. L., Ferreira, D., Silva, C. J., & Rodrigues, L. R. (2021). Novel Biorecognition Elements against Pathogens in the Design of State-of-the-Art Diagnostics. *Biosensors (Basel), 11*(11), 418. DOI: 10.3390/bios11110418 PMID: 34821636

Sarcina, L., Mangiatordi, G. F., Torricelli, F., Bollella, P., Gounani, Z., Österbacka, R., Macchia, E., & Torsi, L. (2021). Surface Plasmon Resonance Assay for Label-Free and Selective Detection of HIV-1 p24 Protein. *Biosensors (Basel), 11*(6), 180. DOI: 10.3390/bios11060180 PMID: 34204930

Schwartz, S.R., Kavanagh, M.M., Sugarman, J., Solomon, S.S., Njindam, I.M., Rebe, K., Quinn, T. C., Toure-Kane, C., Beyrer, C., & Baral, S. (2017). HIV viral load monitoring among key populations in low- and middle-income countries: challenges and opportunities. *Journal of the International AIDS Society, 20 Suppl 7*(Suppl 7), e25003. DOI: 10.1002/jia2.25003

Searight, H. R. (2018). Counseling patients in primary care: Evidence-based strategies. *American Family Physician, 98*(12), 719–728. PMID: 30525356

Seboka, B. T., Yehualashet, D. E., & Tesfa, G. A. (2023). Artificial intelligence and machine learning based prediction of viral load and CD4 status of people living with HIV (PLWH) on anti-retroviral treatment in Gedeo Zone Public Hospitals. *International Journal of General Medicine*, , 435–451. PMID: 36760682

Sekandi, J. N., Shi, W., Zhu, R., Kaggwa, P., Mwebaze, E., & Li, S. (2023). Application of artificial intelligence to the monitoring of medication adherence for tuberculosis treatment in Africa: Algorithm development and validation. *JMIR AI, 2*(1), e40167. PMID: 38464947

Senel, B., & Beka, H. (2025). Artificial Intelligence in HIV Diagnosis and Treatment: A Comprehensive review. *Cumhuriyet Tıp Dergisi/Cumhuriyet ÜNiversitesi Tıp FaküLtesi Dergisi, 47*(1), 10–21. https://doi.org/DOI: 10.7197/cmj.1630164

Senel, B., & Beka, H. (2025). Artificial Intelligence in HIV Diagnosis and Treatment: A Comprehensive Review. *Cumhuriyet Medical Journal*, *47*(1), 10–21.

Serrano, D. R., Luciano, F. C., Anaya, B. J., Ongoren, B., Kara, A., Molina, G., Ramirez, B. I., Sánchez-Guirales, S. A., Simon, J. A., Tomietto, G., Rapti, C., Ruiz, H. K., Rawat, S., Kumar, D., & Lalatsa, A. (2024). Artificial intelligence (AI) applications in drug discovery and drug delivery: Revolutionizing personalized medicine. *Pharmaceutics*, *16*(10), 1328. DOI: 10.3390/pharmaceutics16101328 PMID: 39458657

Shafik, W. (2024b). Dissecting the Role of Women in Cybersecurity and Information Technology: A Medical Perspective. In *Next-Generation Cybersecurity: AI, ML, and Blockchain* (pp. 325–350). Springer. https://doi.org/DOI: 10.1007/978-981-97-1249-6_15

Shafik, W. (2025a). Revolutionizing Skin Cancer Diagnosis With Artificial Intelligence: Insights Into Machine Learning Techniques. In *Impact of Digital Solutions for Improved Healthcare Delivery* (pp. 167–194). IGI Global.

Shafik, W. (2024a). Artificial Intelligence-Enabled Internet of Medical Things for Enhanced Healthcare Systems. In *Smart Healthcare Systems* (pp. 119–134). CRC Press., DOI: 10.1201/9781032698519-9

Shafik, W. (2024c). The Future of Healthcare: AIoMT—Redefining Healthcare with Advanced Artificial Intelligence and Machine Learning Techniques. In *Artificial Intelligence and Machine Learning in Drug Design and Development* (pp. 605–634). Wiley., DOI: 10.1002/9781394234196.ch19

Shafik, W. (2024d). The Future of Healthcare: Data-Driven Trends and Innovation. In *Advancing Healthcare through Data-driven Innovations* (pp. 166–185). CRC Press.

Shafik, W. (2025b). Smart biomedical devices for smart healthcare. In *Machine Learning Models and Architectures for Biomedical Signal Processing* (pp. 421–448). Elsevier.

Sheira, L. A., Ryan, K. P., Fahey, C. A., Katabaro, E. D., Sabasaba, A. N., Njau, P. F., & McCoy, S. I. (2024). The impact of cash incentives on mental health among adults initiating antiretroviral therapy in Tanzania. *AIDS Care*, *36*(2). Advance online publication. DOI: 10.1080/09540121.2023.2222576 PMID: 37321981

Shelton, R. C., Lee, M., Brotzman, L. E., Crookes, D. M., Jandorf, L., Erwin, D., & Gage-Bouchard, E. A. (2019). Use of social network analysis in the development, dissemination, implementation, and sustainability of health behavior interventions for adults: A systematic review. *Social Science & Medicine*, *220*, 81–101. DOI: 10.1016/j.socscimed.2018.10.013 PMID: 30412922

Shi, J., Ying, G., Zheng, R., & Zhang, Z. (2024). Clinical significance and management of low-level HIV viremia in the era of integrase strand transfer inhibitors. *HIV Medicine*, *25*(3). Advance online publication. DOI: 10.1111/hiv.13585 PMID: 37990782

Shi, L., Tang, W., Hu, H., Qiu, T., Marley, G., Liu, X., Chen, Y., Chen, Y., & Fu, G. (2021). The impact of COVID-19 pandemic on HIV care continuum in Jiangsu, China. *BMC Infectious Diseases*, *21*(1), 768. DOI: 10.1186/s12879-021-06490-0 PMID: 34364383

Shimura, M., Higashi-Kuwata, N., Fujiwara, A., Taniguchi, M., Ichinose, T., Hamano, F., Uematsu, M., Inoue, T., Matsuyama, S., Suzuki, T., Ghosh, A. K., Shindou, H., Shimuzu, T., & Mitsuya, H. (2024). A lipid index for risk of hyperlipidemia caused by anti-retroviral drugs. *Antiviral Research*, *223*. Advance online publication. DOI: 10.1016/j.antiviral.2024.105819 PMID: 38272319

Shrestha, R. K., Chavez, P. R., Noble, M., Sansom, S. L., Sullivan, P. S., Mermin, J. H., & MacGowan, R. J. (2020). Estimating the costs and cost-effectiveness of HIV self-testing among men who have sex with men, United States. *Journal of the International AIDS Society*, *23*(1), e25445. DOI: 10.1002/jia2.25445 PMID: 31960580

Singh, A. K., Srinivasan, S., & Jyoti, B. (2025). Implications of Digitalization on Public Health Sector Across Countries. In *Digitalization and the Transformation of the Healthcare Sector* (pp. 359–394). IGI Global Scientific Publishing., DOI: 10.4018/979-8-3693-9641-4.ch013

Singh, Y., Jackson, D., Bhardwaj, S., Titus, N., & Goga, A. (2019). National surveillance using mobile systems for health monitoring: Complexity, functionality and feasibility. *BMC Infectious Diseases*, *19*, 1–10. DOI: 10.1186/s12879-019-4338-z PMID: 31526387

Sivaram, S., Johnson, S., Bentley, M. E., Srikrishnan, A. K., Latkin, C. A., Go, V. F., Solomon, S., & Celentano, D. D. (2007). Exploring "wine shops" as a venue for HIV prevention interventions in urban India. *Journal of Urban Health*, *84*, 563–576. DOI: 10.1007/s11524-007-9196-0 PMID: 17486455

Sivaram, S., Zelaya, C., Srikrishnan, A. K., Latkin, C., Go, V. F., Solomon, S., & Celentano, D. (2009). Associations between social capital and HIV stigma in Chennai, India: Considerations for prevention intervention design. *AIDS Education and Prevention*, *21*(3), 233–250. DOI: 10.1521/aeap.2009.21.3.233 PMID: 19519238

Siyamayambo, C., Phalane, E., & Phaswana-Mafuya, R. N. (2025). Diagnosis and Management of Sexually Transmitted Infections Using Artificial Intelligence Applications Among Key and General Populations in Sub-Saharan Africa: A Systematic Review and Meta-Analysis. *Algorithms*, *18*(3), 151.

Siyamayambo, C., Phalane, E., & Phaswana-Mafuya, R. N. (2025). Diagnosis and management of sexually transmitted infections using artificial intelligence applications among key and general populations in Sub-Saharan Africa: A systematic review and meta-analysis. *Algorithms*, *18*(3), 151. Advance online publication. DOI: 10.3390/a18030151

Slogrove, A. L., Bovu, A., De Beer, S., Phelanyane, F., Williams, P. L., Heekes, A., Kalk, E., Mehta, U., Theron, G., Abrams, E. J., Cotton, M. F., Myer, L., Davies, M. A., & Boulle, A. (2024). Maternal and birth outcomes in pregnant people with and without HIV in the Western Cape, South Africa. *AIDS*, *38*(1). Advance online publication. DOI: 10.1097/QAD.0000000000003728 PMID: 37720974

Sousa, L. R. M., Elias, H. C., Fernandes, N. M., Gir, E., & Reis, R. K. (2021). Knowledge of PEP and PrEP among people living with HIV/aids in Brazil. *BMC Public Health*, *21*, 1–9. DOI: 10.1186/s12889-020-10135-3 PMID: 33413241

Srinivasan, S. (2025). Patient-Centric Care in Tuberculosis Management: Addressing Challenges and Improving Health Outcomes. In *Convergence of Population Health Management, Pharmacogenomics, and Patient-Centered Care* (pp. 265-282). IGI Global. doi: DOI: 10.4018/979-8-3693-3260-3.ch012

Srinivasan, S., & Praba Lama (2025). Patient-Centered Care for TB Patients: An Effective Approach to Corporate Social Responsibility. In Corporate Social Responsibility in Health and Social Care (pp. 183-218).IGI Global. doi:DOI: 10.4018/979-8-3693-5991-4.ch008

Srinivasan, S., Vallipriya, R., & Singh, A. K. (2025). Integrated Public-Private Partnerships to Combat Tuberculosis for Improving Economic Development. In *Public Private Partnership Dynamics for Economic Development* (pp. 323–356). IGI Global Scientific Publishing., DOI: 10.4018/979-8-3693-9153-2.ch015

Srivastava, S. (2018, February 15). How is AI in Healthcare Transforming the Industry? *Appinventiv*. https://appinventiv.com/blog/ai-in-healthcare/

Stojanovski, K., Naja-Riese, G., King, E. J., & Fuchs, J. D. (2021). A systematic review of the social network strategy to optimize HIV testing in key populations to end the epidemic in the United States. *AIDS and Behavior*, *25*, 2680–2698. DOI: 10.1007/s10461-021-03259-z PMID: 33871730

Stone, M., Bainbridge, J., Sanchez, A. M., Keating, S. M., Pappas, A., Rountree, W., Todd, C., Bakkour, S., Manak, M., Peel, S. A., Coombs, R. W., Ramos, E. M., Shriver, M. K., Contestable, P., Nair, S. V., Wilson, D. H., Stengelin, M., Murphy, G., Hewlett, I., & Busch, M. P. (2018). Comparison of Detection Limits of Fourth- and Fifth-Generation Combination HIV Antigen-Antibody, p24 Antigen, and Viral Load Assays on Diverse HIV Isolates. *Journal of Clinical Microbiology*, *56*(8), e02045–e17. DOI: 10.1128/JCM.02045-17 PMID: 29793968

Stoner, M. C., Maragh-Bass, A. C., Sukhija-Cohen, A. C., & Saberi, P. (2022). Digital directly observed therapy to monitor adherence to medications: A scoping review. *HIV Research & Clinical Practice*, *23*(1), 47–60. PMID: 35904111

Sun, Q., Akman, A., & Schuller, B. W. (2025). Explainable artificial intelligence for medical applications: A review. *ACM Transactions on Computing for Healthcare*, *6*(2), 1–31.

Tandon, A., & Feist, W. (2022). Applications of crispr-cas9 technology to treat ccr5 tropic hiv-1. *Journal of Student Research*, *11*(4). Advance online publication. DOI: 10.47611/jsrhs.v11i4.3464

Tao, J., Maguire-Wilkerson, A., Rusley, J., Wray, T., & Chan, P. A. (2025). Implementing conversational artificial intelligence technology for the prevention of HIV and other sexually transmitted infections in real-world settings. *AIDS*, *39*(3), 324–327. PMID: 39878675

Teixeira da Silva, D., Bouris, A., Voisin, D., Hotton, A., Brewer, R., & Schneider, J. (2020). Social networks moderate the syndemic effect of psychosocial and structural factors on HIV risk among young Black transgender women and men who have sex with men. *AIDS and Behavior*, *24*(1), 192–205. DOI: 10.1007/s10461-019-02575-9 PMID: 31289985

Tekle, A., Tsegaye, A., & Ketema, T. (2024). Adherence to Anti-Retroviral Therapy (ART) and Its Determinants Among People Living with HIV/ AIDS at Bonga, Kaffa, South-West Ethiopia. *Patient Preference and Adherence*, *18*. Advance online publication. DOI: 10.2147/PPA.S445164 PMID: 38476589

Thirumalai, D. (2017). *Association between intimate partner violence and HIV infection among married Indian women in Theni District, Tamil Nadu, India.* University of California., https://www.proquest.com/openview/f183d8cb585715b3ca0cc12a54f5f791/1?cbl=18750&pq-origsite=gscholar

Thongkum, W., Klayprasert, P., Semakul, N., Jakmunee, J., Kasinrerk, W., Setshedi, M., Sayed, Y., & Tayapiwatana, C. (2023). Semi-quantification and Potency Verification of the HIV Protease Inhibitor Based on the Matrix-Capsid Protein Immobilized Nickel (II)/NTA-Tol/Graphene Oxide/SPCE Electrochemical Biosensor. *ACS Omega*, *8*(20), 17932–17940. DOI: 10.1021/acsomega.3c01031 PMID: 37251123

Threats, M., & Bond, K. (2021). HIV information acquisition and use among young black men who have sex with men who use the internet: Mixed methods study. *Journal of Medical Internet Research*, *23*(5), e22986. DOI: 10.2196/22986 PMID: 33960953

Tiffin, N., George, A., & LeFevre, A. E. (2019). How to use relevant data for maximal benefit with minimal risk: Digital health data governance to protect vulnerable populations in low-income and middle-income countries. *BMJ Global Health*, *4*(2), e001395. PMID: 31139457

Tiwari, A. K., Aggarwal, G., Pabbi, S., Mitra, S., Yadav, N., Verma, V., & Cheirmaraj, K. (2023). Analytical and clinical performance evaluation of enhanced chemiluminescence-based fourth-generation HIV combo assay: Report from tertiary health-care setup in North India. *Asian Journal of Transfusion Science*, *17*(2), 175–181. DOI: 10.4103/ajts.ajts_128_22 PMID: 38274959

Tosiano, M. A., Jacobs, J. L., Shutt, K. A., Cyktor, J. C., & Mellors, J. W. (2019). A Simpler and More Sensitive Single-Copy HIV-1 RNA Assay for Quantification of Persistent HIV-1 Viremia in Individuals on Suppressive Antiretroviral Therapy. *Journal of Clinical Microbiology*, *57*(3), e01714–e01718. DOI: 10.1128/JCM.01714-18 PMID: 30626659

Treves-Kagan, S., Steward, W. T., Ntswane, L., Haller, R., Gilvydis, J. M., Gulati, H., Barnhart, S., & Lippman, S. A. (2015). Why increasing availability of ART is not enough: A rapid, community-based study on how HIV-related stigma impacts engagement to care in rural South Africa. *BMC Public Health*, *16*, 1–13. DOI: 10.1186/s12889-016-2753-2 PMID: 26823077

Trickey, A., Glaubius, R., Pantazis, N., Zangerle, R., Wittkop, L., Vehreschild, J., Grabar, S., Cavassini, M., Teira, R., D'Arminio Monforte, A., Casabona, J., Van Sighem, A., Jarrin, I., Ingle, S. M., Sterne, J. A. C., Imai-Eaton, J. W., & Johnson, L. F. (2024). Estimation of Improvements in Mortality in Spectrum among Adults with HIV Receiving Antiretroviral Therapy in High-Income Countries. *Journal of Acquired Immune Deficiency Syndromes*, *95*(1). Advance online publication. DOI: 10.1097/QAI.0000000000003326 PMID: 38180742

Tshimula, J. M., Kalengayi, M., Makenga, D., Lilonge, D., Asumani, M., Madiya, D., . . . Kasoro, N. M. (2024). Artificial Intelligence for Public Health Surveillance in Africa: Applications and Opportunities. *arXiv preprint arXiv:2408.02575*.

Tso, L. S., Tang, W., Li, H., Yan, H. Y., & Tucker, J. D. (2016). Social media interventions to prevent HIV: A review of interventions and methodological considerations. *Current Opinion in Psychology*, *9*, 6–10. DOI: 10.1016/j.copsyc.2015.09.019 PMID: 26516632

Tsondai, P. R. (2016). *HIV viral load monitoring in HIV-infected pregnant women established on antiretroviral therapy in Cape Town*.

Tun, W., Conserve, D. F., Bunga, C., Jeremiah, K., Apicella, L., & Vu, L. (2024). Quality of Care is Perceived to be High with Community-based Antiretroviral Therapy (ART) Services for Female Sex Workers in Tanzania: Qualitative Findings from a Pilot Implementation Science Study. *AIDS and Behavior*, *28*(1). Advance online publication. DOI: 10.1007/s10461-023-04155-4 PMID: 37632605

Ukoaka, B. M., Ugwuanyi, E. A., Ukueku, K. O., Ajah, K. U., Udam, N. G., Daniel, F. M., Wali, T. W., & Gbuchie, M. A. (2024). Digital tools for improving antiretroviral adherence among people living with HIV in Africa. *Journal of Medicine, Surgery, and Public Health*, •••, 100077.

Vallée, A., & Arutkin, M. (2024). The Transformative Power of Virtual Hospitals for Revolutionising Healthcare Delivery. *Public Health Reviews*, *45*, 1606371. DOI: 10.3389/phrs.2024.1606371 PMID: 38962359

Van der Berg, A. (2021). *Investigating the effects of treatment in HIV disease models* (Doctoral dissertation, Stellenbosch: Stellenbosch University). https://scholar.sun.ac.za/items/7e137126-b5d0-4652-8000-d391fbe7b097

Vashisht, S., Jha, S., Thakur, N., Khaitan, A., Rai, S., Haldar, P., Kant, S., Kardam, P., & Sangral, M. (2022). Comparing the Effects of Oral HIV Self-Testing With Those of Standard HIV Testing for Men Who Have Sex With Men (MSM): A Systematic Review and Meta-Analysis. *Cureus*, *14*(8), e28157. DOI: 10.7759/cureus.28157 PMID: 36158381

Veenstra, R., Dijkstra, J. K., Steglich, C., & Van Zalk, M. H. (2013). Network–behavior dynamics. *Journal of Research on Adolescence, 23*(3), 399–412. DOI: 10.1111/jora.12070

Veinot, T. C. (2009). Interactive acquisition and sharing: Understanding the dynamics of HIV/AIDS information networks. *Journal of the American Society for Information Science and Technology, 60*(11), 2313–2332. DOI: 10.1002/asi.21151

Verdikt, R., Darcis, G., Ait-Ammar, A., & Van Lint, C. (2019). Applications of CRISPR/Cas9 tools in deciphering the mechanisms of HIV-1 persistence. *Current Opinion in Virology, 38*, 63–69. DOI: 10.1016/j.coviro.2019.07.004 PMID: 31509794

Vlad, G. (2019). Sources of errors in flow cytometry. In *Accurate Results in the Clinical Laboratory* (pp. 401–422). Elsevier., DOI: 10.1016/B978-0-12-813776-5.00027-3

Vogel, M., Schwarze-Zander, C., Wasmuth, J., Spengler, U., Sauerbruch, T., & Rockstroh, J. K. (2010). The treatment of patients with HIV. *Deutsches Ärzteblatt International*. Advance online publication. DOI: 10.3238/arztebl.2010.0507 PMID: 20703338

Wagner, G. J., Bogart, L. M., Klein, D. J., Lawrence, S. J., Goggin, K., Gizaw, M., & Mutchler, M. G. (2024). Culturally Relevant Africultural Coping Moderates the Association Between Discrimination and Antiretroviral Adherence Among Sexual Minority Black Americans Living with HIV. *AIDS and Behavior, 28*(2). Advance online publication. DOI: 10.1007/s10461-023-04233-7 PMID: 38060112

Wambaire, M. N. (2019). *Determinants of Social Network Site Preferences for Accessing Reproductive Health Information among Students in Public Universities in Nairobi, Kenya* (Doctoral dissertation, JKUAT-COHRED). http://ir.jkuat.ac.ke/handle/123456789/5041

Wang, C., Cheng, W., Li, C., Tang, W., Ong, J. J., Smith, M. K., Fu, H., Marks, M., Nie, J., Zheng, H., Tucker, J. D., & Yang, B. (2020). Syphilis Self-testing: A Nationwide Pragmatic Study Among Men Who Have Sex With Men in China. *Clinical Infectious Diseases, 70*(10), 2178–2186. DOI: 10.1093/cid/ciz603 PMID: 31260513

Wang, L., Muwonge, T. R., Simoni, J. M., Nambi, F., Nakabugo, L., Kibuuka, J., Thomas, D., Katz, I. T., Feutz, E., Thomas, K. K., Ware, N. C., Wyatt, M. A., Kadama, H., Mujugira, A., & Heffron, R. (2024). Behavioral Modeling and its Association with PrEP and ART Use in Ugandan HIV-Serodifferent Couples. *AIDS and Behavior, 28*(5). Advance online publication. DOI: 10.1007/s10461-024-04286-2 PMID: 38361169

Ward, P. R., & Fauk, N. K. (2025). Structural conditions, social networks, and the HIV vulnerability among Indonesian male labour migrants and motorbike taxi drivers. *International Journal for Equity in Health, 24*(1), 61. DOI: 10.1186/s12939-025-02420-7 PMID: 40033297

Waterfield, K. C., Shah, G. H., Etheredge, G. D., & Ikhile, O. (2021). Consequences of COVID-19 crisis for persons with HIV: The impact of social determinants of health. *BMC Public Health, 21*, 1–7. DOI: 10.1186/s12889-021-10296-9 PMID: 33546659

West, B. S. (2019). Social networks of substance-using populations: Key issues and promising new approaches for HIV. *Current HIV/AIDS Reports, 16*, 48–56. DOI: 10.1007/s11904-019-00425-w PMID: 30659477

Westerdijk, T. (2024). *Decoding HIV Dynamics: The Role of Modeling in Understanding Viral Load Decay under Retroviral Therapy* (Master's thesis). https://studenttheses.uu.nl/handle/20.500.12932/47716

West, R. E., Oberly, P. J., Riddler, S. A., Nolin, T. D., & Devanathan, A. S. (2024). Development and validation of an ultra-high performance liquid chromatography-tandem mass spectrometry method to quantify antiretroviral drug concentrations in human plasma for therapeutic monitoring. *Journal of Pharmaceutical and Biomedical Analysis, 240*. Advance online publication. DOI: 10.1016/j.jpba.2023.115932 PMID: 38198884

Whiteley, L. B., Olsen, E. M., Haubrick, K. K., Odoom, E., Tarantino, N., & Brown, L. K. (2021). A review of interventions to enhance HIV medication adherence. *Current HIV/AIDS Reports, 18*(5), 443–457. PMID: 34152554

Wiche Salinas, T. R., Zhang, Y., Gosselin, A., Rosario, N. F., El-Far, M., Filali-Mouhim, A., Routy, J. P., Chartrand-Lefebvre, C., Landay, A. L., Durand, M., Tremblay, C. L., & Ancuta, P. (2024). Alterations in Th17 Cells and Non-Classical Monocytes as a Signature of Subclinical Coronary Artery Atherosclerosis during ART-Treated HIV-1 Infection. *Cells, 13*(2). Advance online publication. DOI: 10.3390/cells13020157 PMID: 38247848

Williams, E., Moso, M., Lim, C., Chibo, D., Nicholson, S., Jackson, K., & Williamson, D. A. (2023). Laboratory diagnosis of HIV: A contemporary overview in the Australian context. *Pathology, 55*(5), 610–620. PMID: 37302942

Wolf, P. J. (2022). American Young Adults' Self-Perception of Interpersonal Communication with Family and Friends Online through Social Media and In-Person. https://digitalcommons.liberty.edu/doctoral/3754/

Wong, C. C., Lim, S. H., Tan, C. T., Lui, S. Y., Lee, Y. L., & Chan, K. P. (2018). Performance of the HIV Blot 2.2, INNO-LIA HIV I/II Score, and Geenius HIV 1/2 Confirmatory Assay for use in HIV confirmation. *PLoS One*, *13*(6), e0199502. DOI: 10.1371/journal.pone.0199502 PMID: 29928045

World Health Organization. (2021). *Consolidated guidelines on HIV prevention, testing, treatment, service delivery and monitoring: recommendations for a public health approach*. World Health Organization.

Wratil, P. R., Rabenau, H. F., Eberle, J., Stern, M., Münchhoff, M., Friedrichs, I., Stürmer, M., Berger, A., Kuttner-May, S., Münstermann, D., Lucht, A., Meixenberger, K., Bannert, N., & Keppler, O. T. (2020). Comparative multi-assay evaluation of determine™ hiv-1/2 ag/ab combo rapid diagnostic tests in acute and chronic hiv infection. *Medical Microbiology and Immunology*, *209*(2), 139–150. DOI: 10.1007/s00430-019-00655-0 PMID: 32036450

Wulandari, L. P. L., Ruddick, A., Guy, R., & Kaldor, J. (2019). "Self-testing sounds more private, rather than going to the clinic and everybody will find out": Facilitators and barriers regarding HIV testing among men who purchase sex in Bali, Indonesia. *PLoS One*, *14*(4), e0214987. DOI: 10.1371/journal.pone.0214987 PMID: 30958845

Wu, S., Gao, M., Zheng, J., Yan, P., Wang, W., Lu, X., Qiu, Y., & Yan, Y. (2019). Prevalence of HIV Indeterminate Western Blot Tests and Follow-up of HIV Antibody Sero-Conversion in Southeastern China. *Virologica Sinica*, *34*(4), 358–366. DOI: 10.1007/s12250-019-00130-3 PMID: 31190120

Xiang, Y., Du, J., Fujimoto, K., Li, F., Schneider, J., & Tao, C. (2021). Application of artificial intelligence and machine learning for HIV prevention interventions. *The Lancet. HIV*, *9*(1), e54–e62. DOI: 10.1016/s2352-3018(21)00247-2 PMID: 34762838

Yang, X., Fang, T., Mobarak, S. A., Wang, J., Wang, C., Huang, S., Jiang, L., Chen, Xi., Li, H., Chang, W., Zhang, L., Mo, J., & Ning, C. (2020). Social network strategy as a promising intervention to better reach key populations for promoting HIV prevention: A systematic review and meta-analysis. *Sexually Transmitted Infections*, *96*(7), 485–491. DOI: 10.1136/sextrans-2019-054349 PMID: 32209639

Yigit, I., Wilson, T. E., Taylor, T. N., Kassaye, S. G., Weiser, S. D., Cohen, M. H., & Turan, B. (2025). Association of Experienced Stigma in Healthcare Settings with Health outcomes among Black women living with HIV: Mediating roles of internalized stigma, anticipated Stigma, and trust in HIV Care. *Social Science & Medicine*, *366*, 117699. PMID: 39823813

Yoder, K. (2019). A crispr/cas9 library to map the hiv-1 provirus genetic fitness. *Acta Virologica. English Ed.*, *63*(02), 129–138. DOI: 10.4149/av_2019_201 PMID: 31230441

Yüksel, P., Sarıbaş, S., & Kuşkucu, M. (2018). Problems encountered in conventional hiv 1/2 algorithms: Lack of necessity for immunoblot assays to confirm repeated elisa reactive results. *African Health Sciences*, *18*(2). Advance online publication. DOI: 10.4314/ahs.v18i2.26 PMID: 30602968

Zeng, D., Cao, Z., & Neill, D. B. (2021). Artificial intelligence–enabled public health surveillance—from local detection to global epidemic monitoring and control. In *Artificial intelligence in medicine* (pp. 437–453). Academic Press.

Zeytinoğlu, A., Kayın, M., Altuğlu, İ., Gökengin, D., & Sertöz, R. (2020). İ Comparison of two anti-HIV confirmatory assays: Recombinant HIV 1/2 line immunoassay and Geenius HIV 1/2 confirmatory test. *Mikrobiyoloji Bulteni*, *54*(4), 613–618. DOI: 10.5578/mb.69786 PMID: 33107290

Zhang, B., Wang, Y., Vasilakos, A. V., & Ma, J. (2013). Mobile social networking: Reconnect virtual community with physical space. *Telecommunication Systems*, *54*, 91–110. DOI: 10.1007/s11235-013-9718-x

Zhang, L., Ni, Z., Liu, Y., & Chen, H. (2023). The effectiveness of e-health on reducing stigma, improving social support and quality of life among people living with HIV: A systematic review and meta-analysis of randomized controlled trials. *International Journal of Nursing Studies*, *148*, 104606. DOI: 10.1016/j.ijnurstu.2023.104606 PMID: 37801937

Zhao, A. V., Crutchley, R. D., Guduru, R. C., Ton, K., Lam, T., & Min, A. C. (2022). A clinical review of HIV integrase strand transfer inhibitors (INSTIs) for the prevention and treatment of HIV-1 infection. *Retrovirology*, *19*(1), 22. DOI: 10.1186/s12977-022-00608-1 PMID: 36273165

Zhou, Y., Chen, Y., & Liu, Y. (2021). Controlled copper in situ growth-amplified lateral flow sensors for sensitive, reliable, and field-deployable infectious disease diagnostics. *Biosensors & Bioelectronics*, *171*, 112753. DOI: 10.1016/j.bios.2020.112753 PMID: 33120235

Zolopa, A. R. (2010). The evolution of HIV treatment guidelines: Current state-of-the-art of ART. *Antiviral Research*, *85*(1), 241–244. DOI: 10.1016/j.antiviral.2009.10.018 PMID: 19883695

Zuckoff, A. (2012). "Why won't my patients do what's good for them?" Motivational interviewing and treatment adherence. *Surgery for Obesity and Related Diseases*, *8*(5), 514–521. DOI: 10.1016/j.soard.2012.05.002 PMID: 22704048

About the Contributors

Adnène Arbi is a distinguished academic affiliated with the University of Carthage in Tunisia, where he has contributed significantly to the fields of mathematics and engineering. His tenure at the university spans over a decade, during which he has held various positions, including roles at the Ecole Polytechnique de Tunisie and the National Institute of Applied Sciences and Technology. He served as director of studies and vice-director in the National School of Advanced Sciences and Technologies from 2020 to 2024. His research interests primarily focus on neural networks, dynamical systems, and mathematical modeling, with a particular emphasis on the stability and controllability of complex systems. Arbi's recent publications reflect his commitment to advancing knowledge in applied mathematics, particularly through innovative approaches such as wavelet neural networks and the dynamics of nonlinear systems. His work has been published in reputable journals, contributing to the understanding of mathematical phenomena in both theoretical and practical contexts. In addition to his academic pursuits, Arbi has collaborated with various prestigious institutions globally, including the University of the Witwatersrand and Imperial College London, showcasing his dedication to fostering international research partnerships. His contributions to the academic community continue to inspire emerging scholars and practitioners in the field. Actually, Dr. Arbi served as editor of various journal: Frontiers in Applied Mathematics and Statistics, Journal of Algorithms & Computational Technology, Neural Computing and Applications, Discover Artificial Intelligence, Current Artificial Intelligence, Journal of Innovative Applied Mathematics and Computational Sciences, International Journal of Sustainable Business and Management, Karshi Multidisciplinary International Scientific Journal. Besides, he is author of more than 40 scientific peer- reviewed papers in international journals and conference proceedings, and he served as reviewer for many international conferences, workshops.

Walid Ben Ameur earned his PhD from the University of Carthage. He currently serves as a teacher-researcher at the Department of Life Sciences, Faculty of Sciences of Gabès, Tunisia, and is a member of the Laboratory of Ecology of Terrestrial Fauna at the University of Gabès, Tunisia. Walid Ben Ameur has authored more than 20 peer-reviewed scientific papers published in international journals. His work has made useful contributions to the field of environmental chemistry, with a particular focus on persistent organic pollutants. He has developed analytical techniques for assessing emerging pollutants and evaluating their effects on both the environment and human health. His research spans a diverse range of samples, including those from environmental, biological, human, and food sources. Dr. Ben Ameur has mentored three Master's students and regularly serves as a reviewer for respected journals such as Science of the Total Environment, Chemosphere, Environmental Science and Pollution Research, Marine Pollution Bulletin, Environmental Pollution, Ecotoxicology and Environmental Safety, and Chemistry Africa.

***

Kashvi Chaturvedi, is studying B.Tech, specialisation in Artificial Intelligence and Data Science at Ajeenkya DY Patil University. She started solidifying her programming skills by completing various certification courses like Data Structures in C, Tableau functions and Operating Systems along with doing few projects using languages like Python, C, C++ and creating Web Page using HTML, CSS and Java Script. She had also attended an Arduino-Based Automation course at Dolphin Labs to enhance her software knowledge. There, she learned how to work with sensors, microcontrollers, and circuit design. She has also written multiple review papers on topics such as Geographic Information Systems, Comparative Analysis of BJT Configurations, Swiss Bank vs. European Central Bank: Data Analysis. She is also researching on and learning many topics such as Small Modular Reactors, Bibliometric Analysis, UNSDGs etc. Because of her interest in latest technologies, she also participated in Global Hyperloop Competition hosted by IIT Madras representing her college as team Vac-Vectoor where she learnt more about various subtopics from the mentors.

Susanta Das is a seasoned educator with a proven record of teaching and mentoring diverse students, working at multiple institutions, and providing service to the various initiatives of organizations. He received his Ph.D. and M.A. degrees from Western Michigan University (WMU), USA, and M.Sc. degree from Banaras Hindu University (BHU), India all in Physics. He continued his research as a Marie-Curie post-doctoral fellow at Stockholm University, Stockholm, Sweden on beam diagnostics for the DESIREE (Double ElectroStatic Ion Ring ExpEriment) in the project DITANET (Diagnostic Techniques for particle Accelerators – a Marie-Curie initial training NETwork), at the Indian Institute of Science Education and Research-Kolkata, India on high-pressure physics as a Project Scientist-B, and at the University of Electro-Communications, Tokyo, Japan on ion-surface interactions as a Post-doctoral fellow. Throughout his career, Dr. Das worked and collaborated with many researchers, Ph.D., master, and visiting students from different countries. He further visited many countries to discuss research and an international conference participant (UK, Italy, Germany, Greece, Belgium, Bulgaria, Romania, Brazil etc.). He worked at several institutions before assuming his current role at Ajeenkya D Y Patil University. He received the Marie-Curie post-doctoral fellowship in Sweden, Science Academies' Summer Research Fellowship in India, Gowen Frostic Doctoral Fellowship, Department Graduate Research and Creative Scholar Award by WMU, and Leo R. Parpart Doctoral Fellowship by Dept. of Physics, WMU, among many others, throughout his academic journey. He co-authored several research articles in WoS/Scopus indexed international journals, conference proceedings, and scholarly book chapters and co-edited several books published by renowned international publishing houses (IGI-Global, Springer Nature, Nova Science Publishers, Wiley, Scrivener-Wiley, Notion Press). At present, Dr. Das continues to delve into cutting-edge fields, with a keen interest in nanotechnology, UN SDGs, and data science. His multifaceted contributions, spanning teaching, research, and administrative leadership, showcase a dedicated professional who is instrumental in advancing the vision and mission of the institutions he serves.

Ida Evangeline, presently working as an Assistant Professor in the Department of Electrical and Electronics Engineering at the Government College of Engineering, Tirunelveli, Tamilnadu, India. She obtained her Bachelor's in Electrical and Electronics Engineering from Manonmaniam Sundaranar University in 2003, and Master's in Power Systems Engineering from Anna University, Chennai, Tamilnadu, India in 2005. She completed her PhD degree in 2023 at Anna University, Chennai, Tamilnadu, India. She has published six research papers in international journals. Her current research interests include optimal power flow, renewable energy, soft computing, machine learning, and deep learning.

Vishal Jain is presently working as a Professor at the Department of Computer Science & Engineering, School of Engineering & Technology, Vivekananda Institute of Professional Studies - Technical Campus, New Delhi. Before that, he worked as Professor at Sharda University, Greater Noida and Associate Professor at Bharati Vidyapeeth's Institute of Computer Applications and Management (BVICAM), New Delhi. He has associated as a member of the Faculty Board, Board of Planning and Management, Executive Council, Academic Council, Curriculum Development and

Review Committee and Academic Audit of various higher education Institutions. He is associated with Kuala Lumpur University of Science and Technology (KLUST), Malaysia, Lincoln University College, Malaysia and Research Institute of IoT Cybersecurity, Department of Electronic Engineering, National Kaohsiung University of Science and Technology, Taiwan for research oriented activities.

Mehak Jonjua is a journalist, researcher, and author. Their professional journey began as a reporter with The Squamish Chief, Canada and later joined Manchester Stalwart Capital Management, US. As an educationist, they have worked with DAV and MCMDAV College, Chandigarh, IP University, New Delhi, and Amity University, Noida. At present, they are a professor at Sharda University, Noida.

Jipson Joseph has a PhD in Ethics from DVK Bangalore. Currently, he is a Research Scholar in the School of Law at Christ University, Bangalore. His research interests encompass the fields of ethics, gender studies, constitutional law, human rights, human security, environmental justice, BRICS countries, development policies, and global poverty. He has published six books, co-edited one book, and contributed scholarly articles to numerous international and national journals and edited volumes, including those published by IGI Global Scientific Publishing.

Arpita Nayak is currently serving as an Assistant Professor, offering courses in management. She completed her Ph.D. in management from the KIIT School of Management. Her MBA and strong interest in Human Resource Management (HRM) led her to pursue further studies in HRM. Her passion for talent management inspired her doctoral research on "A Comparative Study on Talent Management in Private and Public Manufacturing Industries in Odisha." Dr. Nayak has presented research papers at both national and international conferences and has published articles in SCOPUS-listed journals. Over the years, she has taught a variety of subjects, including Human Resource Management, Principles of Management, Business Studies Management, Tribal Entrepreneurship, and Organizational Behaviour. In addition to her academic career, she also has several years of corporate work experience.

Krutika Patre, is an aspiring programmer and technology enthusiast, currently pursuing Engineering in Artificial Intelligence and Data Science. With a passion for learning, she is building experience in a variety of programming languages and technologies, including C, C++, Python, Data Structures (DS), HTML, CSS, and JavaScript, DBMS (My SQL). After learning this programming language, she has created interest in Full Stack Development. She had also attended an Arduino-Based Automation course at Dolphin Labs to improve my software knowledge. There, she learned how to work with sensors, microcontrollers, and circuit design. She has written review paper on Sustainable engineering on build environment. She is doing researching and learning many topics related to AI, Policy and governance and related to my interest. She has taken part in hackathons, workshops, and tech events to explore many fields. She is also working with a group on Hyperloop. Being part of this project has really helped her grow, especially in areas like teamwork, innovation, and systems thinking.

Sunil Sankathala is pursuing B. Tech Computer Science and Engineering at Ajeenkya DY Patil University, with a diverse range of interests that bridge technology, sustainability, and innovation. His academic focus lies in computer science fundamentals like programming, data structures, algorithms, and software development. He actively supplements this with hands-on experience in web development and robotics. Beyond the core curriculum, He has a strong research inclination in emerging and impactful fields. His current research interests include Artificial Intelligence in Healthcare, bioplastics, nano bioplastics, e-waste management, and solid waste management—areas where he believes technology can make a meaningful difference in solving real-world problems. He has been publishing research articles and book chapters in reputed national and international journals and books. He is also part of an ambitious Hyperloop project, which involves interdisciplinary collaboration and cutting-edge engineering aimed at revolutionizing transportation. Working on this project has enhanced his skills in teamwork, innovation, and systems thinking. In the tech domain, he has developed proficiency in web development using technologies such as HTML, CSS, JavaScript, and React. His interests in robotics further reflect building smart, responsive systems that interact with the physical world. Throughout his course, he has helped strengthen problem-solving and collaborative skills. He is proficient in languages such as Python, C, C++, MySQL, Ubuntu, Machine Learning and familiar with frameworks and tools like React, Git. He actively participates in hackathons, coding competitions, and tech events to challenge himself and learn from peers. He is also a quick learner and highly adaptable, with an eagerness to stay updated with the latest trends in the tech world. He aspires to become a skilled software engineer and contribute to building innovative solutions that have a positive impact on society. The long-term goal is to work in a dynamic environment where knowledge, grow professionally, and make meaningful contributions to the field of technology. Driven by a spirit of exploration and sustainability, he aims to contribute to technological solutions that address both human and environmental needs. The long-term goal is to become a versatile engineer and researcher, working at the intersection of computer science, environmental innovation, and human well-being.

Ipseeta Satpathy is a senior professor at KIIT University. Specializes in Psychology, Behavioral Science, and Organisational Behaviour.

Wasswa Shafik received a Bachelor of Science degree in information technology from Ndejje University, Uganda, a Master of Engineering degree in Information Technology (Computer and Communication Networks) from Yazd University, Iran, and a PhD in Computer Science with the School of Digital Science, Universiti Brunei Darussalam, Brunei Darussalam. He is also the Founder and Research Director of the Dig Connectivity Research Laboratory (DCRLab) after serving as a Research Associate at the Network Interconnectivity Research Laboratory at Yazd University. Prior to this, he worked as a Community Data Analyst at Population Services International (PSI-Uganda), a Community Data Officer at the Programme for Accessible Health Communication (PACE-Uganda), a Research Assistant at the Socio-Economic Data Centre (SEDC-Uganda), Uganda, an Assistant Data Officer at TechnoServe, Kampala, Uganda, and Asmaah Charity Organization as Cheif Executive Officer. He has hundreds of publications with renowned publishers. His research interests include Artificial Intelligence, Neural Networks, Computer Vision, Smart Agriculture, Digital Health, and Green Computing.

Aditya Shrivastav is an aspiring technologist currently pursuing a Bachelor of Technology (B. Tech.) in Computer Science and Engineering at Ajeenkya D. Y. Patil University. He holds solid programming expertise in C, C++, and Python, alongside strong command over data and business tools such as Microsoft Excel and Tally software. Aditya is a member of Team Vac-Vectoor Hyperloop and participated with the team in the Global Hyperloop Competition organized by IIT Madras, contributing to cutting-edge transportation solutions. He actively engages in hackathons and various technical events to expand his skills and contribute to innovative problem-solving. He has authored and co-authored book chapters in the domains of solid waste management, bioplastics, nanotechnology applications, and artificial intelligence, showcasing his multidisciplinary approach and research acumen. Aditya is also working on an innovative project on predictive e-waste management. The project is targeted toward IT departments, schools, and colleges, aiming to support sustainable practices and resource optimization. In parallel with his academic journey, Aditya is serving as a faculty intern at Disha Computer Institute, where he teaches C, C++, basic Python, basic Java, Excel formulas, and Tally software. His dedication and teaching proficiency earned him a Letter of Appreciation and the opportunity to conduct a workshop on Advanced Excel at G. H. Raisoni College of Arts, Commerce and Science. With a strong foundation in technology, a passion for sustainability, and hands-on experience in both teaching and project development, Aditya Shrivastav is committed to driving impact through research, education, and innovation.

Ajay K. Singh is working as an Associate Professor (Research) in the Department of Humanities and Social Sciences, Graphic Era (Deemed to be University) Dehradun. He has worked as Assistant Professor (Economics) in the School of Liberal Arts & Management, DIT University Dehradun for 6 years. He did Post-Doctorate Research with EDI of India, Ahmedabad, Gujarat (India). He received MPhil (Economics) from DAVV Indore (India), and PhD (Economics) from IIT Indore (India. He has published several research papers in the diversified area such as climate change, agricultural productivity, assessment of food security; estimation of GFSI, development of environmental sustainability index (ESI) and its association with socio-economic indicators; measurement and determinants of entrepreneurship ecosystem, and dimension of sustainable development and its interlinkages with economic development.

R. Vallipriya has been working in the Department of Physical Sciences at the Institute of Education (Affiliated to Tamilnadu Teacher Education University) as an Assistant Professor. With a wealth of experience, Mrs. R.Vallipriya has accumulated 12 years of extensive teaching. Her scholarly contributions include publishing 15 papers, with 1 peer review in various UGC-CARE, SCOPUS, and peer-reviewed journals.

Srinivasan Vasan is an Assistant Professor in the Department of Humanities and Social Sciences at Graphic Era (Deemed to be University), with 14 years of teaching and field expertise. He has served in the Ministry of Health and Family Welfare, as a Guest Faculty, and as a Mobilization Training Specialist with the State Government. Recently, he contributed to a tuberculosis project funded by GFATM and USAID. He has published 60 papers, with 20 more under peer review in UGC-CARE and SCOPUS journals.

Index

V

W

www.ingramcontent.com/pod-product-compliance
Lightning Source LLC
LaVergne TN
LVHW080859300926
849162LV00003B/477